OBSESSIVE COMPULSIVE DISORDER

OBSESSIVE COMPULSIVE DISORDER

Elements, History, Treatments, and Research

LESLIE J. SHAPIRO

Health and Psychology
Sourcebooks

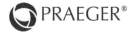 PRAEGER®

An Imprint of ABC-CLIO, LLC
Santa Barbara, California • Denver, Colorado

Library of Congress Cataloging-in-Publication Data

Names: Shapiro, Leslie, author.
Title: Obsessive compulsive disorder : elements, history, treatments, and research / Leslie J. Shapiro.
Description: Santa Barbara, California : Praeger, an imprint of ABC-CLIO, LLC, [2020] | Series: Health and psychology sourcebooks | Includes bibliographical references and index.
Identifiers: LCCN 2020007757 (print) | LCCN 2020007758 (ebook) | ISBN 9781440871306 (hardcover) | ISBN 9781440871313 (ebook)
Subjects: LCSH: Obsessive-compulsive disorder. | Obsessive-compulsive disorder—Treatment.
Classification: LCC RC533 .S528 2020 (print) | LCC RC533 (ebook) | DDC 616.85/227—dc23
LC record available at https://lccn.loc.gov/2020007757
LC ebook record available at https://lccn.loc.gov/2020007758

ISBN: 978-1-4408-7130-6 (print)
        978-1-4408-7131-3 (ebook)

24 23 22 21 20   1 2 3 4 5

This book is also available as an eBook.

Praeger
An Imprint of ABC-CLIO, LLC

ABC-CLIO, LLC
147 Castilian Drive
Santa Barbara, California 93117
www.abc-clio.com

This book is printed on acid-free paper ∞

Manufactured in the United States of America

This book is dedicated to all the lives who are touched by OCD and their courage and strength to endure.

Contents

Series Foreword

An understanding of both physical diseases and mental disorders is vital to each of us, as sickness of body and mind touch every one of us throughout our lives—personally; among family, friends, and associates; and in our immediate and greater society. Yet the cacophony of existing information sources—from piecemeal and poorly-sourced Web sites to dense academic tomes—can make acquiring accurate, accessible, and objective facts a complicated venture. This series is a solution to that dilemma.

The Health and Psychology Sourcebooks series addresses physical, psychological, and environmental conditions that threaten human health and well-being. These books are designed to accessibly and reliably fulfill the needs of students and researchers at community and undergraduate college levels, whether they are seeking vetted information for core or elective courses, papers and publications, or personal enlightenment.

Each volume presents a topic in health or psychology and explains the symptoms, diagnosis, incidence, development, causes, treatments, and related theory. "Up Close" vignettes illustrate how the disease or disorder and its associated difficulties present in varied people and scenarios. History and classic as well as emerging research are detailed. Where controversy is present, it is discussed. Each volume also offers a glossary of terms, references, and resources for further reading.

Introduction

"What if . . ." "What if I left the coffeepot on?" "What if I made the wrong decision and someone gets hurt?"

Did these thoughts cause your heart to beat a little faster? Did you think about going to check the coffeepot or let the thought go? Did you think about changing your mind when you doubted the choice you made?

Although the nature of obsessive compulsive disorder (OCD) is serious and the odds seem stacked against recovery, OCD is a very treatable disorder. There are key elements that will enable people with OCD to have a stable and functional lifestyle. When people with OCD recognize they have a problem, understand what the problem is, seek appropriate help in a timely manner, adhere to treatment, create a support structure, and maintain healthy routines, they can fulfill and achieve their life goals and create their optimal quality of life. Often, people will live their lives with OCD but not be held back by it.

There are, however, numerous potential obstacles that can complicate the treatment and recovery process, and they are addressed throughout the book.

The hallmark of OCD is obsessive doubt; OCD is often referred to as "the doubting disease." When you are treating a patient* with OCD, it seems like the doubts never end and before you know it, you are caught up in them. As you listen to the parsing of unbeknown potential

---

* I use the term patient(s) instead of client(s) because OCD has medical parity and is a neurobiological disorder. Most patients prefer using the medical context for the disorder, rather than a service-based one.

catastrophic outcomes from anxiety-provoking thoughts, you suddenly become aware of the infinite ways that patients fear their germs can cause people to get sick or that someone who thinks a girl is cute can fear that she is a pedophile.

You may try to reason with these irrational thoughts, but it won't work. The truth is, anything *is* possible. Germs do cause illness. There are pedophiles in the world. Cars do kill people. But those without OCD handle and touch things without a thought about who else has handled them and what they might have left on them. Even though car accidents happen on a daily basis, we drive ourselves to where we need to go. That is why when you are listening to a person's symptoms, it is *critical* to understand that the content of obsessions is not important. Obsessions even change from time to time, rendering what seemed so urgent and important then insignificant now. The common denominator of OCD is the *doubt*.

This book has many features that will help readers understand what the symptoms and subtypes of OCD are, how to make a diagnosis, and how to differentiate between OCD and the various related disorders (chapters 1 and 2). The rich history, theories, and research of OCD will be presented through accounts dating back from ancient times to the present, including how OCD was considered to be a religious problem and how we now understand the neurobiological etiology of the disorder (chapters 3 and 4). Readers will learn the how OCD develops and its causes (chapter 5), and the effects and costs OCD has on the individual sufferer's and family's quality of life, as well as the financial costs to society (chapters 5 and 6).

There are two treatment chapters (chapters 7 and 8). Chapter 7 includes important considerations for assessing psychological factors that may affect the treatment process, the various treatment options with an emphasis on behavior therapy that includes tips for effective delivery, and a case study. Family issues and relapse prevention are also addressed, as they can impact how recovery is maintained. Chapter 8 reviews adjunctive therapies that enhance and augment the behavioral work, as well as provides differential treatment approaches for some of the related disorders. The following three chapters (chapters 9, 10, and 11) describe societal, vocational and employment issues and the way that OCD factors into dating, partner, child, and parental relationships.

The end of the book provides a glossary of common terms used in OCD treatment, suggestions for further reading, websites, and organizational resources.

Research on OCD is prolific and informs clinical practice. This book provides the most current knowledge on the topics it covers, but it is likely that new information will be available from ongoing research, technologies, and psychosocial studies that share the common goal of eradicating the all-too-often devastating effects the disorder has on the lives of all those whom it touches.

CHAPTER 1

Diagnosis, Symptoms, Phenomenology, and Incidence

Diagnosis

OCD has been incorporated into the broader *DSM-V* category Obsessive-Compulsive and Related Disorders (OCRDs), which also includes hoarding disorder, excoriation disorder (skin picking), body dysmorphia (reverse anorexia), and trichotillomania (hair pulling; American Psychiatric Association, 2013). OCRDs have similar and overlapping obsessive and compulsive characteristics as well as their own distinct features. These will be covered in the next chapter.

The hallmark of OCD is obsessive doubt. The problem is not a matter of indecision or forgetting, which is what many undiagnosed sufferers may believe. Most obsessions are based in doubts people without OCD typically have (i.e., "Did I shut off the oven?" or "Did I say something annoying to the person I had dinner with last night?"). The difference is that when doubt is triggered in people with OCD, it feels more urgent due to the increasing level of anxiety and urgency the OCD sufferer experiences. OCD provokes doubt about unverifiable past or future events, since time can't be rewound or forwarded as a means of checking what happened or will happen. Even if this were possible, people would likely still doubt whatever "proof" they found.

According to *DSM-V*, the diagnosis consists of obsessive thoughts that are considered intrusive, distressing, and unwanted and that provoke anxiety and discomfort. It also includes compulsions and rituals, mental or physical behaviors performed with the intention of reducing the anxiety or discomfort. For the episode to be considered clinical, the symptoms will add up to at least one hour per day and will interfere with aspects of functioning. There may be a range of insight between good, fair, and poor (American Psychiatric Association, 2013).

Symptoms

Obsessions

As noted, obsessions are defined as recurrent and persistent thoughts, urges, or images that are experienced as intrusive and unwanted and that trigger noticeable anxiety or distress. The content of obsessions is characteristically taboo in nature and ego-dystonic, meaning that they are experienced as distressing, unacceptable, and inconsistent with the person's true personality or values. Understandably, people with OCD would make efforts to push the obsessions away in order to avoid the anxiety and negative emotional experiences they cause. Sufferers often ask, "Why am I having these thoughts? What do they mean? What do they say about me?" This leads to questions and doubts about their true motives or morality. They also try to find some kind of explanation and look for meaning about why they are having them. Additionally, they might wonder if the OCD is a defense mechanism against unconscious wishes that they wish to act out, as was an accepted theory in the early days of psychoanalysis (Freud, 1924).

Since we all experience almost the same intrusive thoughts that turn into obsessions for people with OCD, is there really any difference between a normal bad thought and an obsession? With OCD, the difference is a matter of hard wiring in the brain. We know that having any kind of thought is different from acting on it. Another difference is *how* we react to the thoughts. People without OCD do not experience the same anxiety surge or excessive guilt that these unwanted thoughts cause others, even if they experience discomfort over them.

There are two types of obsessions: *autogenous obsessions* are internally generated and occur spontaneously (sexual, aggressive, blasphemous, and immoral/repugnant thoughts), while *reactive obsessions* are triggered in response to external stimuli (contamination, mistakes, accidents, and asymmetry/disarray; Garcia-Soriano & Belloch, 2013). Studies found that people with autogenous obsessions had a higher belief in the importance of the obsessive thoughts and their ability to control them. Those with reactive obsessions were concerned with having a higher sense of responsibility and were found to use thought avoidance or thought-control strategies to cope (Berry & Laskey, 2012; Lee & Kwon, 2003).

In order to understand the nature of obsessions, researchers have examined the content of intrusive and unwanted thoughts of people in the general population. Rachman and de Silva (1978) originated a survey that elicited the intrusive thoughts of nonclinical participants. They found that 88 percent of the sample endorsed at least one intrusive thought and had virtually the same content as clinical obsessions. Other researchers reported that 99 percent of their nonclinical samples experienced having at least one specific obsession-like intrusive thought, but these occurred less frequently than in those with the disorder (Belloch, Morillo, Lucero, Cabedo, & Carrió, 2004; Purdon & Clark, 1994). Subsequent studies replicated these findings (Berry & Laskey, 2012; Bouvard, Fournet, Denis, Sixdenier, & Clark, 2016; Rachman & de Silva, 1978; Rassin, Cougle, & Muris, 2007). These studies' consistent themes were unacceptable sexual thoughts, fear of causing accidents, and harming/aggressive thoughts about self and others (Berry & Laskey, 2012).

Rachman and de Silva (1978) conducted a unique community-based study that sampled the public about their intrusive thoughts. Table 1.1 provides the outcome of a study by Purdon and Clark (1994) on the prevalence of these intrusive thoughts in their nonclinical sample.

Compared to clinical subjects, found that people without OCD had an easier time accepting and dismissing their thoughts, that the thoughts occurred less frequently, that their duration was shorter, and that they were less intense and distressing.

Compulsions/Rituals

Compulsions or rituals (used interchangeably) are deliberate physical or mental behaviors that are performed to reduce or avoid the anxiety, distress, and emotions provoked by obsessions, created by brain signals as an overresponse in the absence of danger or threat (Boyer, 2003; Li & Mody, 2016). To meet diagnostic criteria, the behaviors must be performed for more than an hour per day (American Psychiatric Association, 2013) or must cause a routine daily task to take several times longer than the norm (Goodman et al., 1989a). Empirically, the tasks take at least three times longer than the norm, based on author's clinical experience.

Analyzing obsessions (mental compulsions) has a rebound effect; attending to them exaggerates their importance, escalates the intensity,

Table 1.1 List of Intrusive Thoughts from Nonclinical Sample (N = 293)

Aggressive/Harming	%
Driving into window	14
Running car off road	60
Hitting animals, people	50
Swerving into traffic	54
Smashing into objects	34
Slitting wrist/throat	21
Cutting off finger	18
Jumping off high place	43
Fatally pushing—stranger	23
Fatally pushing—friend	16
Jumping—train, car	27
Pushing stranger—train, car	14
Pushing family—train, car	10
Hurting strangers	33
Hurting family	55
Choking family member	40
Stabbing family member	41
Throwing something	46
Scratching car paint	16
Breaking window	9
Wrecking something	32
Shoplifting	27
Grabbing money	35
Holding up bank	35
Safety	
Heat/stove on, accident	73
Home unlocked, intruder	73
Taps left on, flood	26
Contamination	
Catching STD	52
Contamination—doors	30

Table 1.1   (Continued)

Contamination	
Contamination—phones	23
Fatal disease—strangers	21
Fatal disease—transmission	21
Dust on the floor	30
Dirt in unseen places	35

Sexual	
Sex with stranger	56
Sex with authority figure	50
Kissing authority figure	41
Seeing authority figures naked	48
Homosexual acts	20
Seeing strangers naked	66
Sex in public	64
Disgusting sex act	48
Exposing self	15

Social	
Breaking wind in public	40
Causing a public scene	45
Insulting stranger	55
Bumping into people	40
Insulting authority	41
Swearing in public	32
Insulting family	57

Source: Purdon and Clark (1994).

and then demands more and more attention (Gillihan, Williams, Malcoun, Yadin, & Foa, 2012). With more attention, the episode becomes more debilitating, as the person begins to neglect other aspects of daily functioning and responsibilities.

Goal-directed, habitual, repetitive, and ritualized behaviors exist in everyday life, often without conscious awareness (Adams et al., 2018). Their purpose is to organize the flow of task completion. They exist in a variety of contexts, including childhood routines, religious and cultural practices, and performance of everyday habitual tasks.

Starting around age two, children begin to display rituals around daily routines that provide a sense of security, order, comfort, and control. Some of these consist of reading the same book every night, insisting that food not touch each other, eating in a certain order, arranging stuffed animals, having a special blanket, checking under the bed or closet for monsters, and sleeping with a light on. Others that are common but appear more like OCD are not leaving the house until things feel "just right," perfectionism, concerns about dirt and cleanliness, ordered household routines, counting and repeating an action to a certain number or number of times, eating rituals, and bedtime rituals (Leonard, Goldberger, Rapoport, Cheslow, & Swedo, 1990). Should these rituals persist beyond age four, they may be signs of early onset OCD (Abed & de Pauw, 1998; Evans & Leckman, 1997).

What role do normal, cultural, and religious rituals play in OCD? Taking one's shoes off before entering a home, washing and praying before eating, checking one's conscience, and confessing are examples of routine cultural and religious practices that transform into compulsions when they are excessive, cause distress if unable to be performed, and go beyond their intended purpose.

In a similar vein, cultural and religious rituals serve to provide cognitive and prosocial community and moral structure, commemorate life-cycle events, and placate forces that may control fate, death, and the unknown (Feygin, Swain, & Leckman, 2006). Evolutionary psychology explains OCD as an extreme manifestation of evolved harm-avoidance strategies (Brüne, 2006). Boyer and Liénard (2006) suggested that ritualized behavior is an evolved precaution system designed to detect and react to threats to safety. Activation of the precaution system explains intrusions and ritual behaviors in normal adults. Within this model, they suggest that the precaution system in those with OCD misappraises potential threats, resulting in doubts about the proper performance of precautions and repetition of action. A lengthier description of culture and religion in OCD, discussing assessment and treatment, will be covered in chapter 11.

Symptomatology

The Yale-Brown Obsessive Compulsive Scale (Y-BOCS) Symptom Checklist presents the varying OCD subtypes (Goodman et al., 1989b). Many individuals present with more than one subtype.

Aggressive/Harming

Common obsessions:

- Experiencing and being afraid of acting on violent, horrific, sexually taboo intrusive thoughts (thoughts of pedophilia, killing loved one)
- Fear of losing control or acting on an impulse (blurting out offensive words)
- Fear of acting socially inappropriately (staring at someone's groin)
- Fear of unintentionally harming others as a result of being careless (accidentally running over someone with car)
- Fear of being responsible for something terrible happening (fire, burglary)
- Fear of harming oneself or others (ego-dystonic thoughts of suicide, homicide)
- Fear of stealing
- Fear of acting out in public places (causing a scene, going crazy)

Common compulsions:

- Checking behaviors (visually checking to be certain nothing is wrong, physically checking for wallet, pressing switches in off position when already off)
- Seeking reassurance from others that nothing is wrong
- Trying to push thoughts away
- Mental reviewing the triggering event (reviewing conversations for mistakes, mentally retracing steps to recall turning something off)
- Avoiding sharp objects, driving, going to public places/parks (keeping away from children)
- Engaging in social avoidance or isolation to keep others safe
- Reassuring oneself that everything is okay
- Using wishing or "should" statements (wishing something to be different)
- Silently repeating special words, images, or numbers
- Counting and recounting
- Making mental lists
- Reviewing thoughts, feelings, conversations, or actions
- Erasing unpleasant mental images
- Undoing something in one's mind

For example, Taylor is driving home from work after sunset and suddenly becomes anxious that the bump he drove over was a hit-and-run accident. He immediately drives back to where he thinks it happened but doesn't see anything. As he is driving off, he thinks that maybe he's seen something out of his peripheral vision and goes back to check. Because there is no evidence, he can't prove with certainty that nothing has happened, so he resigns himself to driving home. He watches the news to see if the police have found a dead body and are looking for him. There is nothing in the news, but he still feels upset and sleeps fitfully. He checks the news in the morning with the same results. Even though he tries to let it go, the doubt and anxiety linger.

Safety

Common obsessions:

- Fear of being responsible for something catastrophic happening
- Fear of accidentally burning down the house by leaving the stove on or appliances plugged in
- Fear of giving someone advice that ends up being harmful
- Fear of poisoning someone by using household products (not seeing warning labels, skull-and-crossbones symbol)

Common compulsions:

- Repeatedly checking appliances, locks, and pockets, and repeatedly retracing steps
- Seeking reassurance
- Reviewing mentally
- Checking that they did or will not harm others
- Checking that they did not or will not harm themselves
- Checking that they did not make mistakes
- Checking body for signs of abnormalities or unwanted symptoms (taking temperature, visually checking throat, physically checking for soreness)

For example, Morgan is frustrated about and stressed by her heavy workload. She hears about a school shooting that has just occurred in a different part of the country and begins to have images of this happening at her kids' school. She tries to shrug it off and not call the school to make sure that everything is safe. She tries to refocus back to her work, but her anxiety rises and she can't get the image out of her head. She worries that having this image means that something bad is happening, and she feels irresponsible if she doesn't go to the school and check. Torn between her workload and her children's safety, she goes to the school, where she sees that everything is normal. She feels anxious, confused, and relieved, but she still can't get rid of the violent images in her head.

Contamination

Common obsessions:

- Fear of dirt, germs, and body fluids (urine, feces, saliva)
- Fear of contracting a disease
- Fear of being poisoned (asbestos, radiation, anthrax)
- Fear of contaminating someone else
- Fear of being contaminated by someone's bad qualities (emotional contamination)
- Excessive concern with environmental contaminants (asbestos, radiation, toxic waste)
- Excessive concern with household items (cleansers, solvents)
- Excessive concern about animals (insects)
- Excessive concern with sticky substances or residues
- Excessive concern with becoming ill because of feared contaminants
- Excessive concern with making others ill by spreading contamination
- Lack of concern about consequences of contamination other than how it might feel (fear of stickiness, feelings of disgust)
- Need to be pure

Common compulsions:

- Excessive hand washing and use of antibacterial gel or hand wipes
- Excessive showering
- Excessive grooming habits
- Excessive use of personal care products (shampoo, soap, toilet paper, disinfectants)
- Excessive cleaning of household items or other inanimate objects
- Unnecessary use of caustic substances to remove germs (bleach)
- Use of physical barriers to avoid touching contaminated surfaces (gloves, paper towels)
- Mental reviewing
- Avoidance of touching others and public items (water fountains, doorknobs)

For example, Lee and his family are eating at a restaurant, and he is suddenly bothered by a dark spot on the wooden table. Not being sure of what it is, he's afraid it is blood. He asks the server to wipe the table down again, but the spot is still there. He can't stop thinking about it and worries that he and his family are going to contract a disease. He puts a napkin over it so that he can't see it. He knows his thoughts are irrational, but he is still tempted to take his family somewhere else to eat.

Intrusive Violent Thoughts

Common obsessions:

- Fear of harming a family member
- Fear of harming a vulnerable person or animal
- Fear of running over a pedestrian with one's car
- Fear of becoming a serial killer

Common compulsions:

- Checking
- Neutralizing
- Thought suppression
- Mental reviewing
- Seeking reassurance
- Avoidance of violent material
- Avoidance of possible "victims"

For example, Blair has been frustrated at work by his heavy workload and has recently been having repetitive thoughts about stabbing a much-older coworker. Blair is so upset by these thoughts that he has requested to be moved to another part of the office. He tries to avoid being around his coworker, but he is required to attend meetings where they are both present. In an attempt to avoid his obsessive thoughts, he sits on the same side of the table so that he doesn't have to look at his coworker.

Intrusive Sexual Thoughts

Common obsessions:

- Excessive concern with pedophilia
- Excessive concern with incest
- Excessive concern with homosexuality

- Excessive concern with bestiality
- Excessive concern with "unnatural" sex acts

Common compulsions:

- Checking
- Neutralizing
- Thought suppression
- Mental reviewing
- Seeking reassurance
- Avoidance of sexual material
- Avoidance of possible "victims"

For example, Roger has severe OCD symptoms and resides in a group home with others who have mental illnesses. He worries that the other residents think he is attracted to them, so he limits his contact with them. He constantly seeks information on the internet about how a person's sexual orientation becomes established and persistently asks his therapist if this behavior means he is gay.

Scrupulosity

Common obsessions:

- Fear of offending God
- Fear of committing blasphemy
- Fear of the devil or some malevolent force
- Fear of going to hell
- Fear of committing a sin
- Fear of having a stain on one's soul
- Need to be pure
- Preoccupation with completing religious rituals "perfectly"
- Excessive concern with sacrilege or blasphemy (taking the Lord's name in vain, fear of making a pact with the devil, calling religious icons sexually explicit names)
- Excessive concern with right and wrong
- Excessive concern with religion or morality

Common compulsions:

- Excessive praying
- Excessive confessing

- Going from church to church or priest to priest for confession or reassurance
- Excessive washing rituals for purification
- Reassurance seeking with family
- Special prayers (short and long) silently repeated in a set manner (God is good)
- Urges to ask, tell, or confess (including reassurance)

For example, Alexa is very involved with her church and dutifully attends services several times a week. Lately, however, she's been having intrusive thoughts and images about having sex with Christ and cursing God. Mortified, she attends confession several times a week to atone for her thoughts, but she never feels absolved and is considering not going to church.

Perfectionism, Symmetry, Exactness, and Not-Just-Right-Experiences

Common obsessions:

- Fear of making mistakes
- Need to achieve unrealistically high standards
- Need to know or remember trivial facts or the exact thing someone has said
- Fear of not saying just the right thing
- Fear of losing things
- Sense of clutter if things are not in perfect order or space
- Wanting things to look right (symmetrical)
- Insistence on certainty and absolutes
- Fear of not saying just the right thing

Common compulsions:

- Adhering to rigid rules for organization and excessive organization
- Lining up papers/objects squarely
- Putting things in order
- Arranging according to subjective rules (alphabetically, chronologically, by color, by size)
- Rigidly following rules or doing tasks perfectly according to a set standard
- Repeating a task until if feels "just right"

- Being overly thorough
- Rereading
- Rewriting until achieving a right, completed, or perfect feeling
- Repeating an activity to undo an obsession
- Ending a task on an even number
- Needing to repeat routine activities (going in or out through a door, getting up from or sitting down in a chair)
- Excessive list making (writing or verbalizing aloud)
- Mental reviewing
- Needing to touch, tap, or rub
- Blinking or staring rituals
- Ritualized eating behaviors

For example, Lee is an administrative assistant at a busy lawyer's office. He has been reprimanded several times for organizing the lawyer's desk while he is at lunch so that the papers he is working on are ordered alphabetically and lined up squarely. Lee worries that his boss will lose track of the important papers he needs for the case he is working on and that he will be blamed for losing them.

Superstitions

Common obsessions:

- Fear of "bad" numbers (13 or 666)
- Belief in lucky or unlucky numbers
- Concern that something bad will happen if a ritual is not completed on the right number
- Fixation on numbers associated with religion/religious practices
- Fixation on numbers associated with birthdays, life events, multiples of a "bad" number (6 + 7 = 13; 3 × 6 = 24)
- Fear of cemeteries
- Fear of black cats
- Attribution of special significance to certain colors (fear or comfort)

Common compulsions:

- Ending on an even number
- Counting to or using a safe number and multiples of that number (brushing each tooth five times, tapping a foot three times, knocking on wood six times)

- Avoiding numbers associated with negative events
- Neutralizing or undoing behaviors (knocking on wood)
- Praying
- Avoidance
- Mentally repeating special words, images, or numbers to neutralize something bad (lucky numbers)

For example, Ali counts in threes while she walks, since she considers this to be a lucky number. If she loses count, she goes back to where she started and tries again. She is often late for work, since she has the need to make sure she performs this ritual correctly so that no harm comes to her loved ones.

Somatic Concerns

Common obsessions:

- Concern with illness or disease
- Excessive concern with a part of the body or aspect of appearance (other than weight)
- Other body-related obsessions

Common compulsions:

- Checking
- Web surfing
- Seeking reassurance from family or doctors

For example, while showering, Pat notices a bump on the back of her neck. Not knowing what it is, she becomes highly anxious and goes on WebMD look for information. Not finding a symptom that exactly matches hers, she makes an appointment with her doctor to see if the bump is cancer. In the meantime, Pat keeps physically checking the bump, which causes irritation and more noticeable redness. At the appointment, the doctor tries to reassure her that it is nothing to worry about and to let it run its course. Still anxious with doubt, Pat makes an appointment with another doctor, who also reassures her that the bump is nothing. Meanwhile, Pat's thoughts are stuck on having a terminal illness and its effect on her family, and her checking behavior continues.

Miscellaneous Symptoms

Common obsessions

- Fear of saying certain things or words
- Fear of losing things
- Intrusive nonviolent images
- Intrusive nonsense sounds, words, or music
- Being bothered by certain sounds/noises to a greater extent than other people
- Pathological doubting (not trusting senses)

Common compulsions:

- Measures other than checking to prevent harm to oneself or others, or to prevent terrible consequences (such as putting an item from the triggering environment into a pocket/purse, not changing clothes until the sense of danger has passed, even for days)
- Mentally finding the right words
- Mentally rehearsing what to say
- Overly or thoroughly explaining

For example, Jordan searches for the perfect words before she speaks in class because she worries that she will embarrass herself by saying something stupid or that she could be misunderstood and feel like she has lied. In order to make sure she is clearly understood, she overexplains her point but is interrupted when her teacher tries to reassure her that he already understands what she is saying.

Other Diagnostic Factors

Symptom Dimensions

Empirical experience and research findings have found predictable and consistent themes among the heterogeneous symptoms of OCD, which have been consolidated into four discrete dimensions: contamination (obsessions with washing and cleaning compulsions); responsibility for harm, injury, bad luck, and mistakes (fear of causing harm obsessions with checking compulsions); unacceptable thoughts (aggressive, sexual, religious, obsessions with mental or undoing rituals); and symmetry, incompleteness, exactness (repeating behaviors until they feel right, ordering, and counting compulsions; Abramowitz et al., 2010; Cordeiro, Sharma, Thennarasu, & Reddy, 2015; Garcia-Soriano & Belloch, 2013). Hoarding was included as a fifth dimension until it was classified as its own disorder in the *DSM-V* (American Psychiatric Association, 2013).

This classification has proven useful for a few reasons. It can help streamline the diagnostic process and facilitate treatment by creating treatment plans that generalize gains within the symptom clusters rather than address one symptom at a time (i.e., conducting exposures for fear of making harmful mistakes can transfer to moral or conscience-related obsessions). They are also said to have genetic, neurobiological, and neurocognitive commonalities, which may help researchers predict what medications, cognitive behavioral therapy (CBT) strategies, or augmentations will be most effective for the presenting symptom dimension (Hashimoto et al., 2011; Mataix-Cols, Rosario-Campos, & Leckman, 2005). A specific genetic marker, BDNF rs3763965, was associated with the symmetry/order/repeating/checking, contamination/cleaning, and somatic dimensions. Another gene, DLGAP1 rs8096794, was identified for aggressive, sexual, and religious dimension (Zai, James, & Richter, 2016).

Not-Just-Right-Experiences (NJREs)/Incompleteness

Paired with symmetry and exactness, not-just-right-experiences are also known as *incompleteness*. While they are a consistent and pervasive OCD trait, they have not been given their own dimensional category even though they have distinct aspects that drive compulsive behaviors. In OCD phenomenology, many patients perform the same compulsions for differing reasons. In the case of NJREs, these behaviors are *task*, rather than *harm*, driven, in that the goal is to feel complete before moving on instead of eliminating anxiety associated with obsessive feared consequences (Coles, Frost, Heimberg, & Rheaume, 2003; Summerfeldt, Kloosterman, Antony, & Swinson, 2014). For instance, Han sits down and stands up in multiples of fours until a complete set provides him the relief to finally settle down into his chair. Ray performs the same behaviors but is motivated by his obsessive fear that his daughter will die in a car crash.

In a similar fashion, perfectionism is another feature in OCD that drives incompletion/NJREs (Coles et al., 2003). Bobby keeps a perfectly ordered home, free of dust and germs. So does Kim. Bobby becomes upset when he notices anything that disrupts the environment because it has become imperfect and begins his extensive cleaning routine. When Kim notices the same disruption, she becomes anxious that her family will become ill unless she restores the household to being free of dust and dirt.

Table 1.2 **Prevalence of OC Symptom Dimensions by Country**

	United States	Italy	Japan	Egypt	Iran	Bahrain	Taiwan
Obsessions							
Contamination	58	60	48	60	60	38	37
Aggressive	45	56	36	41	39	8	12
Sexual	13	17	10	48	41	32	3.5
Religious	26	22	8	60	30	40	-
Symmetry	48	32	42	43	55	-	14
Compulsions							
Washing	60	59	47	63	72	42	45
Checking	69	72	47	58	58	16	50
Repeating	56	58	31	68	-	22	-
Counting	26	16	14	47	44	12	8
Ordering	43	25	22	47	57	-	14

Source: Hollender (1978); Pinto et al. (2007)

Culture

Culture appears to affect prevalence of symptom dimensions according to the prominent values and beliefs within a given society (Cordeiro et al., 2015; Li, Marques, Hinton, Wang, & Xiao, 2009). Table 1.2 presents the prevalence per reported country.

Of note, Japan reported a low rate of religious obsessions supposedly due to the predominance of a Buddhist philosophical lifestyle. It is unclear why the Taiwan study did not report religious obsessions or why Bahrain did not report symmetry obsessions or ordering compulsions in their findings. Taiwan and Bahrain also reported lower levels of aggressive obsessions compared to the other countries. A more thorough examination of ethnic and cultural factors will be reviewed in chapter 11. Symptom dimensions will also be a topic of assessment in chapter 11.

Psychosocial Factors

Family and genetic studies support the heritability of OCD. Rates of OCD heritability are reported to be between 45 and 65 percent (Mataix-Cols et al., 2013; Nestadt et al., 2000).

Age of onset and family history appear to correlate. Early onset was related to high rates of family history (Nestadt et al., 2000). Results of late onset and family history are mixed. Two studies reported no prevalence of family history in their study samples of late onset in first-degree relatives (Nestadt et al., 2000; Sharma, Sundar, Thennarasu, & Reddy, 2015). However, other studies found that relatives of adults with OCD were about two to five times the rate of normal controls and ten times the rate among relatives of children and adolescents of having OCD (Chabane et al., 2005; Nestadt et al., 2000; Pauls, 2010).

There is growing evidence of genetic markers that predispose individuals to inheriting OCD (Burchi & Pallanti, 2019; Rajendram, Kronenberg, Burton, & Arnold, 2017). A glutamate transporter gene has identified early age of OCD onset (Dallaspezia, Mazza, Lorenzi, Benedetti, & Smeraldi, 2014; Dickel et al., 2007; Walitza et al., 2010; Wu et al., 2013).

Age of Onset and Precipitants

Advances in research have stirred several debates about the role age of onset plays in OCD. The debates are important, as there are wide implications for changes in how research findings have reported on the phenomenology, course of illness, treatment outcome, and prognosis. Age of onset may also distinguish a homogeneous aspect of the disorder (Millet et al., 2004).

The first debate is how *onset* is defined. One view considers age of onset as the time symptoms first appear (Butwicka & Gmitrowicz, 2010), often relying on retrospective and subjective recall (Rosario-Campos et al., 2001). The other view determines onset at the first clinically significant episode or when the diagnosis is made (Maina, Albert, Salvi, Pessina, & Bogetto, 2008). Either way, detection and treatment as early as possible can positively affect the overall course and prognosis of the OCD.

The second debate is about the age ranges for early versus late onset, now considered to be distinct subtypes (Sobin, Blundell, & Karayiorgou, 2000; Taylor, 2011). Studies report early onset as beginning at age three or earlier (Garcia et al., 2009; Kenyon & Eaton, 2015; Nestadt et al., 2000) and up to age eighteen (de Mathis et al., 2012; Taylor, 2011). Late onset has ranged from over thirteen to twenty-three years old (Roth, Milovan, Baribeau, & O'Connor, 2005). An intermediate onset subgroup ranging from nine to seventeen has also appeared in the literature (Albert et al., 2015; de Mathis et al., 2012).

Until recently, the course of illness for those with early onset OCD has been considered more impairing (Rosario-Campos et al., 2001; Taylor, 2011). Although recent improvements in early diagnosis and interventions have improved the prognostic outcome (Burchi & Pallanti, 2019), delays in diagnosis and treatment are still common and can have long-term consequences on development, education, interpersonal relationships, and functionality (Moore, Mariaskin, & March, 2007; Westwell-Roper & Stewart, 2019). Diagnosis can take between three to eleven years after the onset of symptoms, due to nonrecognition of the disorder by patients or clinicians, denial or poor insight into the disorder, or issues around stigma (Fenske & Petersen, 2015; Fireman, Koran, Leventhal, & Jacobson, 2001). Of adults with OCD, 30–50 percent reported that their OCD onset occurred before they were eighteen years old (March, Franklin, Nelson, & Foa, 2001).

Table 1.3 provides the differential symptomatology at age of onset.

Stress is known to exacerbate the onset of a first clinically significant OCD episode (Adams et al., 2018). A stressful life event (excluding

Table 1.3   Symptom Prevalence of Early and Late Onset

Obsessions	Early Onset %	Late Onset %
Number of obsessions	3.6	4.9
Aggressive	82	79
Contamination	74	82
Symmetry	45	65
Somatic fears	42	69
Religion	29	57
Superstitions	29	53
Sexual	24	48
Compulsions		
Number of compulsions	3.6	4.7
Repeating	74	86
Cleaning	61	79
Checking	55	91
Tapping/rubbing	55	57
Arranging	42	45
Counting	37	72

Source: Sobin et al. (2000)

trauma) was reported in 25–67 percent of OCD patients at the time of onset of their first episode, characterized as abrupt and not related to having a family history of OCD (Real et al., 2011).

Phenomenologically, women tend to experience subclinical or non-interfering symptoms before their first clinical episode brought on by a significant life event (Frydman et al., 2014). The age of onset for women may coincide with hormonal or reproductive events. The prevalence of a first OCD episode during or after pregnancy occurred in 2–11 percent of women (Sharma & Sommerdyk, 2015). OCD onset has also occurred in new fathers, as reported by Abramowitz and colleagues (2001) in their report of four case studies. They reported that the men had similar obsessive fears and compulsions as the women.

Losses, such as employment or death, developing an illness, and other circumstances that involve a sense of responsibility or duty have been stressful enough to provoke an OCD onset (Rosso, Albert, Asinari, Bogetto, & Maina, 2012). Exposure to danger and being in vulnerable situations can also precipitate OCD (Real et al., 2016).

Gender

The incidence of OCD according to gender is not significantly different, although studies have found a higher rate of early onset in males, with 25 percent occurring before the age of ten (Ruscio, Stein, Chiu, & Kessler, 2010; Sobin et al., 2000). Findings show a higher rate in male children and adolescents (Fineberg et al., 2013).

Phenomenologically, men appear to have a higher frequency of aggressive sexual, religious, and symmetry/exactness obsessions, in addition to checking, ordering/arranging, and hoarding compulsions, while women had obsessions related to contamination and washing/cleaning compulsions, as well as somatic obsessions and compulsions (Labad et al., 2008; Tükel, Polat, Genç, Bozkurt, & Atli, 2004). Table 1.4 outlines clinical differences between the sexes (Bogetto, Venturello, Albert, Maina, & Ravizza, 1999).

Misdiagnosis/Delayed Diagnosis and Referrals

Fortunately, improved recognition of the early signs of OCD has helped facilitate treatment in a more time-sensitive manner. Still, many sufferers may be misdiagnosed, unnecessarily hospitalized, and given inappropriate treatment. People may not understand the nature of their intrusive

Table 1.4   **Differences between Sexes**

	Males	Females
Symptom dimensions	Aggressive, sexual, religious, symmetry/exactness obsessions	Somatic and contamination obsessions and washing/cleaning compulsions
Onset	Gradual	Abrupt/acute stressful life event
Course	Chronic	Episode
Age onset	Earlier	Later
Severity	Greater	Less

Source: Bogetto, Venturello, Albert, Maina, and Ravizza (1999); Torresan et al. (2013)

thoughts or be unwilling to disclose them for fear that their thoughts may be mistaken for homicidal or suicide, that they may be considered a pedophile, or that they suffer from delusions.

Over half of 208 physicians who read clinical OCD vignettes in an online survey misidentified symptoms for homosexuality (84%), aggression (80%), pedophilia (71%), somatic concerns (40%), religious problems (38%), and contamination worries (32%), and they were more likely to prescribe antipsychotic medication (Glazier, Swing, & McGinn, 2015). Level of poor insight may contribute to a misdiagnosis of psychosis in adults (Jacob, Larson, & Storch, 2014). People seeking medical attention for somatic obsessions may be overtreated by physicians who prescribe medication for mild physical symptoms of complaint, or be prescribed medications for symptoms they are afraid of having (Stein, Fineberg, & Harvey, 2001).

Given that the prevalence of childhood OCD is 1–2 percent, improved recognition of OCD by pediatricians will help reduce the burden of OCD and improve the course of normal development and quality of life much sooner (Fenske & Petersen, 2015). Historically, early onset OCD was often mistaken for attention-deficit/hyperactivity disorder (ADHD) and assumed to account for behavioral problems in the classroom. Children were unwittingly prescribed stimulants that are effective for ADHD, which actually exacerbate OCD symptoms (Dar & Abramovitch, 2012). OCD has also been mistaken for autism spectrum disorder due to repetitive behaviors and single-minded focus and preoccupation on thoughts common to both disorders (Brasic & Farhadi, 2018).

Chapter 6 will provide more insights into the burden and costs of delayed diagnosis and treatment.

Incidence

The high prevalence of subthreshold OCD symptoms may help explain past inconsistencies in prevalence estimates across surveys and suggests that the public health burden of OCD may be greater than its low prevalence implies. Evidence of a preponderance of early onset cases in men, high comorbidity with a wide range of disorders, and reliable associations between disorder severity and key outcomes may have implications for how OCD is classified in *DSM-V* (Ruscio et al., 2010).

Findings from epidemiological and phenomenological studies on the incidence of common OCD symptoms are provided in table 1.5. The columns list the percent of obsessions and compulsions separately and do not correspond to each other across the columns (Ruscio et al., 2010). Table 1.6 provides information about the differences between sexes on the age of onset, course of illness, and the presence of a precipitating event (Ruscio, et al., 2010).

OCD comes in many different forms. It can be tempting for clinicians to analyze the content of obsessions with clients in order to formulate the case. Once clinicians providing psychoeducation and redirecting patients away from the catastrophic "what if" thoughts will also help patients to understand that the priority is to focus on the treatment, not on the imaginative consequences of their fears.

Table 1.5   Prevalence of OCD Subtypes and Course of Illness

Obsessions	%	Compulsions	%
Aggressive	71	Checking	69
Contamination	58	Cleaning	60
Pathological doubt	56	Washing	50
Sexual	13	Repeating	56
Symmetry	48	Ordering	43
Religious	26	Counting	36
Somatic	26	Confessing	31
Miscellaneous	57	Symmetry	28
		Multiple	48

Sources: Pinto, Mancebo, Eisen, Pagano, and Rasmussen (2006); Ruscio et al. (2010)

Table 1.6   Age of Onset, Course, and Presence of Precipitant

Age of Onset	
Male	17 (±6.8)
Female	20.8 (±8.5)
Course Type	
Continuous	85%
Deteriorative	10%
Episodic	2%
Precipitant	
Not present	71%
Present	29%

Source: Ruscio et al. (2010)

References

Abed, R. T., & de Pauw, K. W. (1998). An evolutionary hypothesis for obsessive compulsive disorder: A psychological immune system? *Behavioural Neurolology, 11*(4), 245–250. Retrieved from https://www.ncbi.nlm.nih.gov/pubmed/11568426

Abramowitz, J., Moore, K., Carmin, C., Wiegartz, P. S., & Purdon, C. (2001). Acute onset of obsessive-compulsive disorder in males following childbirth. *Psychosomatics, 42*(5), 429–431. doi:10.1176/appi.psy.42.5.429

Abramowitz, J. S., Deacon, B. J., Olatunji, B. O., Wheaton, M. G., Berman, N. C., Losardo, D., . . . Hale, L. R. (2010). Assessment of obsessive-compulsive symptom dimensions: Development and evaluation of the Dimensional Obsessive-Compulsive Scale. *Psychological Assessment, 22*(1), 180–198. doi:10.1037/a0018260

Adams, T. G., Kelmendi, B., Brake, C. A., Gruner, P., Badour, C. L., & Pittenger, C. (2018). The role of stress in the pathogenesis and maintenance of obsessive-compulsive disorder. *Chronic Stress (Thousand Oaks), 2.* doi:10.1177/2470547018758043

Albert, U., Manchia, M., Tortorella, A., Volpe, U., Rosso, G., Carpiniello, B., & Maina, G. (2015). Admixture analysis of age at symptom onset and age at disorder onset in a large sample of patients with obsessive-compulsive disorder. *Journal of Affective Disorders, 187,* 188–196. doi:10.1016/j.jad.2015.07.045

American Psychiatric Association. (2013). *Diagnostic and statistical manual of mental disorders* (5th ed.). Washington, DC: American Psychiatric Publishing.

Belloch, A., Morillo, C., Lucero, M., Cabedo, E., & Carrió, C. (2004). Intrusive thoughts in non-clinical subjects: The role of frequency and unpleasantness on appraisal ratings and control strategies. *Clinical Psychology & Psychotherapy, 11*(2), 100–110. doi:10.1002/cpp.397

Berry, L.-M., & Laskey, B. (2012). A review of obsessive intrusive thoughts in the general population. *Journal of Obsessive-Compulsive and Related Disorders, 1*(2), 125–132. doi:10.1016/j.jocrd.2012.02.002

Bogetto, F., Venturello, S., Albert, U., Maina, G., & Ravizza, L. (1999). Gender-related clinical differences in obsessive-compulsive disorder. *European Psychiatry, 14*(8), 434–441. Retrieved from https://www.ncbi.nlm.nih.gov/pubmed/10683629

Bouvard, M., Fournet, N., Denis, A., Sixdenier, A., & Clark, D. (2016). Intrusive thoughts in patients with obsessive compulsive disorder and non-clinical participants: A comparison using the International Intrusive Thought Interview Schedule. *Cognitive Behaviour Therapy, 46*(4), 287–299.

Boyer, P. (2003). Religious thought and behaviour as by-products of brain function. *Trends in Cognitive Sciences, 7*(3), 119–124. doi:10.1016/S1364-6613(03)00031-7

Boyer, P., & Liénard, P. (2006). Why ritualized behavior?: Precaution systems and action parsing in developmental, pathological and cultural rituals. *Behavioral and Brain Sciences, 29*(6), 595–613, discussion 613–550.

Brasic, J. R., & Farhadi, F. (2018). Pediatric obsessive-compulsive disorder differential diagnosis. Medscape. Retrieved from https://emedicine.medscape.com/article/1826591-differential

Brüne, M. (2006). The evolutionary psychology of obsessive-compulsive disorder: The role of cognitive metarepresentation. *Perspectives in Biology and Medicine, 49*(3), 317–329. doi:10.1353/pbm.2006.0037

Burchi, E., & Pallanti, S. (2019). Diagnostic issues in early-onset obsessive-compulsive disorder and their treatment implications. *Current Neuropharmacology, 178*, 672–680. doi:10.2174/1570159X16666180426151746

Butwicka, A., & Gmitrowicz, A. (2010). Symptom clusters in obsessive-compulsive disorder (OCD): Influence of age and age of onset. *European Child & Adolescent Psychiatry, 19*(4), 365–370. doi:10.1007/s00787-009-0055-2

Chabane, N., Delorme, R., Millet, B., Mouren, M. C., Leboyer, M., & Pauls, D. (2005). Early-onset obsessive-compulsive disorder: A subgroup with a specific clinical and familial pattern? *Journal of Child Psychology and Psychiatry, 46*, 881–887. doi:10.1111/j.1469-7610.2004.00382.x

Coles, M. E., Frost, R. O., Heimberg, R. G., & Rheaume, J. (2003). "Not just right experiences": Perfectionism, obsessive-compulsive features and general psychopathology. *Behaviour Research and Therapy, 41,* 681–700.

Cordeiro, T., Sharma, M. P., Thennarasu, K., & Reddy, Y. C. (2015). Symptom dimensions in obsessive-compulsive disorder and obsessive beliefs. *Indian Journal of Psychological Medicine, 37*(4), 403–408. doi:10.4103/0253-7176.168579

Dallaspezia, S., Mazza, M., Lorenzi, C., Benedetti, F., & Smeraldi, E. (2014). A single nucleotide polymorphism in SLC1A1 gene is associated with age of onset of obsessive-compulsive disorder. *European Psychiatry, 29*(5), 301–303. doi:10.1016/j.eurpsy.2014.02.006

Dar, R., & Abramovitch, A. (2012). OCD for ADHD has serious consequences. *Science Daily.* Retrieved from https://www.sciencedaily.com/releases/2012/12/121218121423.htm

de Mathis, M. A., Diniz, J. B., Hounie, A. G., Shavitt, R. G., Fossaluza, V., Ferrão, Y., . . . Miguel, E. C. (2012). Trajectory in obsessive-compulsive disorder comorbidities. *European Neuropsychopharmacology.* doi: 10.1016/j.euroneuro.2012.08.006

Dickel, D. E., Veenstra-VanderWeele, J., Bivens, N. C., Wu, X., Fischer, D. J., Van Etten-Lee, M., . . . Hanna, G. L. (2007). Association studies of serotonin system candidate genes in early-onset obsessive-compulsive disorder. *Biological Psychiatry, 61*(3), 322–329. doi:10.1016/j.biopsych.2006.09.030

Evans, D. W., & Leckman, J. F. (1997). Ritual, habit, and perfectionism: The prevalence and development of compulsive-like behavior in. *Child Development, 68*(1), 58–68. doi:10.1111/1467-8624.ep9707256799

Fenske, J. N., & Petersen, K. (2015). Obsessive-compulsive disorder: Diagnosis and management. *American Family Physician, 92*(10), 896–903. Retrieved from https://www.ncbi.nlm.nih.gov/pubmed/26554283

Feygin, D. L., Swain, J. E., & Leckman, J. F. (2006). The normalcy of neurosis: Evolutionary origins of obsessive-compulsive disorder and related behaviors. *Progress in Neuro-Psychopharmacology & Biological Psychiatry, 30*(5), 854–864. doi:10.1016/j.pnpbp.2006.01.009

Fineberg, N. A., Hengartner, M. P., Bergbaum, C., Gale, T., Rössler, W., & Angst, J. (2013). Lifetime comorbidity of obsessive-compulsive disorder and sub-threshold obsessive-compulsive symptomatology in the community: Impact, prevalence, socio-demographic and clinical characteristics. *International Journal of Psychiatry in Clinical Practice, 17*(3), 188–196. doi:10.3109/13651501.2013.777745

Fireman, B., Koran, L. M., Leventhal, J. L., & Jacobson, A. (2001). The prevalence of clinically recognized obsessive-compulsive disorder in a large health maintenance organization. *American Journal of Psychiatry, 158*(11), 1904–1910. doi:10.1176/appi.ajp.158.11.1904

Freud, S. (1924). Obsessive actions and religious practices. In *The standard edition of the complete psychological works of Sigmund Freud* (Vol. 9, pp. 117–127) (A. F. Strachey, Trans.). London: Hogarth Press.

Frydman, I., Pedro, E., Torres, A. R., Shavitt, R. G., Ferrão, Y. A., Rosário, M. C., . . . Fontenelle, L. F. (2014). Late-onset obsessive-compulsive disorder: Risk factors and correlates. *Journal of Psychiatric Research, 49*, 68–74.

Garcia, A. M., Freeman, J. B., Himle, M. B., Berman, N. C., Ogata, A. K., Ng, J., . . . Leonard, H. (2009). Phenomenology of early childhood onset obsessive compulsive disorder. *Journal of Psychopathology and Behavioral Assessment, 31*(2), 104–111. doi:10.1007/s10862-008-9094-0

Garcia-Soriano, G., & Belloch, A. (2013). Symptom dimensions in obsessive-compulsive disorder: Differences in distress, interference, appraisals and neutralizing strategies. *Journal of Behavior Therapy and Experimental Psychiatry, 44*(4), 441–448. doi:10.1016/j.jbtep.2013.05.005

Gillihan, S. J., Williams, M. T., Malcoun, E., Yadin, E., & Foa, E. B. (2012). Common pitfalls in exposure and response prevention (EX/RP) for OCD. *Journal of Obsessive-Compulsive and Related Disorders, 1*(4), 251–257. doi:10.1016/j.jocrd.2012.05.002

Glazier, K., Swing, M., & McGinn, L. K. (2015). Half of obsessive-compulsive disorder cases misdiagnosed: Vignette-based survey of primary care physicians. *Journal of Clinical Psychiatry, 76*(6), e761–767. doi:10.4088/JCP.14m09110

Goodman, W. K., Price, L. H., Rasmussen, S. A., Mazure, C., Fleischmann, R. L., Hill, C. L., . . . Charney, D. S. (1989a). The Yale-Brown Obsessive Compulsive Scale (YBOCS): Part I. Development, use, and reliability. *Archives of General Psychiatry, 46*, 1012–1016.

Goodman, W. K., Price, L. H., Rasmussen, S. A., Mazure, C., Fleischmann, R. L., Hill, C. L., . . . Charney, D. S. (1989b). The Yale-Brown Obsessive Compulsive Scale (YBOCS): Part I. Development, use, and reliability. Part II. Validity. *Archives of General Psychiatry, 46*, 1012–1016.

Hashimoto, N., Nakaaki, S., Omori, I. M., Fujioi, J., Noguchi, Y., Murata, Y., . . . Furukawa, T. A. (2011). Distinct neuropsychological profiles of three major symptom dimensions in obsessive-compulsive disorder. *Psychiatry Research, 187*(1–2), 166–173. doi:10.1016/j.psychres.2010.08.001

Hollender, M. (1978). Perfectionism, a neglected personality trait. *Journal of Clinical Psychiatry, 39*(5), 384. Retrieved from http://www.ncbi .nlm.nih.gov/entrez/query.fcgi?cmd=Retrieve&db=PubMed&dopt =Citation&list_uids=641018

Jacob, M. L., Larson, M. J., & Storch, E. A. (2014). Insight in adults with obsessive-compulsive disorder. *Comprehensive Psychiatry, 55*(4), 896–903. doi:10.1016/j.comppsych.2013.12.016

Kenyon, K. M., & Eaton, W. O. (2015). Age at child obsessive-compulsive disorder onset and its relation to gender, symptom severity, and family functioning. *Archives of Scientific Psychology, 3*(1), 150–158. doi:10.1037/arc0000022

Labad, J., Menchon, J. M., Alonso, P., Segalas, C., Jimenez, S., Jaurrieta, N., . . . Vallejo, J. (2008). Gender differences in obsessive-compulsive symptom dimensions. *Depression and Anxiety, 25*(10), 832–838. doi:10.1002/da.20332

Lee, H. J., & Kwon, S. M. (2003). Two different types of obsession: Autogenous obsessions and reactive obsessions. *Behaviour Research and Therapy, 41*(1), 11–29. Retrieved from https://www.ncbi.nlm.nih .gov/pubmed/12488117

Leonard, H. L., Goldberger, E. L., Rapoport, J. L., Cheslow, D. L., & Swedo, S. E. (1990). Childhood rituals: Normal development or obsessive-compulsive symptoms? *Journal of the American Academy of Child & Adolescent Psychiatry, 29*(1), 17–23. doi:10.1097 /00004583-199001000-00004

Li, B., & Mody, M. (2016). Cortico-striato-thalamo-cortical circuitry, working memory, and obsessive-compulsive disorder. *Frontiers in Psychiatry, 7*, 78. doi:10.3389/fpsyt.2016.00078

Li, Y., Marques, L., Hinton, D. E., Wang, Y., & Xiao, Z. P. (2009). Symptom dimensions in Chinese patients with obsessive-compulsive disorder. *CNS Neuroscience & Therapeutics, 15*(3), 276–282. doi:10 .1111/j.1755-5949.2009.00099.x

Maina, G., Albert, U., Salvi, V., Pessina, E., & Bogetto, F. (2008). Early-onset obsessive-compulsive disorder and personality disorders in adulthood. *Psychiatry Research, 158*(2), 217–225.

March, J. S., Franklin, M., Nelson, A., & Foa, E. (2001). Cognitive-behavioral psychotherapy for pediatric obsessive-compulsive disorder. *Journal of Clinical Child & Adolescent Psychology, 30*(1), 8–18. doi:10.1207/S15374424JCCP3001_3

Mataix-Cols, D., Boman, M., Monzani, B., Rück, C., Serlachius, E., Långström, N., & Lichtenstein, P. (2013). Population-based, multigenerational family clustering study of obsessive-compulsive disorder. *JAMA Psychiatry, 70*(7), 709–717. doi:10.1001/jamapsychiatry.2013.3

Mataix-Cols, D., Rosario-Campos, M. C., & Leckman, J. F. (2005). A multidimensional model of obsessive-compulsive disorder. *American Journal of Psychiatry, 162*(2), 228–238. doi:10.1176/appi.ajp.162.2.228

Millet, B., Kochman, F., Gallarda, T., Krebs, M. O., Demonfaucon, F., Barrot, I., . . . Hantouche, E. G. (2004). Phenomenological and comorbid features associated in obsessive-compulsive disorder: Influence of age of onset. *Journal of Affective Disorders, 79*(1–3), 241–246. doi:10.1016/S0165-0327(02)00351-8

Moore, P. S., Mariaskin, A., & March, J. (2007). Obsessive-compulsive disorder in children and adolescents: Diagnosis, comorbidity, and developmental factors. In E. A. G. Storch, G. R. Gefken, & T. Murphy (Eds.), *Handbook of child and adolescent obsessive-compulsive disorder* (pp. 17–45). New York: Lawrence Erlbaum Associates.

Nestads. G., Samuels, J., Riddle, M., Bienvenu, O. J., Liang, K. Y., LaBuda, M., Grados, M., & Hoehn-Saric, R. A. (2000). A family study of obsessive-compulsive disorder. *Archives of General Psychiatry, 57*(4), 358–363. doi:10.1001/archpsyc.57.4.358

Pauls, D. L. (2010). The genetics of obsessive-compulsive disorder: A review. *Dialogues in Clinical Neuroscience, 12*(2), 149–163. Retrieved from https://www.ncbi.nlm.nih.gov/pubmed/20623920

Pinto, A., Eisen, J. L., Mancebo, M. C., Greenberg, B. D., Stout, R. L., & Rasmussen, S. A. (2007). Taboo thoughts and doubt/checking: A refinement of the factor structure for obsessive-compulsive disorder symptoms. *Psychiatry Research, 151*(3), 255–258.

Pinto, A., Mancebo, M. C., Eisen, J. L., Pagano, M. E., & Rasmussen, S. A. (2006). The Brown Longitudinal Obsessive Compulsive Study: Clinical features and symptoms of the sample at intake. *Journal of Clinical Psychiatry, 67*(5), 703–711. Retrieved from https://www.ncbi.nlm.nih.gov/pubmed/16841619

Purdon, C., & Clark, D. A. (1994). Obsessive intrusive thoughts in nonclinical subjects: II. Cognitive appraisal, emotional response and thought control strategies. *Behaviour Research and Therapy, 32*(4), 403–410. doi:10.1016/0005-7967(94)90003-5

Rachman, S., & de Silva, P. (1978). Abnormal and normal obsessions. *Behaviour Research and Therapy, 16*(4), 233–248. Retrieved from https://www.ncbi.nlm.nih.gov/pubmed/718588

Rajendram, R., Kronenberg, S., Burton, C. L., & Arnold, P. D. (2017). Glutamate genetics in obsessive-compulsive disorder: A review. *Journal* of the Candian Academy of Child and Adolescent Psychiatry, 26(3), 205–213. Retrieved from https://www.ncbi.nlm.nih.gov/pubmed /29056983

Rassin, E., Cougle, J. R., & Muris, P. (2007). Content difference between normal and abnormal obsessions. *Behaviour Research and Therapy,* 45(11), 2800–2803. doi:10.1016/j.brat.2007.07.006

Real, E., Labad, J., Alonso, P., Segalàs, C., Jiménez-Murcia, S., Bueno, B., . . . Menchón, J. M. (2011). Stressful life events at onset of obsessive-compulsive disorder are associated with a distinct clinical pattern. *Depression and Anxiety, 28*(5), 367–376. doi:10.1002/da.20792

Real, E., Subirà, M., Alonso, P., Segalàs, C., Labad, J., Orfila, C., . . . Menchón, J. M. (2016). Brain structural correlates of obsessive-compulsive disorder with and without preceding stressful life events. *World Journal of Biological Psychiatry, 17*(5), 366–377. doi:10.3109 /15622975.2016.1142606

Rosario-Campos, M. C., Leckman, J. F., Mercadante, M. T., Shavitt, R. G., Prado, H. S., Sada, P., . . . Miguel, E. C. (2001). Adults with early-onset obsessive-compulsive disorder. *American Journal of Psychiatry, 158*(11), 1899–1903. doi:10.1176/appi.ajp.158.11.1899

Rosso, G., Albert, U., Asinari, G. F., Bogetto, F., & Maina, G. (2012). Stressful life events and obsessive-compulsive disorder: Clinical features and symptom dimensions. *Psychiatry Research, 197*(3), 259–264. doi:10.1016/j.psychres.2011.10.005

Roth, R. M., Milovan, D., Baribeau, J., & O'Connor, K. (2005). Neuropsychological functioning in early- and late-onset obsessive-compulsive disorder. *Journal of Neuropsychiatry and Clinical Neurosciences, 17*(2), 208–213. doi:10.1176/appi.neuropsych.17.2.208

Ruscio, A. M., Stein, D. J., Chiu, W. T., & Kessler, R. C. (2010). The epidemiology of obsessive-compulsive disorder in the National Comorbidity Survey Replication. *Molecular Psychiatry, 15*(1), 53–63. doi:10.1038/mp.2008.94

Sharma, E., Sundar, A. S., Thennarasu, K., & Reddy, Y. C. (2015). Is late-onset OCD a distinct phenotype?: Findings from a comparative analysis of "age at onset" groups. *CNS Spectrums, 20*(5), 508–514. doi:10.1017/S1092852914000777

Sharma, V., & Sommerdyk, C. (2015). Obsessive-compulsive disorder in the postpartum period: Diagnosis, differential diagnosis and management. *Women's Health, 11*(4), 543–552.

Sobin, C., Blundell, M. L., & Karayiorgou, M. (2000). Phenotypic differences in early- and late-onset obsessive-compulsive disorder. *Comprehensive Psychiatry, 41*(5), 373–379. doi:10.1053/comp.2000.9009

Stein, D. J., Fineberg, N. A., & Harvey, B. (2001). Unusual symptoms of OCD. In N. Fineberg, D. Marazziti, & D. J. Stein (Eds.), *Obsessive compulsive disorder: A practical guide* (pp. 37–50). London: Martin Dunitz.

Summerfeldt, L. J., Kloosterman, P. H., Antony, M. M., & Swinson, R. P. (2014). Examining an obsessive-compulsive core dimensions model: Structural validity of harm avoidance and incompleteness. *Journal of Obsessive-Compulsive and Related Disorders, 3*(2), 83–94. doi:10.1016/j.jocrd.2014.01.003

Taylor, S. (2011). Early versus late onset obsessive-compulsive disorder: Evidence for distinct subtypes. *Clinical Psychology Review, 31*(7), 1083–1100.

Torresan, R. C., Ramos-Cerqueira, A. T. A., Shavitt, R. G., do Rosário, M. C., de Mathis, M. A., Miguel, E. C., & Torres, A. R. (2013). Symptom dimensions, clinical course and comorbidity in men and women with obsessive-compulsive disorder. *Psychiatry Research, 209*(2), 186–195.

Tükel, R., Polat, A., Genç, A., Bozkurt, O., & Atli, H. (2004). Gender-related differences among Turkish patients with obsessive-compulsive disorder. *Comprehensive Psychiatry, 45*(5), 362–366. doi:10.1016/j.comppsych.2004.06.006

Walitza, S., Wendland, J. R., Gruenblatt, E., Warnke, A., Sontag, T. A., Tucha, O., & Lange, K. W. (2010). Genetics of early-onset obsessive-compulsive disorder. *European Child & Adolescent Psychiatry, 19*(3), 227–235. doi:10.1007/s00787-010-0087-7

Westwell-Roper, C., & Stewart, S. E. (2019). Challenges in the diagnosis and treatment of pediatric obsessive-compulsive disorder. *Indian Journal of Psychiatry, 61*(Suppl 1), S119–S130. doi:10.4103/psychiatry.IndianJPsychiatry_524_18

Wu, H., Wang, X., Xiao, Z., Yu, S., Zhu, L., Wang, D., . . . Fralick, D. (2013). Association between SLC1A1 gene and early-onset OCD in the Han Chinese population: A case-control study. *Journal of Molecular Neuroscience, 50*(2), 353–359. doi:10.1007/s12031-013-9995-6

Zai, G. A. K., James, L., & Richter, M. P. A. (2016). *Genetics of obsessive-compulsive disorder: From phenotypes to pharmacogenetics* (Doctoral dissertation). University of Toronto, Canada.

CHAPTER 2

Obsessive Compulsive Related and Comorbid Disorders

Because the *DSM-V* category Obsessive Compulsive and Related Disorders includes diagnoses that have obsessive and compulsive traits, it is essential that practitioners be able to distinguish them from each other, especially if a person has more than one diagnosis.

Likewise, it is also important to distinguish between compulsivity and impulsivity. The chapter will begin with this topic to provide an understanding of the different mechanisms that drive these two factors and then will move on to delineating the spectrum of related disorders that have elements of compulsive or impulsive urges and behaviors.

Differentiating Impulsivity and Compulsivity

Before delving into aspects of OCD comorbid and related disorders, a review of how to distinguish compulsive and impulsive behaviors is provided, as these conditions are misidentified in the culture. It is important that an accurate diagnosis is made in order to provide appropriate differential treatment, as some people have behaviors that lie along the compulsive-impulsive spectrum. A recent prevalence rate of OCD and any impulse control was found to be 36 percent (Torres et al., 2016). Having this understanding will help readers when discussing the related diagnoses throughout this chapter.

Compulsive behaviors are motivated out of fear, and while they are being performed, they are experienced as distressing. Some behaviors, such as beginning and ending a walk with the left foot, have no obvious relationship to the overall goal to protect someone from harm, are driven by the desire to alleviate fear and anxiety, and often result in avoiding triggering situations.

Unlike compulsions, impulsive behaviors are often carried out with poor judgment that provides pleasure, reward, and immediate gratification. Many people are driven by thrill-seeking urges reinforced by a euphoric feeling, which is why they are so difficult to control. As a result, impulsive behaviors such as eating, shopping, gambling, and electronic gaming are typically mislabeled *compulsive*. Impulsivity might include a self-destructive risk-taking relationship, while compulsivity is risk averse and serves to keep things safe. Impulsivity differs from spontaneity, which is driven by a sense of love, freedom, creativity, self-expression, and innovation.

Table 2.1 presents the differing characteristics that seem to underlie the two constructs. Table 2.2 describes the differing experiences and physiological processes between compulsive and impulsive urges.

For example, Myra has obsessive fears about blaspheming God. She is a practicing Christian and ritualistically prays when she goes about her day, due to having the intrusive thought that she may have committed the unpardonable sin of rejecting God. While out shopping, she goes on shopping binges that provide an emotional high and an escape from the challenges of reality. Her OCD causes anxiety, and the binges set off

Table 2.1 Characteristics of Compulsive and Impulsive Behavior

Compulsive	Impulsive
Inability or unwillingness to tolerate distress	Inability to delay gratification
Decisions are made with the goal of alleviating anxiety	Decisions are made with the goal of attaining an immediate reward regardless of outcome
Intention of behavior is to neutralize threat or reduce anxiety	Intention of behavior is to increase arousal, pleasure, or gratification
Symptoms are ego-dystonic	Symptoms are ego-syntonic
Behavior prevents fear of causing harm	Behavior has real potential to be harmful to self or others
Risk averse	Risk affinity; risk taking/thrill seeking

Table 2.2   Experience and Process of Resisting Compulsive and Impulsive Urges

	Compulsive	Impulsive
Subjective Experience	Fear	Building tension
Function of Behavior	Decrease of fear	Pleasant sensation
Maintained by	Negative reinforcement (ending aversive sensation)	Positive reinforcement (engaging in the behavior is strengthened by occurrence of pleasant sensation)
Resolution of Urges	Decrease through habituation	Increase over time until completion

endorphins, but at the end of the day, both the OCD and the emotional consequences of spending money that add to her debt leave her feeling hopeless and depressed.

Obsessive Compulsive Spectrum and Related Disorders

An accurate diagnosis of OCD is challenging, as its symptomatology has some characteristics that overlap with other disorders now considered to be on the OC spectrum, as reflected by the category established in the *DSM-V* (American Psychiatric Association, 2013) Obsessive Compulsive and Related Disorders.

Obsessive compulsive spectrum disorder (OCSD) was created to identify disorders that have confounding obsessive-compulsive traits (Hollander, Mucci, & Mucci, 2000). It is not a validated construct, but it has clinical utility because it helps conceptualize the differential and overlapping qualities of several discrete disorders. Table 2.3 provides the prevalence ratings of OCD and comorbidities.

Body-Focused Repetitive and Impulsive Behaviors

Body-focused repetitive behavior disorders (BFRBs) refer to a group of behaviors, usually nervous habits or grooming behaviors that are performed to the point of self-injury. These include nail biting (onychophagia), nose picking (rhinotillexis), skin/scab picking (dermatillomania), hair pulling (trichotillomania), and lip/cheek biting or skin chewing (dermatophagia). The subsequent consequences are not only physical pain

Table 2.3   **Common Comorbid Disorders with OCD**

Axis I	Prevalence %
MAJOR DEPRESSION	12–68 (Altıntaş & Taşkıntuna, 2015) 37 (Torres et al., 2006)
SOCIAL PHOBIA	15–44 (Altıntaş & Taşkıntuna, 2015) 30 (Frías, Palma, Farriols, & González, 2015) 17 (Torres et al., 2006)
PANIC DISORDER	2–25 (Altıntaş & Taşkıntuna, 2015) 22 (Torres et al., 2006)
BODY DYSMORPHIC DISORDER	28 BDD primary (Frías et al., 2015) 10 OCD primary (Frías et al., 2015) 0.1–15 (Altıntaş & Taşkıntuna, 2015) 12 (Lochner et al., 2014)
BIPOLAR DISORDER	4–8 (Saraf et al., 2017; Shashidhara, Sushma, Viswanath, Math, & Janardhan Reddy, 2015) 1–15 (Altıntaş & Taşkıntuna, 2015)
ATTENTION-DEFICIT/ HYPERACTIVITY DISORDER	0–60 (Lochner et al., 2014)
GENERALIZED ANXIETY DISORDER	1–35 (Lochner et al., 2014) 31 (Torres et al., 2006)
EATING DISORDER	2–5 (Altıntaş & Taşkıntuna, 2015)
POST-TRAUMATIC STRESS DISORDER	30 primary OCD (Dykshoorn, 2014) 30–82 primary PTSD (Dykshoorn, 2014)
SUBCLINICAL AUTISM SPECTRUM DISORDER	10–17 (Arildskov et al., 2016)
TOURETTE'S SYNDROME	50 (Hirschtritt et al., 2015) 4 (Lochner et al., 2014)
TIC DISORDERS	13 (Lochner et al., 2014)
TRICHOTILLOMANIA (HAIR PULLING)	19 (Keuthen et al., 2016) 5 (Lochner et al., 2014)
EXCORIATION (SKIN PICKING)	20 (Keuthen et al., 2016)
Axis II	
OBSESSIVE COMPULSIVE PERSONALITY DISORDER	10 (Bulli, Melli, Cavalletti, Stopani, & Carraresi, 2016)
NARCISSISTIC PERSONALITY DISORDER	6 (Bulli et al., 2016)

but also emotional and psychological pain, shame, remorse, damages to appearance, and medical problems, such as infection from open wounds (Leung & Robson, 1990; Teng, Woods, Twohig, & Marcks, 2002).

Because these disorders are self-soothing, regulate emotion, reduce anxiety or tension, and can distract from starting or completing a task (Maraz, Griffiths, & Demetrovics, 2016), they are difficult to stop. The release of endorphins produces a feeling of euphoria that reinforces the behavior when the next urge arises, and the cycle is repeated (Nock, Prinstein, & Sterba, 2009).

A study of 1,618 people found that one out of three people met the clinical diagnosis of at least one grooming disorder (Bienvenu et al., 2009).

Trichotillomania

Trichotillomania (TTM), hair pulling, like other impulsive behaviors, is self-soothing and pleasurable (Swedo & Leonard, 1992). The criteria outlined in the *DSM-V* for TTM are ongoing episodes of hair pulling that the person attempts to resist and that, while pleasurable at the time, are also distressing and can interfere with social, work, and daily functioning (American Psychiatric Association, 2013).

There are two types of hair pulling: *automatic*, which is unconscious and produced by internal cues (sensations on scalp, building urges, stress, etc.), and *focused*, which is conscious, is usually provoked by external cues (hair-pulling implements, mirrors, particular settings, certain visual or tactile stimuli, etc.) and can be planned (Christenson, Pyle, & Mitchell, 1991; Duke, Bodzin, Tavares, Geffken, & Storch, 2009).

Hair can be pulled from the head, face, eyebrows, eyelashes, armpits, legs, and pubic hair. Many hair pullers have ritualistic behaviors, such as feeling for hairs that have a bumpy texture, inspecting the hair and the follicle, biting/chewing the follicle, and sometimes eating the hair (trichophagy). The latter can lead to health problems, such as hair balls (trichobezoars) that can cause severe digestive and pancreatic problems, repetitive movement injuries, scalp bleeding or irritation, or dental damage from chewing the root of the pulled hair (Begotka, Woods, & Wetterneck, 2004).

Other consequences of TTM are bald spots that are covered by hairstyles, wigs, scarves, hats, or hair weaves. Eyebrows are often penciled in, or sunglasses are worn to hide the lack of eyelashes or eyebrows. Emotional consequences of shame and guilt are experienced because of the self-inflicted and destructive nature of the behaviors, as well as the feeling of having something to hide. Sufferers may go to great lengths to not undress or take their hair down in front of spouses.

The prevalence of TTM was found to be 1–3 percent of adults in the United States (Johnson & El-Alfy, 2016). A study of 2,524 college students found that 3 percent of females and 2 percent of males had subclinical trichotillomania; they created bald spots in the area from which they pulled their hair, perhaps indicating more a "bad" habit than a diagnostic level of severity (Christenson et al., 1991).

For example, Brenda lives alone. While watching TV a night, Brenda feels around her scalp for bumps and coarse hairs. She does this almost mindlessly and feels comfort and relief from the behavior. When she becomes aware of how long she has been at it, she goes to the mirror and sees a bald patch on her scalp and then sees the pile of hair around her couch, further evidence of her loss of control. She feels shame for what she has done and what she looks like, and she gets very down on herself. She has to decide if she will wear a wig or a scarf to school tomorrow, hoping that no one will comment on her appearance.

Excoriation Disorder (Skin Picking Disorder)

Excoriation is defined as recurrent skin picking and has been classified as its own distinct disorder in *DSM-V* (American Psychiatric Association, 2013). Common skin picking sites include the face, fingers, back of arms, thighs, scalp, and back. Patients will visually or physically check for bumps, acne, ingrown hair follicles, and other imperfections. Excessive skin picking results in scabs and sores that never heal, holes in the skin, need for stitches, and scarring (Odlaug & Grant, 2008).

Similar to self-injurious behaviors, these behaviors may serve to regulate emotions. Patients often report being in a trancelike state or experiencing depersonalization or derealization during long picking episodes.

Undiagnosed people who pick their skin often seek dermatological help (Grant et al., 2012). With repeated visits, dermatologists may recognize the pattern of self-imposed skin problems, but few refer the person for psychiatric help (Jafferany, Vander Stoep, Dumitrescu, & Hornung, 2010).

The rate of patients attending dermatology outpatient treatment is approximately 2 percent; many have other primary skin conditions, like acne, that complicate the problem (Nirmal, Shenoi, Rai, Sreejayan, & Savitha, 2013). The overall prevalence of excoriation disorder is relatively common and affects between 1 and 5 percent of the general population (Lochner, Roos, & Stein, 2017). Comorbid skin picking and trichotillomania was found to be between 6 and 23 percent (Odlaug, Kim, & Grant, 2010).

For example, Bobbie is working on a hard problem at work. She goes for a bathroom break and, as usual, checks her face in the mirror, unfortunately lit by fluorescent lights. Seeing a blemish she didn't notice that morning, she squeezes it with her fingernails. Not satisfied, she digs further, aware that she is creating a noticeable red mark on her face. Embarrassed and distressed, she sneaks back to her desk to get her cover-up stick and tries her best to hide it. Her coworkers know what she is doing, but Bobbie remains in denial.

Other BFRBs

Other BFRBs consist of what are considered nervous habits, such as nail and/or cuticle biting (onychophagia), which causes bleeding or infected fingertips; blemish picking or squeezing, which that causes scarring and infections; and biting the inside of the cheek (morsicatio buccarum), which can be so severe that the person bites off a chunk of skin, leading to difficult medical problems; and biting lips.

These behaviors are typically performed when the individual is stressed, excited, bored, or inactive. Hours may be spent in these activities, taking individuals away from family or work activities. Depression, shame, and isolation can also result. BFRBs most often begin in late childhood or in the early teens and may affect at least one out of twenty people.

The prevalence of nail biting was found to be 20–30 percent (Halteh, Scher, & Lipner, 2017). Excessive nail biting can erode teeth and damage the roots (Ghanizadeh, 2011). Cheek biting was reported to occur in 1–7 percent in adolescents and young adults (Flaitz & Felefli, 2000). Consequences are inflammation or lesions of the cheek and grinding down of teeth (Bhatia, Goyal, & Kapur, 2013).

For example, Ray begins biting his nails in middle school. When he is thinking, stressed, or bored, he looks at his nails for any new white growth to bite off. When there isn't anything, he goes after his cuticles. Most of the time, Ray only stops when he starts bleeding, but sometimes the pain he feels isn't enough and he keeps going. He hides his fingers with Band-Aids, and he shrugs when people ask him what happened. When his wounds become infected, his physician prescribes antibiotics but expresses his concerned at the frequency of these episodes.

Body Sensation Focus, Body Appearance Disorders, and Somatic/Health Anxiety

These disorders include somatic symptom disorder (health anxiety), body dysmorphic disorder (BDD), and muscle dysmorphia.

Body Dysmorphic Disorder

Appearance seems to have a high value in almost every society. Body dysmorphic disorder, also referred to as *imagined ugliness*, is an obsessive concern with an imagined or slight defect in appearance (Phillips, 2005). If there is a slight "defect" in appearance, the person assumes others notice it and are judgmental about it or are critical of that person.

Although many symptoms of OCD and BDD overlap, people with BDD seem to have less insight than people with OCD, because they experience their symptoms as more ego-syntonic, overvalued (a higher belief that the thought is true), or even delusional (Phillips, 2004; Yılmaz, İzci, Mermi, & Atmaca, 2016).

Most symptoms involve the face and head, because that is what people see. The most common BDD symptoms are concerns with complexion, size and position of facial features, nose, and ears; frequent mirror-checking behaviors of long duration; worries about too much facial or body hair; camouflaging skin with makeup applied perfectly; wearing hats to cover thinning hair; and avoidance of public situations due to the sense that they are being negatively scrutinized and feeling as if they lived in a fish bowl (Perugi et al., 1997). BDD does not include body-image concerns such as anorexia or being overweight, and it can be considered a severe form of social anxiety (Fang & Hofmann, 2010).

Psychoeducation of medical doctors, specifically dermatologists and plastic surgeons, has increased over the past decade, since the mental health community has become more aware of BDD and its symptomatology. As a result, referrals to mental health clinicians are being made so that people can be helped to understand that the problem is less about the physical feature of concern and more about the distorted image they have and the negative perception they think people have of them (Dufresne, Phillips, Vittorio, & Wilkel, 2001). The Body Dysmorphic Disorder Questionnaire–Dermatology Version is a convenient validated questionnaire available for screening patients in dermatology practice (Dufresne et al., 2001). There are no statistics available for how often patients are referred for mental health treatment, but 70 percent of 173 physicians surveyed reported that they refused to perform surgery on those screened for BDD (Bouman, Mulkens, & van der Lei, 2017).

BDD and Aesthetics: Cosmetic, Dermatology, and Dental Settings

The prevalence of BDD in cosmetic surgery practices was reported to be as high as 14 percent (Bouman, Mulkens, & van der Lei, 2017), and 26–40 percent of people with BDD were found to seek cosmetic surgery. Cosmetic rhinoplasty (nose job) is one of the most commonly sought-after procedures, as the nose is front and center on the face (Reichert, Scheithauer, Hoffmann, Hellings, & Picavet, 2014). A study was conducted of people requesting rhinoplasty in a cosmetic surgery practice, and 21 percent either met criteria or were likely to have BDD (Veale, De Haro, & Lambrou, 2013). In a study of those seeking breast augmentation surgery, BDD was found in 7–16 percent of the sample (Crerand, Franklin, & Sarwar, 2006; Sarwer et al., 2003).

Similarly, the prevalence of BDD was found to be 12–14 percent in dermatology practice (Conrado et al., 2010). For facial blemishes, dermabrasion and topical agents were the most common dermatological treatment sought and received (Bjornsson, Didie, & Phillips, 2010).

BDD and Cosmetic Dentistry

People with BDD also seek to remedy their obsessive appearance concerns through dentistry. Teeth whitening, braces, and teeth filling are commonly requested by BDD patients (Sarwer & Spitzer, 2012). In general dentistry, 4 percent met BDD criteria (De Jongh, Aartman, Parvaneh, & Ilik, 2009), and in orthodontics, 8 percent did (Hepburn & Cunningham, 2006).

BDD and Nonmedical Interventions

Other cosmetic methods of improving appearance are available by nonphysicians. BDD patients seek methods such as electrolysis, hair plugs, Botox, facials, eyebrow dye or tattoos, hair removal (waxing), and mesotherapy, which is injections of vitamins, enzymes, hormones, and plant extracts to rejuvenate and tighten skin, as well as to remove excess fat (Hunt, Thienhaus, & Ellwood, 2008).

Outcome and Consequences of Modifying Appearance

Dissatisfaction or New Preoccupation

The literature is clear and consistent that patients who underwent cosmetic surgery or dermatology treatments were more likely to become depressed due to being dissatisfied with the treatment outcome or believing that the procedure made them look worse (Phillips & Menard, 2006). Patients have unrealistic expectations and high hopes that their appearance will be fixed and that the interventions will solve the problem. Unfortunately, the problem is an issue of internal suffering, anxiety, distorted self-image, and low self-worth (Buhlmann, Teachman, Naumann, Fehlinger, & Rief, 2009). In some patients, BDD symptoms may become more severe following cosmetic treatments, or the patient's appearance concern may shift to another physical feature (Higgins & Wysong, 2017).

Suicide and Violence

The medication isotretinoin has a warning label that it is linked with depression and suicidality. In a study of two hundred BDD patients who received dermatological treatments, twenty of the twenty-four patients who received isotretinoin reported a history of suicidal ideation and five had attempted suicide (Crerand, Phillips, Menard, & Fay, 2005). The authors indicated that this finding was attributed not to risk of the medication but to the patients' BDD diagnosis.

Further, the mean annual suicidal ideation rate of people with BDD is 57 percent, which is approximately ten to twenty-five times higher than in the U.S. population, and the mean annual suicide attempt rate of 3 percent is an estimated three to twelve times higher (Phillips & Menard, 2006). Women who have sought breast augmentation surgery were found to have suicide rates two to three times higher than the general population (Sarwer et al., 2003). The author has also noted incidents of violent behavior toward physicians providing cosmetic treatments. Two percent of cosmetic surgeons indicated that they had been physically threatened by a patient with BDD (Sarwer, 2002).

The prevalence of BDD in the general population is said to be between 1 and 2 percent (Bjornsson et al., 2010). Lifetime comorbidity rates of BDD-OCD are almost three times higher in samples with a primary diagnosis of BDD, 28 percent, than those with primary OCD, 10 percent (Keuthen et al., 2016).

For example, twenty-six-year-old Evan is concerned that he has dark circles under his eyes that make him look old, tired, and unattractive. He sleeps with an eye mask in the hope that blocking out light helps his eyes rest. In the morning, he uses a magnifying mirror to see how his eyes look from many different angles. He has spent a good amount of money on products, including bleach, expensive cover-ups, eye creams and gels, eye pads, and any other items that promise to get rid of his circles. He has used all of the products suggested on the internet, such as cucumbers, cold tea bags, coconut oil, cold milk, tomatoes, lemon juice, rose water, antihistamines, vitamin C, and the list goes on. Sometimes he puts on too much concealer, which attracts more attention to the problem. Whenever he can get away with it, he wears sunglasses not just to block out the sun but also to stop other from seeing what he looks like. When Evan went to a dermatologist, the doctor told him that he would usually consider prescribing a cream with retinol but didn't see the need for it. Frustrated, Evan saw another dermatologist who did prescribe the cream, but using it did not change Evan's level of preoccupation, concealing behaviors, and avoidant body language around others.

Muscle Dysmorphia

Muscle dysmorphia (MD) is also known as the Adonis complex, bigorexia, and reverse anorexia; it consists of the idea that one's body is not sufficiently lean and muscular (Leone, Sedory, & Gray, 2005). Typical behaviors include long hours of lifting weights, use of dietary supplements, excessive detail to diet, and tracking food intake that controls metabolism (Tod, Edwards, & Cranswick, 2016). Enhancing muscle mass through the use of anabolic steroids, overtraining to the point of joint and heart strain, and abusing dietary supplements that disrupt the person's natural constitutional balance can cause severe medical problems (Pope, Gruber, Choi, Olivardia, & Phillips, 1997). The prevalence rate of MD in bodybuilders has been estimated to be as high as 10 percent (Pope, Katz, & Hudson, 1993). Mostly men, but also some women, suffer from MD. Gruber and Pope (1999) reported on ten female bodybuilders who had experienced at least one sexual assault and developed MD. Prior to the assault, two of the women already had MD, whereas after the incident, they all had the condition, illuminating again the role traumatic experiences can play in the development and maintenance of obsessive symptoms.

Similar to BDD, MD is considered more difficult to treat due to poor insight, ego-syntonic symptoms, and overidentification people have about their appearance being the most important feature of their identity. Exposure and response prevention, discussed later in detail, can be useful when insight and motivation are good. Otherwise, a chronic pain model can be helpful in teaching people how to accept the effect of the problem on daily functioning (i.e., that the compulsive behaviors such as overtraining are the problem rather than their beliefs about their body), while still continuing to practice normalized behavior. In addition, the model discourages people from talking about the problem as a way to keep it from being the focal point of daily life. In the case of OCD and related disorders, resisting urges to ask reassuring questions from others would help reduce appearance focused awareness.

Prevalence rates in the general population for MD are largely unknown. Studies have been conducted mostly of bodybuilders in gym or fitness settings, and the rate was found to be between 10 and 53 percent (Nieuwoudt, Zhou, Coutts, & Booker, 2015). Nieuwoudt and colleagues (2015) also found that of the 648 participants, 110 (17%) were at risk of having MD, 69 (11%) were at risk of having BDD, and 219 (33%) were at risk of having an eating disorder. Furthermore, 36 (6%) were found at risk of having both MD and BDD, and 60 (9%) were at risk of having both MD and an eating disorder (Nieuwoudt et al., 2015).

Personal trainers may also be prone to MD. A study comprised of 1,039 male and female fitness trainers found a prevalence rate of MD in 23 percent and a drive from masculinity rate of 28 percent in this population. (Diehl & Baghurst, 2016). The study also found traits such as depression, anxiety, hostility, somatization, interpersonal sensitivity, obsessive-compulsive symptoms were significantly and positively related to MD and DFM (Diehl & Baghurst, 2016). There are currently no prevalence rates of MD available in the literature.

For example, Paul knows exactly how long his gym workouts need to be and how many he needs to do in order to achieve the level of muscle mass he feels would be adequate for his appearance. He has a strict workout schedule for each muscle group, allowing for maximum muscle training and rest. He also has a strict diet set and knows how and when the food will be metabolized. He uses powder supplements to ensure that his body has the optimal level of vitamins and nutrients. He restricts his food and liquid intake according to the rigid rules he has set, even though they go beyond what is considered reasonable by trainers and others with whom he works out. He doesn't have time for social or leisure activities, since he considers them a waste of time. Paul's world has become limited and unsustainable, and he eventually becomes so burned out. With the help of loved ones, he agrees to see a sports psychologist who specializes in DM. Although it takes a lot of grieving for Paul to recover from his sense of failure, his therapist helps him slowly get his life back in balance and back on track.

Health Anxiety/Somatic Symptom Disorder/Illness Anxiety Disorder

While it was formerly known as *hypochondriasis*, the *DSM-V* now identifies health anxiety as somatic symptom disorder and illness anxiety disorder (American Psychiatric Association, 2013). The *DSM-V* included this disorder in the somatic symptom and related disorders category, while the International Code of Diseases classified it as belonging to the section on obsessive compulsive and related disorders section (Lopez-Sola et al., 2018). For practical purposes, the term *health anxiety* (HA) will be used going forward to refer to these disorders.

Health anxiety consists of being preoccupied by persistent and excessive thoughts that somatic experiences are symptoms of a serious or fatal illness (Eastin & Guinsler, 2006). According to Rief and Martin (2014), in people experiencing HA, normal bodily sensations that might not be noticed by others can be interpreted as serious and cause an urgent need to be seen by a medical professional. People may have obsessive doubt about test results that were negative and then pursue second or third opinions. They may also seek reassurance from family members by having them look at areas of concern on their body, as well as performing compulsive checking behaviors themselves. They may avoid physical exertion, such as exercising, heavy lifting, using stairs, and other behaviors that can cause rapid breathing and heart rate, for fear of having a heart attack

Excessive thoughts, feelings, and behaviors can include a high level of worry about potential illness, fear that normal physical sensations are a sign of severe physical illness even when there is no evidence, and doubts about the adequacy of the medical evaluation and treatment. There are also fears that any physical activity may cause damage to the body, compulsive body checking and scanning for abnormalities, overly frequent health care visits for reassurance where concerns are not relieved or are made worse, unresponsiveness to medical treatment or atypical sensitive to medication side effects, and exaggerated fears of having a severe case of a medical condition (http://www.nchmd.org/education/mayo-health-library/details/CON-20124065).

According to Kroenke (2003), 40–50 percent of patients arrive to appointments with medically unexplained symptoms (Kroenke, 2003). Common symptoms are pain related (headache, back pain, painful urination, joint pain, diffuse pain, and extremity pain), gastrointestinal (nausea, vomiting, abdominal pain, bloating, gas, and diarrhea), cardiopulmonary (chest pain, dizziness, shortness of breath, sweating, and palpitations), neurologic (fainting, pseudoseizures, amnesia, muscle weakness, difficulty or painful swallowing, double or blurred vision, difficulty walking, difficulty urinating, deafness, and hoarseness or loss of speech), and reproductive (painful intercourse, painful menstruation, and burning in sex organs (Kroenke, 2003)). Other somatic symptoms of concern are minor physical abnormalities, such as a small sore or an occasional cough, and or vague and ambiguous physical sensations, such as light-headedness and skin discoloration (Abramowitz, Deacon, & Valentiner, 2007).

Checking medical websites is also a common manifestation. Frequent online seekers tend to make more medical appointments based on information found online (Eastin & Guinsler, 2006). Neurology was the most commonly visited medical specialty, with 25 percent of patients having HA, followed by respiratory medicine (21%), gastroenterology (20%), cardiology (19%), and endocrinology (18%) (Tyrer et al., 2011). Further, obsessional thoughts, body dysmorphic concerns, and social anxiety symptoms may have a causal influence on HA and may affect up to 7 percent of individuals during middle adulthood years, as changes in the body become more frequent (López-Solà et al., 2018).

Up to 9 percent of patients in general medical practice clinics and up to 5 percent of the general population meet diagnostic criteria for HA (Creed & Barsky, 2004). A study found an 8 percent comorbidity rate of HA and OCD, and in OCD patients, 10 percent met criteria for HA (Hedman et al., 2017).

For example, Jesse is home alone watching TV and suddenly experiences heart palpitations. Worried he is having a heart attack, he calls an ambulance and is taken to the nearest hospital emergency room. A thorough work-up is conducted, and Jesse is released as the results come back normal. Jesse is relieved, but he wants to know why he had the palpitations and wonders if they will happen again. In order to know what to do, Jesse begins searching the internet to see what causes relate to heart palpitations. Jesse becomes fearful of running and stops doing any kind of aerobics.

Orthorexia Nervosa (ON)

A cultural health-focused trend has emerged over the last few decades consisting of eating organically grown foods and avoiding eating foods that are processed, caged, and fed with growth hormones. As with many lifestyle choices, issues around perfectionism can turn good intentions into rigid, rule-based, and perfectionistic behaviors. As a result, although it is not officially a diagnosis, orthorexia will be included in this section of body-focused disorders. Orthorexia nervosa initially was defined as a "fixation on righteous eating" (Bratman, 2017). Once considered motivated by a focus on eating a healthy diet, it is now said to include obsessive thoughts about food purity, extreme fasting or overexercising, and restrictive rules and behaviors around eating (Tremelling, Sandon, Vega, & McAdams, 2017). As such, it is being recommended for classification as a *DSM* mental disorder.

Moroze and colleagues (Moroze, Dunn, Holland, Yager, & Weintraub, 2015) have proposed specific criteria for orthorexia nervosa: obsessional preoccupation with eating "healthy foods"; focusing on the quality and composition of meals even if they are nutritionally unbalanced due to concerns about food "purity"; rigid avoidance of "unhealthy" foods that may contain any fat, preservatives, food-additives, animal products, or other ingredients considered by the subject to be unhealthy; excessive amounts of time (e.g., three or more hours per day) spent reading about, acquiring, and/or preparing specific types of foods based on their perceived quality and composition; having guilty feelings and worries after "indulging" in "unhealthy" or "impure" foods; exhibiting intolerance of others' food beliefs or practices; and spending excessive amounts on unaffordable food because of their perceived quality and composition. With ON, nutritional imbalances may compromise physical health, and the preoccupation can negatively impact social, academic or vocational functioning (Moroze et al., 2015).

It is unclear how many personal trainers or fitness professionals have ON themselves, but among a study of 2,500 dieticians, 50 percent were at risk for ON (Tremelling et al., 2017). Prevalence of ON in the general population was determined at 7 percent (Donini, Marsili, Graziani, Imbriale, & Cannella, 2004; Håman, Barker-Ruchti, Patriksson, & Lindgren, 2015).

For example, Ruth is very health conscious and has been a vegetarian for most of her adult life. At one point, she becomes vegan in order to eliminate the health risks of animal-based products, such as eggs and dairy. Ruth becomes obsessive about what she puts into her body and spends longer amounts of time checking food labels, even though she is shopping in the vegan section of the health food store. After a while, she stops going to parties, and her friends become worried about how thin she is getting. They also become weary of Ruth's focus on talking about the virtues of her vegan diet and proselytizing about the risks they are taking by eating processed food and drinking alcohol. Basically, Ruth is not fun. When Ruth's health begins to suffer, she rationalizes that she isn't eating the perfect food regimen and sees a nutritionist. The nutritionist is alarmed by Ruth's weight and appearance and orders her to have her blood tested. Ruth has been malnourished for quite some time and will need rehabilitative interventions in order to restore her health.

Emetephobia/Specific Phobia of Vomiting

Emetophobia is the fear of vomiting. Considered a specific phobia, it has not been classified as an OC spectrum or related disorder, but it has similar characteristics and behaviors of the somatic/health anxiety/disgust type (van Hout & Bouman, 2012). Emetophobia has been found to be a common comorbid disorder with OCD (Sykes, Boschen, & Conlon, 2016) and is more prominent in women (Veale et al., 2013). Empirically, individuals with emetophobia avoid food, smells, social situations, and other anticipated situations that they fear will trigger the physiological response. A case study was written about a woman who wanted to become pregnant but delayed due to her fear of having morning sickness (Maack, Deacon, & Zhao, 2013).

People with emetophobia avoid some situations or activities, such as being near people who are ill or drunk; drinking alcohol; fairground rides; traveling by boats, airplanes, or public transportation; crowded places; eating from salad bars or buffets; and using public toilets (Lipsitz, Fyer, Paterniti, & Klein, 2001; Veale & Lambrou, 2006). They may also avoid certain foods or restrict their eating in order to reduce the risk of vomiting or the amount of food vomited, check sell dates on food products, hand wash, and seek reassurance (Veale, Costa, Murphy, & Ellison, 2012). Other behaviors may be making sure that they know where the bathrooms or exits are wherever they go, keeping very still or trying to keep tight control of their body if they are having stomach problems, taking anti-nausea medication prophylactically, or trying to distract themselves away from worrying about vomiting (Veale et al., 2012).

The prevalence of emetophobia ranges from 0.1 to 7 percent (Becker et al., 2007). A fear of vomiting is common in the community, affecting up to 7 percent of women and 2 percent of men (van Hout & Bouman, 2012). The most common comorbidity in emetophobia was found to be OCD, in 12 percent of eighty-three cases (Veale, Hennig, & Gledhill, 2015).

For example, Hana begins having trouble getting to and staying at school. She is anxious and feels nauseous frequently throughout the day. She becomes afraid that at any moment she might vomit, which by itself is disgusting, but she's also afraid that she will cause a sickening scene should it occur in class or during activities. She stops going to the cafeteria due to the risk that the smells there will turn her stomach and cause her to get sick.

Behavioral Addictions and Non-Body-Focused Repetitive Behaviors

Behavioral addictions and non-body-focused impulsive behaviors, often mistakenly referred to as compulsive, include shopping, gambling, eating, excessive computer/gaming use, sexual impulsivity, and pornography. They differ from substance addiction in that no drugs are ingested to produce the reinforcing high. There are, however, common brain functions and neurotransmitter activity between substance and behavioral addictive behaviors (Leeman & Potenza, 2013). Neurofunctionally, they are the same as problems with impulse control.

Buying/Shopping

It is so easy to buy and shop, because stores and malls try to provide an atmosphere of ease and stimulation at the same time. Shopping can be reinforced as a social activity and a means of escaping reality for a while.

Compulsive buying and shopping happen around the world and across cultures. They are actually impulsive behaviors; they are performed without planning and are experienced as self-soothing. The behaviors become problematic when people buy things they don't need or can't afford, go into debt, shop as an avoidance behavior, and accumulate material items that take up unavailable space at home.

The prevalence rate of compulsive buying has been reported as 7 percent (Mueller et al., 2011) and comorbid with OCD at 8 percent (Torres et al., 2016).

For example, David is upset by his boss. On his way home, he stops at the mall just to walk around, as he often does in an unconscious attempt to numb out his feelings. Already maxed out on a few of his credit cards, his permission-giving statement to justify his behavior is "My niece's birthday is coming up soon, so I'll look around and see what I can get her." Unable to make up his mind, he buys $150 worth of different-size toddler clothes since she will likely grow out of some of them within the year. Like always, he justifies that he could always return items, even though he never does.

Stealing/Kleptomania

Shoplifting and stealing also have differing functions and are also impulsive. Those who steal compulsively experience similar urges as other impulsive behaviors, in that a buildup of tension is relieved by acting on those urges. A plan is usually made ahead of time and carried out. During the episode, there is an experience of pleasure and gratification as well as a relief of stress, and there may even be an acting out of anger as a component of reinforcement.

Individuals with kleptomania give much less thought to their behavior and act on impulsive urges. Little or no negative emotions are experienced, and they may even throw away the item(s). People with this problem, obviously, can be arrested and have legal problems.

The overall lifetime prevalence of shoplifting in the general population was 1–11.3 percent (Blanco et al., 2008). Rates of co-occurring OCD in samples of individuals who have kleptomania have ranged from 7 to 60 percent (Grant, 2003; Presta et al., 2002). Conversely, rates of kleptomania in OCD samples were 2–6 percent (Fontenelle, Mendlo-wicz, & Versiani, 2005; Matsunaga et al., 2005). In those arrested for shoplifting, the prevalence of kleptomania is 4–24 percent and found to be three times more likely in women (Talih, 2011).

For example, Madi has a secret. Even though her OCD revolves around fear of offending others, she engages in stealing small items from stores. In the example above, David soothes himself by buying things, but when Madi is stressed, she takes thrilling risks by acquiring items without paying for them. She also lies when people ask her about the items and comment about how much money she must spend. She has taken to hiding things, and at times, her girlfriend finds them. She does feel some remorse after these episodes when the thrill wears off.

Pathological Gambling

As a source of entertainment, brick-and-mortar and online casinos, lottery tickets, and other small-money gambling have become more convenient, available, and socially acceptable as private and public money-generating ventures. Casinos offer a wide range of diversions, from shows to restaurants and the like. Cities have come to rely on the revenue derived from state-sponsored lotteries to help their communities. Most people participate in these types of gambling for amusement and already know they will lose the money they have budgeted ahead of time.

However, people with gambling problems experience euphoric highs when they win and remorseful, even suicidal, lows when they lose. A common pattern is getting caught in a vicious cycle of people taking their winnings to chase even more thrills and money by "reinvesting" the won money for even more money that they inevitably lose. Remorse and guilt, as well as a building tension, drive them to at least get their initial money back, and the cycle is repeated. They often try to hide their addiction by sneaking time away from work and family, or lie about what they are doing, to win back the debt they have incurred. They often go into more debt, leaving themselves and families in financial ruin or worse.

A study of 43,093 households found a lifetime prevalence rate of gambling to be 1–3 percent (Onur et al., 2016). Two percent of those who experience pathological gambling have comorbid OCD (Hollander, 1996; Mueller et al., 2011).

For example, when Joyce answers the phone, she is confronted by a debt collection agency who wants payment for a default credit card. Joyce is shocked because as far as she knows, there are never any financial problems. What she doesn't know is that her husband, Gus, has maxed out several credit cards due to his gambling addiction. Yes, they have gone to a casino from time to time on a date night, but she has no idea that he has a serious gambling addiction. When she confronts him, he explains to her how he has gotten everything under control and says not to worry about it. He says that he has made the minimum payment on the credit card yesterday and that the phone call was a mistake.

Gus has been busy trying to win back his losses by convincing himself that this time he is going to hit the jackpot. He has so many episodes of exhilaration just thinking about that moment that he loses sight of the inevitable result of losing it all again. Now that it is out in the open how out of control his addiction is, he can no longer hide the reality of the amount of debt he has put his family into. When Joyce refuses to enable him by paying down the credit cards and threatens divorce, Gus agrees to get help. He is able to arrange a payment plan with the credit card companies and goes to Gambler's Anonymous several times a week. Even with that, he still has strong urges to chase the high he felt when he was at the blackjack tables.

Compulsive Sexual Behavior, Hypersexuality, and Sexual Impulsivity

No longer considered an impulse control disorder, sexual impulsivity and addiction share the same traits as the other impulsive addictive behaviors. Previously, compulsive sexual behavior was classified as *sexual impulsivity* because of its similarity to other disorders of impulse control. It was also called *sexual compulsivity* because of its similar behavioral pattern and some neurobiological similarity to OCD. It was also referred to as *sexual addiction* because of the repetitive and escalating patterns of sexual behavior resulting in negative consequences to self and others (Jhanjee, Bhatia, Kumar, & Jindal, 2010).

Obvious negative consequences of excessive sexual behavior are contracting sexually transmitted diseases, pregnancy, safety risks, and physical/sexual abuse. Additionally, emotional distress, employment difficulties, relationship problems, legal issues, and demoralization as a result of hypersexuality have been reported (Reid, Garos, & Fong, 2012).

Research continues to sort out what the biological, psychological, and social causes of behavior addictions are in general (Leeman & Potenza, 2013). Again, it is important to distinguish the behavior as impulsive (pleasure seeking), compulsive (distress avoidance), or addictive (neurophysiological cravings) in order to select the best treatment approach.

The disorder has an estimated prevalence of 3–6 percent (Kuzma & Black, 2008). Lifetime prevalence of compulsive sexual behavior was 6 percent in patients with current OCD and significantly higher in men than women (Fuss, Briken, Stein, & Lochner, 2019).

For example, even though Clay has obsessive moral perfectionism, he engages in watching porn. This behavior causes him much distress and aggravates his OCD, because he feels that he is probably cheating on his wife. Even though he feels guilt and remorse, he also feels intense pleasure and relief that he is unable to experience with his wife. When his wife goes to bed, he escapes into a fantasy world where he can lose himself and be gratified. He always promises to stop, but he never can. He prays to God to help heal him from his lust, but it is too powerful for him to control.

Pathological Jealousy (Unrelated to Relationship OCD)

Once considered *morbid jealousy*, pathological jealousy (PJ) is under consideration for classification as an OC spectrum disorder (Ecker, 2012). Insight into jealousy can lie on a continuum from obsessional to delusional (Insel & Akiskal, 1986). People with obsessional jealousy fear that their partner is being unfaithful and tend to look for ways their partner may be committing unfaithful acts; however, the symptoms are experienced as ego-dystonic, are unwanted, and are viewed as contrary to expression of healthy romantic feelings (Bishay, Petersen, & Tarrier, 1989; Ecker & Gönner, 2006). Common behaviors are trying to control or checking up on the partner's whereabouts, asking repetitive reassuring questions, checking electronic communications, and the like. People with PJ are aware that their fears are without basis and are ashamed of having them (Bishay et al., 1989).

Those with delusional jealousy, on the other hand, have no insight into their beliefs and are convinced that their partner is cheating on them. Their judgment is poor, and they engage in stalking and other unsafe behaviors, such as perpetrating acts of anger like domestic violence toward the partner and violence toward the alleged lover, create legal problems, and commit suicide (Kingham & Gordon, 2004).

Marazziti and colleagues (2003) reported that compared to nonclinical subjects, jealous obsessions negatively impacted relationships in those with OCD (Marazziti et al., 2003). There are no comorbid prevalence rates of PJ and OCD (Kingham & Gordon, 2004).

For example, Isak has no reason to suspect that his partner, Owen, is cheating on him, but he keeps having strong nagging thoughts when Owen is not around that he could be meeting up with someone else. He tries to shrug the thoughts off as ridiculous, as the couple has been getting along just fine. Isak begins questioning Owen about his day with an ear toward finding inconsistencies about what Owen says his day has been like and how he is saying it. Isak begins looking in Owen's pockets and phone for evidence that he is spending time with someone else. Isak is mortified at what he is doing and confesses his jealous feelings to Owen. Owen does his best to reassure Isak about the relationship, but the jealous behavior begins to drive a wedge in the relationship.

Eating Disorders

Anorexia Nervosa (AN)

Anorexia nervosa is the preoccupation and fear of being overweight. Overlapping features of AN and OCD are the need for control and perfection. In AN, usually women, but also men, have a distorted image of themselves; they can become medically compromised in AN's extreme form. Compulsive behaviors in AN consist of calorie counting, cutting food into vary small pieces, nibbling, leaving portions of food on their plate, wearing baggy clothing to hide their bodies, and frequently weighing themselves (Gianini et al., 2015).

Problems with restrictive eating exist in both OCD and anorexia. In OCD, however, it may occur due to fear of eating contaminated food, may be performed as a scrupulosity purification ritual, and may consist of ritualistic eating rules, avoiding certain foods that are considered emotionally contaminated, or avoiding food that the person has had a bad experience eating in the past. None of these behaviors is performed with the goal of losing weight (Halmi et al., 2005).

A study by Cederlöf and colleagues (2015) looked at the overlapping symptoms between OCD (N = 19,814) and AN (N = 8,462) and found that those with a primary diagnosis of AN were ten times more likely to be later diagnosed with OCD, while those with primary OCD were four times as likely to be subsequently diagnosed with AN. They reported that an estimated lifetime prevalence of OCD in patients with eating disorders ranged from 10 to 62 percent and those with eating disorders in OCD samples ranged between 11 and 42 percent (Cederlöf et al., 2015).

For example, Pam is too thin, due to restricting her food intake. She doesn't like food that is red or slimy. The color red reminds her of blood, and the texture of slimy food is associated with something rotten she has eaten earlier in her life. She also doesn't like feeling full and only partially eats what she is served. Concerned about her weight, her parents take her to an eating disorder specialist, who structures a healthy meal plan with which Pam agrees to comply. After several weeks of struggling with her parents and her therapist, Pam discloses that the spaghetti meal on the menu is disgusting and refuses to agree to eat it. After talking more with Pam privately and getting a fuller understanding of the problem, her therapist refers her for OCD treatment.

Binge Eating Disorder (BED)

Binge eating disorder has been categorized as an eating disorder distinct from other eating disorders such as bulimia nervosa (BN; and is defined as recurrent eating of "an amount of food that is definitely larger than most people would eat in a similar period of time under similar circumstances" (American Psychiatric Association, 2013)). According to the criteria, the disorder is marked by "a sense of lack of control over eating during the episode," a characteristic of impulsivity. Its features consist of secret and rapid consumption of large quantities of food until feeling uncomfortably full, often carbohydrates (comfort food), accompanied by feelings of a loss of control about eating. After the episode, the person has feelings of self-disgust, depression, guilt, and remorse for having lost control.

Binge eating disorder is commonly mistaken for compulsive eating. Although categorized as an eating disorder, BED is similar to other problems involving impulse control, in that it is a destructive behavior that is also a form of self-soothing. It is more like an addiction than a compulsion, in that the behavior produces feelings of gratification and elation during the episode but has longer-term negative consequences, especially health-related problems.

Behaviorally, men (26%) were more likely to report overeating in general, while women (30%) were more likely to endorse loss of control while eating (Striegel-Moore et al., 2009). The twelve-month and lifetime prevalence estimates were 4 percent of women and 2.0 percent of men (Hudson, Hiripi, Pope, & Kessler, 2007).

For example, when Valerie feels lonely, sad, or anxious, she craves foods high in carbohydrates (comfort food). If she has eaten the muffins, ice cream, or chips, on impulse she may go to the store and buy more. There is a sense of trying to be comforted and full through eating, even though she knows how out of control and ashamed she feels after an episode. Although she vows to never do it again, it is an endless pattern that has caused her to gain weight, feel bad about the way she looks, and socially isolate. She looks up websites to see what others say about how they have stopped the behavior, and it scares her to learn how many times people relapse because they still feel emotionally empty. One thing catches her attention: to try engaging in creative arts as a means of healthy emotional expression. Having given up on it long ago, Valerie signs up for a sculpture class, where she makes beautiful figurines and healthy social connections.

Bulimia Nervosa

According to the *DSM-V*, bulimia nervosa consists of recurrent episodes of impulsive overeating in one sitting and, in turn, impulsively inducing vomiting or overusing laxatives. People may try to gain control over this behavior by fasting or compulsive exercising (American Psychiatric Association, 2013). Health-related consequences of purging are erosion of tooth enamel, digestive bloating or reflux, enlarged heart, and salivary gland swelling (Rushing, Jones, & Carney, 2003).

Similar to BED, sadness, loneliness, guilt, and feelings of helplessness or hopelessness trigger the episodes (Frayn, Livshits, & Knäuper, 2018). The eating is done as an attempt to fill the emotionally empty space. The purging plays a similar role, as a way to expel emotions (Canetti, Bachar, & Berry, 2002).

Tyagi and colleagues (2015) hypothesized that serotonin dysregulation may be a common biological overlap between OCD and an eating disorder, including BN. They also identified behavioral traits seen in both BN and OCD as repeated checking, reassurance seeking, and ritualistic eating (Tyagi et al., 2015). Comorbid BN and OCD was reported to be up to 40 percent independent of food-related obsessions and compulsions (Godart, Flament, Perdereau, & Jeammet, 2002).

For example, Suri was a little overweight for her size at a young age and was sometimes teased. She was sexually abused by an uncle a few times and used food to stuff her shame and wall people off. Over the years, her weight has gone up and down as she has tried to work on her self-esteem and desire to feel attractive. During a time of being depressed, she starts binge eating comfort food, which she says feels "imperative" and does provide some comfort in the moment. In the aftermath of eating so much that she feels sick, Suri induces vomiting by sticking her fingers down her throat. After several episodes and feeling out of control, Suri begins to feel suicidal and is hospitalized. She is treated with antidepressants and is referred to a residential eating-disorder program to regain her health and to begin dealing with the emotions she is trying to numb out with food.

Delusional and Dissociative Disorders

The connection between dissociation and OCD remains unclear. Dissociative disorders most commonly result from a traumatic experience. However, dissociation or depersonalization may also result from intense physiological states of distress while obsessing (Belli et al., 2012). These states may serve to reduce the level of distress experienced during an intense or high-anxiety episode. During dissociative episodes, people experience feelings of detachment from their mental processes or body, as if they are an outside observer (e.g., the feeling of being in a dream).

Inferential confusion is a particular experience in OCD, during which a person's overthinking creates confusion that leads the person to confuse an imagined possibility with an actual probability (Soffer-Dudek, 2019). Another overthinking phenomenon is dissociative absorption (Rufer, Fricke, Held, Cremer, & Hand, 2006).

The brain regions involved in dissociative absorption lie in the emotion processing and memory areas of the amygdala, hippocampus, parahippocampal gyrus, and middle/superior temporal gyrus, interoception and attention regulation (insula), self-referential processes, cognitive control, and arousal modulation. These functions may be altered during dissociation (Krause-Utz, Frost, Winter, & Elzinga, 2017).

Checking, symmetry, and ordering symptoms were associated with dissociative symptomatology in patients with OCD. Compulsive checking appears to induce dissociative experiences (Grabe et al., 2001).

The delusional somatic disorders reviewed in this section are olfactory reference syndrome and koro, both of which have symptom overlap with OCD.

Olfactory Reference Syndrome (ORS)

Olfactory reference syndrome (hallucinatory odor) is excessive preoccupation with the possibility that one's body odor or breath may be foul or unpleasant (Greenberg, Shaw, Reuman, Schwartz, & Wilhelm, 2016). Most people with ORS actually smell what they perceive and are experiencing a hallucination through their sense of smell. According to Phillips and Menard (2011), common OCD-like behaviors for fear of bad breath include excessive washing, cleaning, toothbrushing, and mouthwash, as well as use of breath mints and chewing gum. For body odor symptoms, people apply too much perfume, cologne, or deodorant, and compulsively spray air fresheners. Ironically, these excessive call attention to themselves, which is the very thing they try to avoid. Others avoiding being around people, going out in public, and other social activities (Phillips & Menard, 2011).

Similarities have been found between ORS and BDD, including constant preoccupation with and checking behaviors about the perceived problem (Phillips, Gunderson, Gruber, & Castle, 2006).

Nearly three-quarters of people with ORS report periods during which they avoided most social interactions because of their ORS symptoms, and about 50 percent report periods during which they avoided most of their important occupational, academic, or life activities because of ORS symptoms. Some people are completely housebound because they feel too distressed, self-conscious, and embarrassed about the perceived odor to be around other people or because they fear offending others with their smell.

Medical professionals whom people with ORS may visit before, or even after, being diagnosed with ORS are dentists, surgeons, and ear, nose, and throat specialists for supposed halitosis; proctologists, surgeons, and gastroenterologists for supposed anal odors; and other physicians such as dermatologists and gynecologists (Greenberg et al., 2018). Treatments such as a tonsillectomy for perceived bad breath or electrolysis of sweat glands for a perceived sweaty smell may also be sought. The outcome of such procedures is similar to BDD, in that patients are often dissatisfied with the results (Phillips & Menard, 2011).

High rates of psychiatric hospitalization, suicidal thoughts, suicide attempts, and completed suicide have been reported, which many individuals attribute primarily to their ORS symptoms (Pryse-Phillips, 1971). Commonly co-occurring disorders are major depressive disorder, social anxiety disorder, drug or alcohol use disorders, obsessive compulsive disorder, and body dysmorphic disorder.

For example, Gary smells like rotten flowers. Wherever he is and whatever he is doing, he smells like flowers that have sat in a vase until their stems were rotten in the water. Although no one whom Gary has ever asked has noticed any rotting smell around him, the odor they do notice is the overpowering cologne he uses to cover up the bad smell he is convinced he emits. He has been asked by very caring and not-so-caring people to cut down or stop using it. On bad days, he calls in sick to work, cancels social plans, or contemplates suicide.

Koro/Genital Retraction Syndrome

Koro, in Chinese called *suo-yang* (Mattelaer & Jilek, 2007), is a rare disorder characterized by a male's fear of or belief that he is experiencing genital retraction. Koro is described as culture-bound and is found most often in Southeast Asia but also occurs in Africa and Europe (Bhatia, Jhanjee, & Kumar, 2011). Koro is said to be a manifestation of an acute anxiety state (Kumar, Phookun, & Datta, 2014) and is characterized by a fear that the penis is shrinking and will retract into the abdomen, resulting in death. Insight is poor to delusional (American Psychiatric Association, 2013).

A small-scale epidemic of genital shrinking occurred in six West African nations between January 1997 and October 2003 (Dzokoto & Adams, 2005). In China, there was the 1984–85 koro epidemic in Hainan Island and Leizhou Peninsula. In India, fifty-five cases have occurred. The first such epidemic occurred in 1968 in North Bengal region of West Bengal State, and the second one in 1982 affected mainly West Bengal (Chowdhury et al., 1988) and Assam (Dutta,1983). The third miniepidemic occurred in a village in the South Twenty-Four Parganas district of West Bengal in 1988 (Chowdhury et al., 1994). A fourth Koro epidemic took place in Tripura in 1998. This time the epicenter of the epidemic was Assam (Roy et al., 2011), then Mumbai, and then it was transmitted by migrant laborers to West Bengal (Ghosh, Nath, Brahma, & Chowdhury, 2013).

Koro may be related to body dysmorphic disorder, but it differs in that it is culture bound in particular geographic areas, is usually brief in duration, and responds positively to reassurance (Cheng, 1997; Mattelaer & Jilek, 2007).

Ghosh and colleagues (2013) described an interesting anecdotal incidence of a koro epidemic in India in 2010. They reported it spread from Assam to Mumbai, then to West Bengal, and totaled fifty-five cases. Hypochondriacal preoccupation with genital symptoms was seen in 56 percent of cases, along with associated moderate-to-severe depression. Definite features of BDD regarding penile size and disfigurement was seen in 6 percent of the male patients (Ghosh et al., 2013). Bhatia and colleagues (2011) reported that 2 percent of fifty men in India with culturally bound syndromes had koro (Bhatia et al., 2011).

For example, Kim believes that he is cursed by from having sexual relations with a prostitute fifteen years ago. He has a sensation that his penis is retracting into his body and performs frequent checking rituals. He makes visits to several urologists, and they run tests with normal results, which makes him even more convinced he is cursed. Kim is having marital problems, and fraught with guilt, he blames himself for failing as a husband. After a particularly severe episode, Kim's wife brings him to the local emergency room, where they assess and diagnose the problem. He is referred to a psychiatrist, who prescribes an antidepressant and also refers them to a couple's therapist.

Movement Disorders

Tourette's Syndrome

Tourette's syndrome (TS) is an involuntary movement disorder that typically consists of motor and vocal tics that can be simple or complex. Similar to impulsive behaviors, tics can be considered as problems with impulse control and are not compulsive, intentional repetitive actions (Petter, Richter, & Sandor, 1998). Criteria for TS are the following:

- Tics are typically sudden, rapid, recurrent, nonrhythmic, and stereotyped motor movement or vocalizations.
- Tics occur episodically throughout the day, nearly every day, or intermittently throughout a period of more than one year.
- There is never a tic-free period of more than three consecutive months.
- The episodes cause marked distress or significant impairment in social, occupational, or other important areas of functioning.
- There may be one or more involuntary vocal tics, although not necessarily all at the same time (Novotny, Valis, & Klimova, 2018).

Simple tics are motor movements from a single muscle or a group of muscles. Cath and colleagues (Cath et al., 2011) have provided the following examples of simple motor tics behaviors:

- Arm jerks
- Eye blinking
- Facial grimacing
- Head jerking
- Mouth opening
- Nose twitching

- Shoulder shrugs
- Teeth tapping
- Throat clearing

They have also given these examples of phonic tics:

- Coughing
- Grunting
- Making animal or bird sounds
- Sniffing
- Throat clearing
- Whistling

Complex motor tics involve contractions in different muscle groups and either a cluster of simple actions or a more coordinated sequence of movements. They also typically involve more elaborate manifestations, appear to have a more purposeful action or utterance, and may be socially inappropriate. Examples include the following:

- Touching/tapping
- Picking
- Rude/obscene finger or hand gestures
- Repetition of the movements of others
- Making obscene gestures
- Facial and body contortions or twirling around
- Hopping, touching, hitting, smelling, jumping, bending, picking
- Holding a position for several seconds
- Touching objects
- Clapping

Complex vocal tics may consist of the following:

- Barks
- Grunts
- Hoots
- Imitation of sounds or words of others
- Involuntary uttering of obscenities
- Moans
- Repetition of one's own sounds and words
- Screeches
- Sniffs

Vocal tics can interfere with the flow of speech and can cause difficulties at the initiation of speech, resembling a stammer/stutter, or at phrase transitions (Felling & Singer, 2011). Problems with labile emotion, anger control, and aggression can be exhibited in some people with TS such as the following:

- Banging oneself against a hard object
- Body punching or slapping
- Destroying objects
- Head banging
- Kicking
- Poking sharp objects into the body
- Punching holes in walls
- Scratching body parts
- Screaming
- Stomping
- Threatening behaviors (Muller et al., 1997)

The prevalence of TS has been found to be 1–5 percent in the general population (Scharf et al., 2015) and 4–20 percent in children, whose symptoms may remit over time (Swain & Leckman, 2005). Comorbid TS and OCD rates have said to be between 11 and 80 percent (Zohar et al., 1992).

For example, Oliver Sacks (1970) described a weekend jazz drummer nicknamed "Witty Ticcy Ray" who was successfully treated for TS with Haldol. He was transformed from frenetic agitation to a calm and patient person. Unfortunately, his drumming became boring; it lacked the idiosyncratic tic movements that made the music so interesting. The solution he found was to take the Haldol on weekdays for his day job and then take a drug "vacation" during the weekends for his drumming.

Other OC-Like Disorders

Misophonia/Selective Sound Sensitivity Syndrome

Misophonia, which literally means dislike or hatred of sound, was initially recognized by audiologist Marsha Jones, who referred to it as *selective sound sensitivity syndrome* (Bernstein, Angell, & Dehle, 2013). It is characterized as a complex neurobiological and behavioral disorder (Jastreboff & Jastreboff, 2002) and is said to describe the condition more accurately, as the emphasis is on the variety of sounds that affect different people (Dozier, 2015). It had been suggested that misophonia be included as an OCRD in the *DSM-V* (Schröder, Vulink, & Denys, 2013).

One theory about the etiology of misophonia is that it is a neurophysiological response tied to the executive functions responsible for emotion, memory, and learning (Jastreboff & Jastreboff, 2002). Another theory is that it becomes a conditioned response by the particular sound that sets off a physical reflex that then provokes a strong emotional response (Dozier, 2015).

People who treat misophonia have learned that the unpredictability, suddenness, and uncertainty about how long the sound will last contribute to anticipatory anxiety and avoidant behavioral choices. Sufferers say that the anger, rage, and urge to cause harm are directed more toward the person who is making the sound than the sound itself (Schröder et al., 2013).

Triggering sounds often include the following:

- Breathing
- Chewing
- Clicking
- Clock ticking
- Consonant sounds
- Dishes clattering or spoons scraping on dishes
- Dogs barking
- Fingernail clipping
- Fingernail tapping
- Footsteps
- Gulping
- Lip smacking
- Kissing
- Nose breathing
- Nose wheezing
- Nose whistling
- Pipes knocking
- Refrigerator humming
- Slurping
- Sneezing
- Sniffing
- Snoring
- Snorting
- Sound through walls
- Tapping

- Typing
- Whistling
- Yawning (Edelstein et al., 2013)

Referral to an audiologist may be considered to rule in or out medical conditions, such as sensitivity to the intensity of volume of sounds or tinnitus. Of note, 60 percent of tinnitus patients have misophonia (Jastreboff & Jastreboff, 2002). Although there is no data, empirical accounts report a substantial rate of misophonia and OCD (Webber, Johnson, & Storch, 2014).

For example, Kyle stops eating dinner with his family. He can't stand the knife scraping, chewing, smacking, and talking with food in in their mouths. He flies into fits of rage and accuses his parents and sister of purposely making those noises, and he is furious that they keep torturing him. He is starting to get bothered by the sound of chairs scaping on the floors in classes and his classmates' sniffling. He tries using earplugs but can't hear his teacher. The stress is beginning to be too much to bear. Kyle's pediatrician recommends that he get his ears checked and refers him to an audiologist, who diagnoses the problem. Kyle and his family agree on the recommendation of using a noise-cancelling device as needed as well as undergoing cognitive-behavior therapy.

Obsessive Compulsive Personality Disorder (OCPD)

In psychoanalytic theory, obsessive compulsive personality disorder was referred to as the "anal retentive character," said to develop due to being chastised for toilet-training accidents or an underindulged libido (Freud, Strachey, Freud, Rothgeb, & Richards, 1953; Hall, 1954).

OCPD and OCD have several common factors, such as the need for control, perfectionism, and black-and-white thinking. OCPD is based on the need for order, perfection, mental and interpersonal control, and fairly rigid rule-based behavior. People with OCPD pay strict attention to details, make copious lists, have perfect organization, and experience distress and disappointment when external factors don't conform to this pattern of behavior. They often have rigid rules around morality, ethics, or values to which they and others should strictly adhere. They are typically task oriented and work bound, often at the expense of social and leisure activities, and the demands of perfection may result in work being turned in late (American Psychiatric Association, 2013).

For all the above reasons, the disorder has a negative effect on the people around the patient with OCPD. Depending on the dynamics, the quality of interpersonal relationships/friendships may suffer, and people may realize they have sacrificed some personal ties due to their level of rigidity and demands. This is common reason for seeking therapy.

Although OCD and OCPD have similar characteristics and may sometimes be comorbid conditions, OCPD should be ruled out during an active OCD episode in order to see what symptoms resolve in treatment (Pato & Zohar, 1991). Unfortunately, motivation for change in people with OCDP is low, since they don't experience distress from their symptoms and seem to have trouble understanding why others find them unreasonable. Longer-term cognitive behavioral therapy (CBT) or psychotherapy may be helpful when the person experiences enough negative consequences from the rigid interpersonal and functional style of living.

The prevalence of OCPD in the general population is 2–8 percent and is said to occur in 8–9 percent of outpatients. According to studies on comorbid OCD and OCPD, the range is between 23 and 36 percent.

For example, Stuart's perfectionism can be seen in all areas of his life. His tools are clean, neat, and organized. As a carpenter, his attention to detail is flawless, and his customers are pleased with his work. However, they also complain about how long it takes for him to finish their projects. If there is a flaw, no matter how slight, he works hard to fix it, or he may throw it in the trash start over. At home, his family is expected to maintain order and cleanliness, and he becomes upset when something is put out of place.

Autism Spectrum Disorder (Formerly Asperger's Syndrome)

Autism spectrum disorder (ASD) is a developmental disorder characterized by significant difficulties in social interaction and nonverbal communication, along with restricted and repetitive patterns of behavior and interests. The *DSM-V* designated Asperger's syndrome as an autism spectrum disorder, along with autism and pervasive developmental disorder not otherwise specified (de Giambattista et al., 2019).

Many people on the autism spectrum display similar behaviors to OCD, such as repetitive and stereotypical behaviors, rigidity in functional tasks, perfectionism, or obsessive interest and time spent on specific themes, such as subway systems or sports trivia (Jiujias, Kelley, & Hall, 2017). Baron-Cohen and Wheelwright (1989) termed the ego-syntonic type of obsessions as *autism obsessive compulsive phenomena* (Baron-Cohen and Wheelwright, 1989). Unlike obsessive thoughts in OCD that trigger anxiety or guilt, obsessional interests in ASD provoke positive emotions and feelings of pleasure (Fischer-Terworth & Probst, 2009). Likewise, the repetitive behaviors in OCD are distressing and do not provide relief, while the restricted repetitive and stereotypic behavior associated with ASD are experienced as soothing and comforting (Rice, 2014).

According to Russell and colleagues (2005), 4 percent of the people in their study of autistic spectrum disorders were diagnosed with comorbid OCD (Russell, Mataix-Cols, Anson, & Murphy, 2005). Some of the most frequent OC symptoms they found included the following:

- Aggressive obsessions (50%)
- Checking compulsions (60%)
- Cleaning (55%)
- Contamination (60%)
- Hoarding (43%)
- Repeating (43%)
- Symmetry (55%)

In *Stuck*, Hoffman (2012) identified other similar obsessive compulsive behaviors in people with ASD, such as picking up random items like hair strands from the floor, rigidly wearing certain colored clothing, following a limited and selective diet, turning lights on and off repeatedly, and only sitting in certain places (Hoffman, 2012).

For example, Gene is a bright student but has rigid repetitive behaviors at school and at home. His current eating rule is grilled cheddar-cheese sandwiches and potato chips from a can, because they are all the same and intact. To his mother's dismay, he only wears white, because it is a light solid color. He has his mother cut the labels off of his shirts and demands that any new shirts have the label stamped on them. He has an obsessive interest in city transit and subway systems and their maps. He does not like being interrupted for things like coming to dinner when he is absorbed in looking things up online.

One of Gene's special education teachers senses that Gene is experiencing more than just ASD challenges, because he becomes upset at having to erase his schoolwork to the point of creating a hole in the paper. His therapist assesses that his rigid rule about wearing white clothes has to do with purity and the need to please God. Gene does some exposure work with his OCD symptoms of perfectionism and needing to feel right and is willing to begin wearing other-color clothing.

Pediatric Autoimmune Neuropsychiatric Disorders
Associated with and without Streptococcus and
Pediatric Acute-Onset Neuropsychiatric Syndrome (PANS)

Pediatric acute-onset neuropsychiatric syndrome disorders may be caused by an infection, but they also include acute-onset neuropsychiatric disorders that do not appear to be caused by environmental or immunology problems.

An abrupt and dramatic onset of OCD or severely restricted food intake are the first diagnostic criteria for PANS. The obsessive compulsive symptoms must be sufficiently frequent and intense, and they must cause significant distress and interference in the child's activities at home, at school, and with peers. For a PANS diagnosis, two of the other neuropsychiatric symptoms from the list below will be present:

- Anxiety
- Behavioral (developmental) regression
- Deterioration in school performance
- Emotional lability and/or depression
- Irritability, aggression, and/or severely oppositional behaviors
- Sensory or motor abnormalities
- Somatic signs and symptoms, including sleep disturbances, enuresis, or urinary frequency (Murphy et al., 2015)

Pediatric autoimmune neuropsychiatric disorders associated with streptococcal (PANDAS) infections occur when a child has a streptococcus infection that causes an inflammation in the brain (Chiarello, Spitoni, Hollander, Matucci Cerinic, & Pallanti, 2017). A sudden acute and dramatic reaction triggers dramatic neuropsychological and motor symptoms such as OCD, anxiety, tics, personality changes, decline in math and handwriting abilities, sensory sensitivities, restrictive eating, and more.

The diagnostic criteria are the following:

- Association with group A beta-hemolytic streptococcal infection (a positive throat culture for strep or history of scarlet fever)
- Association with neurological abnormalities (physical hyperactivity or unusual, jerky movements that are not in the child's control)
- Episodic course of symptom severity
- Pediatric onset of symptoms (age three years to puberty)
- Presence of obsessive compulsive disorder and/or a tic disorder

- Very abrupt onset or worsening of symptoms (https://www.nimh
  .nih.gov/labs-at-nimh/research-areas/clinics-and-labs/pdnb/pandas
  -frequently-asked-questions.shtml)

Children with PANDAS may also experience one or more of the following symptoms in conjunction with their OCD and/or tics:

- Attention-deficit/hyperactivity disorder symptoms (hyperactivity, inattention, fidgety)
- Fine/gross motor changes (changes in handwriting)
- Joint pains
- Mood changes (irritability, sadness, emotional lability)
- Nighttime bed wetting and/or daytime urinary frequency
- Separation anxiety (child is "clingy" and has difficulty separating from caregivers; for example, the child may not want to be in a different room in the house from his or her parents)
- Sleep disturbance (https://www.nimh.nih.gov/health/publications /pandas/index.shtml)

PANDAS Network estimates that PANDAS/PANS affect as many as 1 in 200 children (http://www.pandasnetwork.org/understanding-pan daspans/what-is-pandas/). Among 136 youth with a lifetime OCD diagnosis, 5 percent met proposed criteria for PANDAS and/or PANS, of whom two met PANDAS criteria, four met PANS criteria, and one met criteria for both (Jaspers-Fayer et al., 2017).

For example, Gretchen wakes up with an onslaught of tics, is emotionally out of control, and has repetitive behaviors. She has also been having a sore throat. When she is calm enough to go to school, her performance changes, and her handwriting regresses back to when she was five, not the twelve-year-old she is now. Her parents bring her to doctors and specialists, who prescribe medication for anxiety, tic, and OCD, but nothing works. The family and the household transform into a triage setting, where the focus is on attending to whatever behavior is most out of control and keeping her and the family safe. During one episode, the family takes Gretchen to the emergency room. Gretchen is evaluated, and the resident on staff that night confirms through a throat culture that she has strep throat and that she is likely experiencing a PANDAS episode. Because the strep throat is still active, a course of antibiotics is prescribed, and she gradually regains her normal baseline personality and behavior.

Hoarding Disorder

Once considered an OCD subtype, hoarding disorder is now its own diagnosis and categorized in the Obsessive Compulsive and Related Disorders category of the *DSM-V* (American Psychiatric Association, 2013). Hoarding is the saving, keeping, and accumulation of items that are considered to have some kind of value, even though they might be considered useless, unimportant, and trash to others (Pushkarskaya et al., 2017). Strong emotional attachment, sentimental value, potential usefulness, and fear of running out of supplies (e.g., buying multiples of toilet paper because it's on sale) are some of the rationalizations for the behavior (Frost, Tolin, Steketee, Fitch, & Selbo-Bruns, 2009).

Hoarding has received much media attention, as evidenced by the TV series *Hoarders* on the A&E cable channel, PBS documentaries, and memes found on the internet. Parents who have problems with hoarding have been implicated in child neglect and abuse cases, and public health task forces have been organized due to the impact of hoarding on the home environment. Children of hoarders are usually unable to have play dates at their houses because of the shame and embarrassment of the chaotic household environment.

Hoarding appears to be hardwired and ego-syntonic, which makes it a very difficult problem to treat. It typically involves the acquisition of excessive amounts of material goods that may appear valueless or useless. As a result of the hoarding and associated challenges with making decisions about what to keep and what to throw away, the individual often has difficulty with organization. Hoarders have been considered creative due to their ability to think of clever or creative ways of using discarded or useless items, even though they hardly ever do (Pushkarskaya et al., 2017). Some people have hoarding behaviors not because they want to save items but because they have problems with disorganization and making decisions about what is important to save or throw away (Ayers, Castriotta, Dozier, Espejo, & Porter, 2014). Junk mail, magazines, and newspaper are common items that pile up and are neglected.

Common dysfunctional thoughts of hoarders are the belief that items with sentimental value should be saved, fears of getting rid of something that he or she might "need" later, belief that almost everything has purpose or value, difficulty making decisions about what to save, belief that even common items are irreplaceable, and fear of not having important or useful information for later and mistakenly discarding important things along with unimportant items (Timpano, Muroff, & Steketee, 2016).

Commonly hoarded items are the following:

- Articles
- Books
- CDs
- Clothes
- Collections or sets of favorite things
- Emails
- Magazines
- Mail
- Newspapers
- Pictures
- Post-it Notes and slips of paper to read later
- Receipts (Kyrios, Steketee, Frost, & Oh, 2002)

Behaviors may include sorting through garbage, saving items to recycle or reuse, taking multiples of freebies (e.g., brochures, samples), and churning (moving items around from one pile to the next when trying to organize or sort through items). Extreme distress and a sense of loss of control are experienced if family members attempt to throw things away and sometimes even when others touch the items.

Some serious negative effects of hoarding can be the following:

- Fires caused by piles of papers kept near the stove
- Injuries sustained when piles of items topple down
- Involvement of child services
- Lack of functional living space
- Mold/squalor leading to health problems
- Public health concerns requiring community intervention (Bratiotis, Schmalisch, & Steketee, 2011)

Current environmental concerns can cause "green guilt," which reinforces hoarding. Reusing and recycling make it difficult for hoarders to throw things away. They may even pick up trash they see while out in public and take it home. Hoarders also do not like to waste and keep things until its last shred of utility (Shapiro, 2014).

Finally, hoarding is not the same as collecting. Cognitive behavioral therapy is considered the most effective psychotherapy for treating the dysfunctional beliefs and patterns of functioning that contribute to hoarding (Muroff, Bratiotis, & Steketee, 2011). Motivational interviewing strategies are also effective in helping to improve insight, which is typically limited in this disorder (Tolin, 2011).

The prevalence rate of hoarding is between 1.5 and 5 percent of the general population (Nordsletten et al., 2013; Timpano et al., 2011). The prevalence of co-occurring OCD was 3–24 percent (Frost, Steketee, & Tolin, 2011; Ivanov et al., 2013).

For example, although financially comfortable, Bill picks off a few grapes in the produce section while shopping. He also pulls over to the side of the road to pick up cans that he can redeem for five cents. His wife no longer tolerates saving food until it molds, so Bill has a separate refrigerator in the garage. His interest in cars has created columns of saved magazines he has not yet read but intends to before recycling them. When asked about discarding these and the other hoarded items, his response is "I will lose parts of myself."

Because Bill's marriage is on the line, he begins to see a therapist, who is able to conduct home-based sessions. The therapist sees piles of unread newspapers and magazines. She sees most of the living spaced crammed with categories of collected items, none of which can really be appreciated because they can't be singularly viewed. His wife insists on having hoarded-free zones in the house so that she can have freedom of space, but it is hard to ignore how Bill's things encroach on the very edge of the dividing rooms. Bill is motivated to save his marriage but insists on painstakingly looking at each hoarded item and deciding which to keep, which to donate and which to discard. At one point, seeing how ambivalent Bill is about reducing the quantity of his hoard, Bill's wife decides to get her own apartment where she can live more comfortably.

References

Abramowitz, J. S., Deacon, B. J., & Valentiner, D. P. (2007). The short health anxiety inventory: Psychometric properties and construct validity in a non-clinical sample. *Cognitive Therapy and Research, 31*(6), 871–883.

Altıntaş, E., & Taşkıntuna, N. (2015). Factors associated with depression in obsessive-compulsive disorder: A cross-sectional study. *Nöropsikiyatri Arşivi/Archives of Neuropsychiatry, 52*(4), 346–353. doi:10.5152/npa.2015.7657

American Psychiatric Association. (2013). *Diagnostic and statistical manual of mental disorders* (5th ed.). Washington, DC: American Psychiatric Publishing.

Arildskov, T. W., Højgaard, D. R. M. A., Skarphedinsson, G., Thomsen, P. H., Ivarsson, T., Weidle, B., . . . Hybel, K. A. (2016). Subclinical autism spectrum symptoms in pediatric obsessive-compulsive disorder. *European Child & Adolescent Psychiatry, 25*(7), 711–723. doi:10.1007 /s00787-015-0782-5

Ayers, C. R., Castriotta, N., Dozier, M. E., Espejo, E. P., & Porter, B. (2014). Behavioral and experiential avoidance in patients with hoarding disorder. *Journal of Behavior Therapy and Experimental Psychiatry, 45*(3), 408–414. doi:10.1016/j.jbtep.2014.04.005

Baron-Cohen, S. & Wheelwright, S. (1989). "Obsessions" in children with autism or Asperger syndrome: Content analysis in terms of core domains of cognition. *British Journal of Clinical Psychology, 175*(5), 484–490.

Becker, E. S., Rinck, M., Türke, V., Kause, P., Goodwin, R., Neumer, S., & Margraf, J. (2007). Epidemiology of specific phobia subtypes: Findings from the Dresden Mental Health Study. *European Psychiatry, 22*(2), 69–74. doi:10.1016/j.eurpsy.2006.09.006

Begotka, A. M., Woods, D. W., & Wetterneck, C. T. (2004). The relationship between experiential avoidance and the severity of trichotillomania in a nonreferred sample. *Journal of Behavior Therapy and Experimental Psychiatry, 35*(1), 17–24. doi:10.1016/j .jbtep.2004.02.001

Bernstein, R. E., Angell, K. L., & Dehle, C. M. (2013). A brief course of cognitive behavioural therapy for the treatment of misophonia: A case example. *Cognitive Behaviour Therapist, 6*(e10). doi:10.1017 /S1754470X13000172

Bhatia, M. S., Jhanjee, A., & Kumar, P. (2011). Culture bound syndromes: A cross-sectional study from India. *European Psychiatry, 26,* 448–448. doi:10.1016/S0924-9338(11)72155-1

Bhatia, S. K., Goyal, A., & Kapur, A. (2013). Habitual biting of oral mucosa: A conservative treatment approach. *Contemporary Clinical Dentistry, 4*(3), 386–389. doi:10.4103/0976-237x.118357

Bienvenu, O. J., Wang, Y., Shugart, Y. Y., Welch, J. M., Grados, M. A., Fyer, A. J., . . . Nestadt, G. (2009). Sapap3 and pathological grooming in humans: Results from the OCD collaborative genetics study. *American Journal of Medical Genetics Part B: Neuropsychiatric Genetics, 150B*(5), 710–720. doi:10.1002/ajmg.b.30897

Bishay, N. R., Petersen, N., & Tarrier, N. (1989). An uncontrolled study of cognitive therapy for morbid jealousy. *British Journal of Psychiatry, 154*(3), 386–389.

Bjornsson, A. S., Didie, E. R., & Phillips, K. A. (2010). Body dysmorphic disorder. *Dialogues in Clinical Neuroscience, 12*(2), 221–232.

Retrieved from https://www.ncbi.nlm.nih.gov/pubmed/20623926; https://www.ncbi.nlm.nih.gov/pmc/articles/PMC3181960/

Blanco, C., Grant, J., Petry, N. M., Simpson, H. B., Alegria, A., Liu, S. M., & Hasin, D. (2008). Prevalence and correlates of shoplifting in the United States: Results from the National Epidemiologic Survey on Alcohol and Related Conditions (NESARC). *American Journal of Psychiatry, 165*(7), 905–913.

Bouman, T. K., Mulkens, S., & van der Lei, B. (2017). Cosmetic professionals' awareness of body dysmorphic disorder. *Plastic Reconstructuve Surgery, 139*(2), 336–342.

Bratiotis, C., Schmalisch, C. S., & Steketee, G. (2011). *The hoarding handbook: A guide for human service professionals.* Oxford; New York: Oxford University Press.

Bratman, S. (2017). Orthorexia vs. theories of healthy eating. *Eating and Weight Disorders, 22*(3), 381–385. doi:10.1007/s40519-017-0417-6

Buhlmann, U., Teachman, B. A., Naumann, E., Fehlinger, T., & Rief, W. (2009). The meaning of beauty: Implicit and explicit self-esteem and attractiveness beliefs in body dysmorphic disorder. *Journal of Anxiety Disorders, 23*(5), 694–702. doi:10.1016/j.janxdis.2009.02.008

Bulli, F., Melli, G., Cavalletti, V., Stopani, E., & Carraresi, C. (2016). Comorbid personality disorders in obsessive-compulsive disorder and its symptom dimensions. *Psychiatric Quarterly, 87*(2), 365–376. doi:10.1007/s11126-015-9393-z

Canetti, L., Bachar, E., & Berry, E. M. (2002). Food and emotion. *Behavioural Processes, 60*(2), 157–164.

Cath, D. C., Hedderly, T., Ludolph, A. G., Stern, J. S., Murphy, T., Hartmann, A., . . . Group, E. G. (2011). European clinical guidelines for Tourette syndrome and other tic disorders. Part I: Assessment. *European Child & Adolescent Psychiatry, 20*(4), 155–171. doi:10.1007/s00787-011-0164-6

Cederlöf, M., Thornton, L. M., Baker, J., Lichtenstein, P., Larsson, H., Rück, C., . . . Mataix-Cols, D. (2015). Etiological overlap between obsessive-compulsive disorder and anorexia nervosa: A longitudinal cohort, multigenerational family and twin study. *World Psychiatry, 14*(3), 333–338. doi:10.1002/wps.20251

Cheng, S. T. (1997). Epidemic genital retraction syndrome: Environmental and personal risk factors in southern China. *Journal of Psychology & Human Sexuality, 9*(1), 57–70.

Chiarello, F., Spitoni, S., Hollander, E., Matucci Cerinic, M., & Pallanti, S. (2017). An expert opinion on PANDAS/PANS: Highlights and controversies. *International Journal of Psychiatry in Clinical Practice, 21*(2), 91–98. doi:10.1080/13651501.2017.1285941

Christenson, G. A., Pyle, R. L., & Mitchell, J. E. (1991). Estimated lifetime prevalence of trichotillomania in college students. *Journal of Clinical Psychiatry, 52*(10), 415–417. Retrieved from https://www.ncbi.nlm.nih.gov/pubmed/1938977

Conrado, L. A., Hounie, A., Diniz, J., Fossaluza, V., Torres, A., Miguel, E., & Ararigboia Rivitti, E. (2010). Body dysmorphic disorder among dermatologic patients: Prevalence and clinical features. *Journal of the American Academy of Dermatology, 63,* 235–243. doi:10.1016/j.jaad.2009.09.017

Creed, F., & Barsky, A. (2004). A systematic review of the epidemiology of somatisation disorder and hypochondriasis. *Journal of Psychosomatic Research, 56*(4), 391–408. doi:10.1016/s0022-3999(03)00622-6

Crerand, C. E., Franklin, M. E., & Sarwar, D. B. (2006). Body dysmorphic disorder and cosmetic surgery. *Plastic and Reconstructive Surgery, 118,* 167–180.

Crerand, C. E., Phillips, K. A., Menard, W., & Fay, C. (2005). Nonpsychiatric medical treatment of body dysmorphic disorder. *Psychosomatics, 46*(6), 549–555. doi:10.1176/appi.psy.46.6.549

de Giambattista, C., Ventura, P., Trerotoli, P., Margari, M., Palumbi, R., & Margari, L. (2019). Subtyping the autism spectrum disorder: Comparison of children with high functioning autism and Asperger syndrome. *Journal of Autism and Developmental Disorders, 49*(1), 138–150. doi:10.1007/s10803-018-3689-4

De Jongh, A., Aartman, I. H., Parvaneh, H., & Ilik, M. (2009). Symptoms of body dysmorphic disorder among people presenting for cosmetic dental treatment: A comparative study of cosmetic dental patients and a general population sample. *Community Dentistry and Oral Epidemiology, 37*(4), 350–356. doi:10.1111/j.1600-0528.2009.00469.x

Diehl, B. J., & Baghurst, T. (2016). Biopsychosocial factors in drives for muscularity and muscle dysmorphia among personal trainers. *Cogent Psychology, 3*(1), 1243194. doi:10.1080/23311908.2016.1243194

Donini, L. M., Marsili, D., Graziani, M. P., Imbriale, M., & Cannella, C. (2004). Orthorexia nervosa: A preliminary study with a proposal for diagnosis and an attempt to measure the dimension of the phenomenon. *Eating and Weight Disorders, 9*(2), 151–157. Retrieved from https://www.ncbi.nlm.nih.gov/pubmed/15330084

Dozier, T. H. (2015). Etiology, composition, development and maintenance of misophonia: A conditioned aversive reflex disorder. *Psychological Thought, 8*(1), 114–129. doi:10.5964/psyct.v8i1.132

Dufresne, R. G., Phillips, K. A., Vittorio, C. C., & Wilkel, C. S. (2001). A screening questionnaire for body dysmorphic disorder in a cosmetic dermatologic surgery practice. *Dermatologic Surgery, 27*(5), 457–462.

Duke, D. C., Bodzin, D. K., Tavares, P., Geffken, G. R., & Storch, E. A. (2009). The phenomenology of hairpulling in a community sample. *Journal of Anxiety Disorders, 23*(8), 1118–1125. doi:10.1016/j.janxdis.2009.07.015

Dykshoorn, K. L. (2014). Trauma-related obsessive-compulsive disorder: A review. *Health Psychology and Behavioral Medicine, 2*(1), 517–528. doi:10.1080/21642850.2014.905207

Dzokoto, V. A., & Adams, G. (2005). Understanding genital-shrinking epidemics in West Africa: Koro, juju, or mass psychogenic illness? *Culture, Medicine, and Psychiatry, 29*(1), 53–78.

Eastin, M. S., & Guinsler, N. M. (2006). Worried and wired: Effects of health anxiety on information-seeking and health care utilization behaviors. *CyberPsychology & Behavior, 9*(4), 494–498.

Ecker, W. (2012). Non-delusional pathological jealousy as an obsessive-compulsive spectrum disorder: Cognitive-behavioural conceptualization and some treatment suggestions. *Journal of Obsessive-Compulsive and Related Disorders, 1*(3), 203–210.

Ecker, W., & Gönner, S. (2006). The feeling of incompleteness: Rediscovery of an old psychopathological symptom of obsessive-compulsive disorder. *Nervenarzt, 77*(9), 1115–1120, 1122. doi:10.1007/s00115-006-2070-6

Edelstein, M., Brang, D., Rouw, R. & Ramachandran, V. S. (2013). Misophonia: Physiological investigations and case descriptions. *Frontiers in Human Neuroscience, 7*, 276

Fang, A., & Hofmann, S. G. (2010). Relationship between social anxiety disorder and body dysmorphic disorder. *Clinical Psychology Review, 30*(8), 1040–1048. doi:10.1016/j.cpr.2010.08.001

Felling, R. J., & Singer, H. S. (2011). Neurobiology of Tourette syndrome: Current status and need for further investigation. *Journal of Neuroscience, 31*(35), 12387–12395. doi:10.1523/jneurosci.0150-11.2011

Fischer-Terworth, C., & Probst, P. (2009). Obsessive-compulsive phenomena and symptoms in Asperger's disorder and high-functioning autism: An evaluative literature review. *Life Span and Disability, 12*(1), 5–27.

Flaitz, C. M., & Felefli, S. (2000). Complications of an unrecognized cheek biting habit following a dental visit. *Pediatric Dentistry, 22*(6), 511–512.

Fontenelle, L. F., Mendlowicz, M. V., & Versiani, M. (2005). Impulse control disorders in patients with obsessive-compulsive disorder. *Psychiatry and Clinical Neurosciences, 59*(1), 30–37.

Frayn, M., Livshits, S., & Knäuper, B. (2018). Emotional eating and weight regulation: A qualitative study of compensatory behaviors and concerns. *Journal of Eating Disorders, 6*(1), 23. doi:10.1186 /s40337-018-0210-6

Freud, S., Strachey, J., Freud, A., Rothgeb, C. L., & Richards, A. (1953). *The standard edition of the complete psychological works of Sigmund Freud.* London: Hogarth Press.

Frías, Á., Palma, C., Farriols, N., & González, L. (2015). Comorbidity between obsessive-compulsive disorder and body dysmorphic disorder: Prevalence, explanatory theories, and clinical characterization. *Neuropsychiatric Disease and Treatment, 11*, 2233–2244.

Frost, R. O., Steketee, G., & Tolin, D. F. (2011). Comorbidity in hoarding disorder. *Depression and Anxiety, 28*(10), 876–884. doi:10.1002 /da.20861

Frost, R. O., Tolin, D. F., Steketee, G., Fitch, K. E., & Selbo-Bruns, A. (2009). Excessive acquisition in hoarding. *Journal of Anxiety Disorders, 23*(5), 632–639. doi:10.1016/j.janxdis.2009.01.013

Fuss, J., Briken, P., Stein, D. J., & Lochner, C. (2019). Compulsive sexual behavior disorder in obsessive-compulsive disorder: Prevalence and associated comorbidity. *Journal of Behavioral Addictions, 8*(2), 242–248. doi:10.1556/2006.8.2019.23

Ghanizadeh, A. (2011). Nail biting: Etiology, consequences and management. *Iranian Journal of Medical Sciences, 36*(2), 73–79. Retrieved from https://www.ncbi.nlm.nih.gov/pubmed/23358880; https://www .ncbi.nlm.nih.gov/pmc/articles/PMC3556753/

Ghosh, S., Nath, S., Brahma, A., & Chowdhury, A. N. (2013). Fifth koro epidemic in India: A review report. *World Cultural Psychiatry Research Review,* March, 8–20.

Gianini, L., Liu, Y., Wang, Y., Attia, E., Walsh, B. T., & Steinglass, J. (2015). Abnormal eating behavior in video-recorded meals in anorexia nervosa. *Eating Behaviors, 19*, 28–32. doi:10.1016/j.eatbeh.2015.06.005

Godart, N. T., Flament, M. F., Perdereau, F., & Jeammet, P. (2002). Comorbidity between eating disorders and anxiety disorders: A review. *International Journal of Eating Disorders, 32*(3), 253–270.

Grabe, H. J., Meyer, C., Hapke, U., Rumpf, H.-J., Freyberger, H. J., Dilling, H., & John, U. (2001). Lifetime-comorbidity of obsessive-compulsive disorder and subclinical obsessive-compulsive disorder in northern

Germany. *European Archives of Psychiatry and Clinical Neuroscience, 251*(3), 130–135. doi:10.1007/s004060170047

Grant, J. E. (2003). Family history and psychiatric comorbidity in persons with kleptomania. *Comprehensive Psychiatry, 44*(6), 437–441. doi:10.1016/s0010-440x(03)00150-0

Grant, J. E., Odlaug, B. L., Chamberlain, S. R., Keuthen, N. J., Lochner, C., & Stein, D. J. (2012). Skin picking disorder. *American Journal of Psychiatry, 169*(11), 1143–1149. doi:10.1176/appi.ajp.2012 .12040508

Greenberg, J. L., Berman, N. C., Braddick, V., Schwartz, R., Mothi, S. S., & Wilhelm, S. (2018). Treatment utilization and barriers to treatment among individuals with olfactory reference syndrome (ORS). *Journal of Psychosomatic Research, 105,* 31–36. doi:10.1016/j .jpsychores.2017.12.004

Greenberg, J. L., Shaw, A. M., Reuman, L., Schwartz, R., & Wilhelm, S. (2016). Clinical features of olfactory reference syndrome: An internet-based study. *Journal of Psychosomatic Research, 80,* 11–16. doi:10.1016/j.jpsychores.2015.11.001

Gruber, A. J., & Pope, H. G. (1999). Compulsive weight lifting and anabolic drug abuse among women rape victims. *Comprehensive Psychiatry, 40*(4), 273–277.

Hall, C. S. (1954). *A primer of Freudian psychology* (1st ed.). Cleveland,OH: World.

Halmi, K., Tozzi, F., Thornton, L., Crow, S., Fichter, M., Kaplan, A., . . . Bulik, C. (2005). The relation among perfectionism, obsessive-compulsive personality disorder and obsessive-compulsive disorder in individuals with eating disorders. *International Journal of Eating Disorders, 38*(4), 371–374. doi:10.1002/eat.20190

Halteh, P., Scher, R. K., & Lipner, S. R. (2017). Onychophagia: A nail-biting conundrum for physicians. *Journal of Dermatological Treatment, 28*(2), 166–172. doi:10.1080/09546634.2016.1200711

Håman, L., Barker-Ruchti, N., Patriksson, G., & Lindgren, E.-C. (2015). Orthorexia nervosa: An integrative literature review of a lifestyle syndrome. *International Journal of Qualitative Studies on Health and Well-Being, 10*(1), 26799.

Hedman, E., Ljótsson, B., Axelsson, E., Andersson, G., Rück, C., & Andersson, E. (2017). Health anxiety in obsessive compulsive disorder and obsessive compulsive symptoms in severe health anxiety: An investigation of symptom profiles. *Journal of Anxiety Disorders, 45,* 80–86.

Hepburn, S., & Cunningham, S. (2006). Body dysmorphic disorder in adult orthodontic patients. *American Journal of Orthodontics and Dentofacial Orthopedics, 130*(5), 569–574. doi:10.1016/j .ajodo.2005.06.022

Higgins, S., & Wysong, A. (2017). Cosmetic surgery and body dysmorphic disorder: An update. *International Journal of Women's Dermatology, 4*(1), 43–48. doi:10.1016/j.ijwd.2017.09.007

Hirschtritt, M. E., Lee, P. C., Pauls, D. L., Dion, Y., Grados, M. A., Ill-mann, C., . . . Mathews, C. A. (2015). Lifetime prevalence, age of risk, and genetic relationships of comorbid psychiatric disorders in Tou-rette syndrome. *JAMA Psychiatry, 72*(4), 325–333.

Hoffman, J. (2012). *Stuck: Asperger's syndrome and obsessive-compulsive behaviors.* Weston, FL: Weston Press.

Hollander, E. (1996). Obsessive-compulsive disorder-related disorders: The role of selective serotonergic reuptake inhibitors. *International Clinical Psychopharmacology, 11*(Suppl 5), 75–87. Retrieved from https://www.ncbi.nlm.nih.gov/pubmed/9032004

Hollander, E., Mucci, R., & Mucci, C. (2000). The obsessive compulsive spectrum: Survey of 800 practitioners. *CNS Spectrums, 5*(8), 61–64.

Hudson, J. I., Hiripi, E., Pope, H. G., & Kessler, R. C. (2007). The prevalence and correlates of eating disorders in the National Comor-bidity Survey Replication. *Biological Psychiatry, 61*(3), 348–358. doi:10.1016/j.biopsych.2006.03.040

Hunt, T. J., Thienhaus, O., & Ellwood, A. (2008). The mirror lies: Body dysmorphic disorder. *American Family Physician, 78*(2), 217–222. Retrieved from https://www.ncbi.nlm.nih.gov/pubmed/18697504

Insel, T. R., & Akiskal, H. S. (1986). Obsessive-compulsive disorder with psychotic features: A phenomenologic analysis. *American Journal of Psychiatry, 143*, 1527–1533.

Ivanov, V. Z., Mataix-Cols, D., Serlachius, E., Lichtenstein, P., Anckarsäter, H., Chang, Z., . . . Rück, C. (2013). Prevalence, comorbidity and heritability of hoarding symptoms in adolescence: A population based twin study in 15-year olds. *PLoS ONE, 8*(7), e69140. doi:10.1371 /journal.pone.0069140

Jafferany, M., Vander Stoep, A., Dumitrescu, A., & Hornung, R. L. (2010). The knowledge, awareness, and practice patterns of der-matologists toward psychocutaneous disorders: Results of a sur-vey study. *International Journal of Dermatology, 49*(7), 784–789. doi:10.1111/j.1365-4632.2009.04372.x

Jaspers-Fayer, F., Han, S. H. J., Chan, E., McKenney, K., Simpson, A., Boyle, A., . . . Stewart, S. E. (2017). Prevalence of acute-onset subtypes in pediatric obsessive-compulsive disorder. *Journal of Child and Ado-lescent Psychopharmacology, 27*(4), 332–341.

Jastreboff, M. M., & Jastreboff, P. J. (2002). Decreased sound tolerance and tinnitus retraining therapy (TRT). *Australian and New Zealand Journal of Audiology, 24*(2), 74–84. doi:10.1375/audi.24.2.74.31105

Jhanjee, A., Bhatia, M. S., Kumar, P., & Jindal, A. (2010). Sexual addiction in association with obsessive-compulsive disorder. *German Journal of Psychiatry, 13*(4), 171–174.

Jiujias, M., Kelley, E., & Hall, L. (2017). Restricted, repetitive behaviors in autism spectrum disorder and obsessive-compulsive disorder: A comparative review. *Child Psychiatry & Human Development, 48*(6), 944–959.

Johnson, J., & El-Alfy, A. T. (2016). Review of available studies of the neurobiology and pharmacotherapeutic management of trichotillomania. *Journal of Advanced Research, 7*(2), 169–184. doi:10.1016/j.jare.2015.05.001

Keuthen, N. J., Curley, E. E., Scharf, J. M., Woods, D. W., Lochner, C., Stein, D. J., . . . Grant, J. E. (2016). Predictors of comorbid obsessive-compulsive disorder and skin-picking disorder in trichotillomania. *Annals of Clinical Psychiatry, 28*(4), 280–288.

Kingham, M., & Gordon, H. L. (2004). Aspects of morbid jealousy. *Advances in Psychiatric Treatment, 10*(3), 207–215. doi:10.1192/apt.10.3.207

Kroenke, K. (2003). Patients presenting with somatic complaints: Epidemiology, psychiatric comorbidity and management. *International Journal of Methods in Psychiatric Research, 12*(1), 34–43. Retrieved from https://www.ncbi.nlm.nih.gov/pubmed/12830308

Kumar, R., Phookun, H. R., & Datta, A. (2014). Epidemic of koro in north east India: An observational cross-sectional study. *Asian Journal of Psychiatry, 12*, 113–117. doi:10.1016/j.ajp.2014.07.006

Kuzma, J. M., & Black, D. W. (2008). Epidemiology, prevalence, and natural history of compulsive sexual behavior. *Psychiatric Clinics of North America, 31*(4), 603–611.

Kyrios, M., Steketee, G., Frost, R. O., & Oh, S. (2002). Cognitions in compulsive hoarding. In R. O. Frost & G. Steketee (Eds.) *Cognitive Approaches to Obsessions and Compulsions: Theory, Assessment, and Treatment.*

Leeman, R. F., & Potenza, M. (2013). A targeted review of the neurobiology and genetics of behavioral addictions: An emerging area of research. *Canadian Journal of Psychiatry, 58*, 260–273. doi:10.1177/070674371305800503

Leone, J. E., Sedory, E. J., & Gray, K. A. (2005). Recognition and treatment of muscle dysmorphia and related body image disorders. *Journal of Athletic Training, 40*(4), 352–359. Retrieved from https://www.ncbi .nlm.nih.gov/pubmed/16404458

Leung, A. K., & Robson, W. L. (1990). Nailbiting. *Clinical Pediatrics (Philadelphia), 29*(12), 690–692. doi:10.1177/000992289002901201

Lipsitz, J. D., Fyer, A. J., Paterniti, A., & Klein, D. F. (2001). Emetophobia: Preliminary results of an internet survey. *Depression and Anxiety, 14*(2), 149–152. Retrieved from https://www.ncbi.nlm.nih.gov /pubmed/11668669

Lochner, C., Fineberg, N. A., Zohar, J., van Ameringen, M., Juven-Wetzler, A., Altamura, A. C., . . . Stein, D. J. (2014). Comorbidity in obsessive-compulsive disorder (OCD): A report from the International College of Obsessive-Compulsive Spectrum Disorders (ICOCS). *Comprehensive Psychiatry, 55*(7), 1513–1519. doi:https://doi.org/10.1016 /j.comppsych.2014.05.020

López-Solà, C., Bui, M., Hopper, J. L., Fontenelle, L. F., Davey, C. G., Pantelis, C., . . . Harrison, B. J. (2018). Predictors and consequences of health anxiety symptoms: A novel twin modeling study. *Acta Psychiatrica Scandinavica, 137*(3), 241–251. doi:doi:10.1111/acps.12850

Lopez-Sola, C., Hopper, B. M., Fontenelle, L. F., Davey, C. G., Pantelis, C., Alonso, P., . . . Harrison, B. J. (2018). Predictors and Consequences of Health Anxiety Symptoms: A Novel Twin Modeling Study. *Acta Psychiatrica Scandinavica*, 241-251. doi:10.111.acps.12850

Maack, D., Deacon, B., & Zhao, M. (2013). Exposure therapy for emetophobia: A case study with three-year follow-up. *Journal of Anxiety Disorders, 27*, 527–534. doi:10.1016/j.janxdis.2013.07.001

Maraz, A., Griffiths, M. D., & Demetrovics, Z. (2016). The prevalence of compulsive buying: A meta-analysis. *Addiction, 111*(3), 408–419.

Marazziti, D., Di Nasso, E., Masala, I., Baroni, S., Abelli, M., Mengali, F., . . . Rucci, P. (2003). Normal and obsessional jealousy: A study of a population of young adults. *European Psychiatry, 18*(3), 106–111. doi:10.1016/s0924-9338(03)00024-5

Matsunaga, H., Kiriike, N., Matsui, T., Oya, K., Okino, K., & Stein, D. J. (2005). Impulsive disorders in Japanese adult patients with obsessive-compulsive disorder. *Comprehensive Psychiatry, 46*(1), 43–49.

Mattelaer, J. J., & Jilek, W. (2007). Koro: The psychological disappearance of the penis. *Journal of Sexual Medicine, 4*(5), 1509–1515.

Moroze, R. M., Dunn, T. M., Holland, J. C., Yager, J., & Weintraub, P. (2015). Microthinking about micronutrients: A case of transition from obsessions about healthy eating to near-fatal "orthorexia nervosa" and proposed diagnostic criteria. *Psychosomatics, 56*(4), 397–403.

Mueller, A., Mitchell, J. E., Peterson, L. A., Faber, R. J., Steffen, K. J., Crosby, R. D., & Claes, L. (2011). Depression, materialism, and excessive internet use in relation to compulsive buying. *Comprehensive Psychiatry, 52*(4), 420–424. doi:10.1016/j.comppsych.2010.09.001

Muroff, J., Bratiotis, C., & Steketee, G. (2011). Treatment for hoarding behaviors: A review of the evidence. *Clinical Social Work Journal, 39*(4), 406–423. doi:10.1007/s10615-010-0311-4

Murphy, T. K., Patel, P. D., McGuire, J. F., Kennel, A., Mutch, P. J., Parker-Athill, E. C., Hanks, C. E., Lewin, A. B., Storch, E. A., Toufexis, M. D., Dadlani, G. H., & Rodriguez, C. A. (2015). Characterization of the pediatric acute-onset neuropsychiatric symdrome phenotype. *Journal of Child and Adolescent Psychiatry, 25(1)*, 14–25.

Nieuwoudt, J. E., Zhou, S., Coutts, R. A., & Booker, R. (2015). Symptoms of muscle dysmorphia, body dysmorphic disorder, and eating disorders in a nonclinical population of adult male weightlifters in Australia. *Journal of Strength and Conditioning Research, 29*(5), 1406–1414. doi:10.1519/jsc.0000000000000763

Nirmal, B., Shenoi, S. D., Rai, S., Sreejayan, K., & Savitha, S. (2013). "Look beyond skin": Psychogenic excoriation—A series of five cases. *Indian Journal of Dermatology, 58*(3), 246. doi:10.4103/0019-5154.110885

Nock, M. K., Prinstein, M. J., & Sterba, S. K. (2009). Revealing the form and function of self-injurious thoughts and behaviors: A real-time ecological assessment study among adolescents and young adults. *Journal of Abnormal Psychology, 118*(4), 816–827. doi:10.1037/a0016948

Nordsletten, A. E., Reichenberg, A., Hatch, S. L., de la Cruz, L. F., Pertusa, A., Hotopf, M., & Mataix-Cols, D. (2013). Epidemiology of hoarding disorder. *British Journal of Psychiatry, 203*(6), 445–452.

Novotny, M., Valis, M., & Klimova, B. (2018). Tourette syndrome: A mini-review. *Frontiers in Neurology, 9*, 139. doi:10.3389/fneur.2018.00139

Odlaug, B. L., & Grant, J. E. (2008). Clinical characteristics and medical complications of pathologic skin picking. *General Hospital Psychiatry, 30*(1), 61–66. doi:10.1016/j.genhosppsych.2007.07.009

Odlaug, B. L., Kim, S. W., & Grant, J. E. (2010). Quality of life and clinical severity in pathological skin picking and trichotillomania. *Journal of Anxiety Disorders, 24*(8), 823–829. doi:10.1016/j.janxdis.2010.06.004

Onur, O. S., Tabo, A., Aydin, E., Tuna, O., Maner, A. F., Yildirim, E. A., & Çarpar, E. (2016). Relationship between impulsivity and obsession types in obsessive-compulsive disorder. *International Journal of Psychiatry in Clinical Practice, 20*(4), 218–223. doi:10.1080/13651501.2 016.1220580

Pato, M. T., & Zohar, J. (1991). *Current treatments of obsessive-compulsive disorder.* Washington, DC: American Psychiatric Press.

Perugi, G., Giannotti, D., Frare, F., Vaio, S. D., Valori, E., Maggi, L., . . . Akiskal, H. S. (1997). Prevalence, phenomenology and comorbidity of body dysmorphic disorder (dysmorphophobia) in a clinical population. *International Journal of Psychiatry in Clinical Practice, 1*(2), 77–82. doi:10.3109/13651509709024707

Petter, T., Richter, M. A., & Sandor, P. (1998). Clinical features distinguishing patients with Tourette's syndrome and obsessive-compulsive disorder from patients with obsessive-compulsive disorder without tics. *Journal of Clinical Psychiatry, 59*(9), 456–459.

Phillips, K. A. (2004). Body dysmorphic disorder: recognizing and treating imagined ugliness. *World Psychiatry, 3*(1), 12–17. Retrieved from http://www.ncbi.nlm.nih.gov/pmc/articles/PMC1414653/

Phillips, K. A. (2005). *The broken mirror: Understanding and treating body dysmorphic disorder* (Rev. and expanded ed.). Oxford and New York: Oxford University Press.

Phillips, K. A., Gunderson, C., Gruber, U., & Castle, D. J. (2006). Delusions of body malodour: The olfactory reference syndrome. In W. J. Brewer, D. Castle, & C. Pantelis (Eds.), *Olfaction and the Brain* (pp. 334–353). Cambridge: Cambridge University Press.

Phillips, K. A., & Menard, W. (2006). Suicidality in body dysmorphic disorder: A prospective study. *American Journal of Psychiatry, 163*(7), 1280–1282. doi:10.1176/ajp.2006.163.7.1280

Phillips, K. A., & Menard, W. (2011). Olfactory reference syndrome: Demographic and clinical features of imagined body odor. *General Hospital Psychiatry, 33*(4), 398–406. doi:10.1016/j.genhosppsych.2011.04.004

Pope, H. G., Jr., Gruber, A. J., Choi, P., Olivardia, R., & Phillips, K. A. (1997). Muscle dysmorphia: An underrecognized form of body dysmorphic disorder. *Psychosomatics, 38*(6), 548–557. doi:10.1016 /s0033-3182(97)71400-2

Pope, H. G., Jr., Katz, D. L., & Hudson, J. I. (1993). Anorexia nervosa and "reverse anorexia" among 108 male bodybuilders. *Comprehensive Psychiatry, 34*(6), 406–409.

Presta, S., Marazziti, D., Dell'Osso, L., Pfanner, C., Pallanti, S., & Cassano, G. B. (2002). Kleptomania: Clinical features and comorbidity in an Italian sample. *Comprehensive Psychiatry, 43*(1), 7–12.

Pryse-Phillips, W. (1971). An olfactory reference syndrome. *Acta Psychiatrica Scandinavica, 47*(4), 484–509.

Pushkarskaya, H., Tolin, D., Ruderman, L., Henick, D., Kelly, J. M., Pittenger, C., & Levy, I. (2017). Value-based decision making under uncertainty in hoarding and obsessive-compulsive disorders. *Psychiatry Research, 258*, 305–315. doi:10.1016/j.psychres.2017.08.058

Reichert, M., Scheithauer, M., Hoffmann, T. K., Hellings, P., & Picavet, V. (2014). What rhinoplasty surgeons should know about body dysmorphic disorder (BDD). *Laryngorhinootologie, 93*(8), 507–513. doi:10.1055/s-0034-1371825

Reid, R. C., Garos, S., & Fong, T. (2012). Psychometric development of the hypersexual behavior consequences scale. *Journal of Behavioral Addictions, 1*(3), 115–122. doi:10.1556/JBA.1.2012.001

Rice, R. H. (2014). The repetitive behavior spectrum in autism and obsessive compulsive disorder: From helpful to harmful. *Autonomy, the Critical Journal of Interdisciplinary Autism Studies, 1*(2), 1–17.

Rief, W. & Martin, A. (2014). How to use the new DSM-5 somatic symptom disorder diagnosis in research and practice: A critical evaluation and a proposal for modifications. *Annual Review of Clinical Psychology, 10*, 339–367.

Rufer, M., Fricke, S., Held, D., Cremer, J., & Hand, I. (2006). Dissociation and symptom dimensions of obsessive-compulsive disorder. *European Archives of Psychiatry and Clinical Neuroscience, 256*(3), 146–150.

Rushing, J. M., Jones, L. E., & Carney, C. P. (2003). Bulimia nervosa: A primary care review. *Primary Care Companion to the Journal of Clinical Psychiatry, 5*(5), 217–224. doi:10.4088/pcc.v05n0505

Russell, A. J., Mataix-Cols, D., Anson, M., & Murphy, D. G. M. (2005). Obsessions and compulsions in Asperger syndrome and high-functioning autism. *British Journal of Psychiatry, 186*(June), 525–528.

Sacks, O. (1970). *The man who mistook his wife for a hat.* New York: Harper & Row.

Saraf, G., Paul, I., Viswanath, B., Narayanaswamy, J. C., Math, S. B., & Reddy, Y. C. J. (2017). Bipolar disorder comorbidity in patients with a primary diagnosis of OCD. *International Journal of Psychiatry in Clinical Practice, 21*(1), 70–74. doi:10.1080/13651501.2016.1233344

Sarwer, D. B. (2002). Awareness and identification of body dysmorphic disorder by aesthetic surgeons: Results of a survey of American Society for Aesthetic Plastic Surgery members. *Aesthetic Surgery Journal, 22*(6), 531–535. doi:10.1067/maj.2002.129451

Sarwer, D. B., LaRossa, D., Bartlett, S. P., Low, D. W., Bucky, L. P., & Whitaker, L. A. (2003). Body image concerns of breast augmentation patients. *Plastic and Reconstructive Surgery, 112*(1), 83–90. doi:10.1097/01.PRS.0000066005.07796.51

Sarwer, D. B., & Spitzer, J. C. (2012). Body image dysmorphic disorder in persons who undergo aesthetic medical treatments. *Aesthetic Surgery Journal, 32*(8), 999–1009. doi:10.1177/1090820x12462715

Scharf, J. M., Miller, L. L., Gauvin, C. A., Alabiso, J., Mathews, C. A., & Ben-Shlomo, Y. (2015). Population prevalence of Tourette syndrome: A systematic review and meta-analysis. *Movement Disorders, 30*(2), 221–228. doi:10.1002/mds.26089

Schröder, A., Vulink, N., & Denys, D. (2013). Misophonia: Diagnostic criteria for a new psychiatric disorder. *PLoS ONE, 8*. doi:10.1371/journal.pone.0054706

Shapiro, L. J. (2014). *Understanding OCD: Skills to control the conscience and outsmart obsessive compulsive disorder*. Santa Barbara, CA: Praeger.

Shashidhara, M., Sushma, B. R., Viswanath, B., Math, S. B., & Janardhan Reddy, Y. C. (2015). Comorbid obsessive compulsive disorder in patients with bipolar-I disorder. *Journal of Affective Disorders, 174*, 367–371. doi:10.1016/j.jad.2014.12.019

Soffer-Dudek, N. (2019). Dissociative absorption, mind-wandering, and attention-deficit symptoms: Associations with obsessive-compulsive symptoms. *British Journal of Clinical Psychology, 58*(1), 51–69. doi:10.1111/bjc.12186

Striegel-Moore, R. H., Rosselli, F., Perrin, N., DeBar, L., Wilson, G. T., May, A., & Kraemer, H. C. (2009). Gender difference in the prevalence of eating disorder symptoms. *International Journal of Eating Disorders, 42*(5), 471–474. doi:10.1002/eat.20625

Swain, J. E., & Leckman, J. F. (2005). Tourette syndrome and tic disorders: Overview and practical guide to diagnosis and treatment. *Psychiatry (Edgmont), 2*(7), 26–36. Retrieved from http://www.ncbi.nlm.nih.gov/pmc/articles/PMC3000195/

Swedo, S. E., & Leonard, H. L. (1992). Trichotillomania: An obsessive-compulsive disorder? *Psychiatric Clinics of North America, 15*, 777–790.

Sykes, M., Boschen, M. J., & Conlon, E. G. (2016). Comorbidity in emetophobia (specific phobia of vomiting). *Clinical Psychology & Psychotherapy, 23*(4), 363–367. doi:10.1002/cpp.1964

Talih, F. R. (2011). Kleptomania and potential exacerbating factors: A review and case report. *Innovations in Clinical Neuroscience,*

8(10), 35–39. Retrieved from https://www.ncbi.nlm.nih.gov/pubmed /22132369; https://www.ncbi.nlm.nih.gov/pmc/articles/PMC3225132/

Teng, E. J., Woods, D. W., Twohig, M. P., & Marcks, B. A. (2002). Body-focused repetitive behavior problems: Prevalence in a nonre-ferred population and differences in perceived somatic activity. *Behavior Modification, 26*(3), 340–360.

Timpano, K. R., Exner, C., Glaesmer, H., Rief, W., Keshaviah, A., Brahler, E., & Wilhelm, S. (2011). The epidemiology of the proposed DSM-5 hoarding disorder: Exploration of the acquisition specifier, associated features, and distress. *Journal of Clinical Psychiatry, 72*(6), 780–786.

Timpano, K. R., Muroff, J., & Steketee, G. (2016). A review of the diagnosis and management of hoarding disorder. *Current Treatment Options in Psychiatry, 3*, 394–410. doi:10.1007/s40501-016-0098-1

Tod, D., Edwards, C., & Cranswick, I. (2016). Muscle dysmorphia: Current insights. *Psychology Research and Behavior Management, 9*, 179–188. doi:10.2147/PRBM.S97404

Tolin, D. F. (2011). Understanding and treating hoarding: A biopsycho-social perspective. *Journal of Clinical Psychology, 67*(5), 517–526. doi:10.1002/jclp.20795

Torres, A. R., Fontenelle, L. F., Shavitt, R. G., Ferrao, Y. A., do Rosario, M. C., Storch, E. A., & Miguel, E. C. (2016). Comorbidity variation in patients with obsessive-compulsive disorder according to symptom dimensions: Results from a large multicentre clinical sample. *Journal of Affective Disorders, 190*, 508–516. doi:10.1016/j.jad.2015.10.051

Torres, A. R., Prince, M. J., Bebbington, P. E., Bhugra, D., Brugha, T. S., Farrell, M., . . . Singleton, N. (2006). Obsessive-compulsive disor-der: Prevalence, comorbidity, impact, and help-seeking in the British National Psychiatric Morbidity Survey of 2000. *American Journal of Psychiatry, 163*(11), 1978–1985. doi:10.1176/ajp.2006.163.11.1978

Tremelling, K., Sandon, L., Vega, G. L., & McAdams, C. J. (2017). Orth-orexia nervosa and eating disorder symptoms in registered dietitian nutritionists in the United States. *Journal of the Academy of Nutrition and Dietetics, 117*(10), 1612–1617. doi:10.1016/j.jand.2017.05.001

Tyagi, H., Patel, R., Rughooputh, F., Abrahams, H., Watson, A. J., & Drummond, L. (2015). Comparative prevalence of eating disorders in obsessive-compulsive disorder and other anxiety disorders. *Psychiatry Journal, 2015*, 186927. doi:10.1155/2015/186927

Tyrer, P., Cooper, S., Crawford, M., Dupont, S., Green, J., Murphy, D., . . . Bhogal, S. (2011). Prevalence of health anxiety problems in medical clinics. *Journal of Psychosomatic Research, 71*(6), 392–394.

van Hout, W. J., & Bouman, T. K. (2012). Clinical features, prevalence and psychiatric complaints in subjects with fear of vomiting. *Clinical Psychology & Psychotherapy, 19*(6), 531–539. doi:10.1002/cpp.761

Veale, D., Costa, A., Murphy, P., & Ellison, N. (2012). Abnormal eating behaviour in people with a specific phobia of vomiting (emetophobia). *European Eating Disorders Review, 20*(5), 414–418. doi:10.1002/erv.1159

Veale, D., De Haro, L., & Lambrou, C. (2013). Cosmetic rhinoplasty in body dysmorphic disorder. *British Journal of Plastic Surgery, 56*(6), 546–551.

Veale, D., Hennig, C., & Gledhill, L. (2015). Is a specific phobia of vomiting part of the obsessive compulsive and related disorders? *Journal of Obsessive-Compulsive and Related Disorders, 7*(222), 1–6. doi:10.1016/j.jocrd.2015.08.002

Veale, D., & Lambrou, C. (2006). The psychopathology of vomit phobia. *Behavioural and Cognitive Psychotherapy, 34*, 139–150. doi:10.1017/S1352465805002754

Webber, T. A., Johnson, P. L., & Storch, E. A. (2014). Pediatric misophonia with comorbid obsessive-compulsive spectrum disorders. *General Hospital Psychiatry, 36*(2), 231.e231–232. doi:10.1016/j.genhosppsych.2013.10.018

Yılmaz, S., İzci, F., Mermi, O., & Atmaca, M. (2016). Metacognitive functions in patients who has obsessive compulsive disorder and major depressive disorder: A controlled study. *Anatolian Journal of Psychiatry, 17*(6), 451–458.

Zohar, A., Ratzoni, G., Pauls, D., Apter, A., Bleich, A., Kron, S., . . . Cohen, D. (1992). An epidemiological study of obsessive-compulsive disorder and related disorders in Israeli adolescents. *Journal of the American Academy of Child and Adolescent Psychiatry, 31*(6), 1057–1061. doi:S0890-8567(09)64818-8 [pii] 10.1097/00004583-199211000-00010

CHAPTER 3

History

Reports of OCD span the ages and depict the changes in etiological beliefs and treatment strategies over the eras. Historical references of OCD have been traced back to the second millennium in Sumeria and Akkadia areas of Babylonia. Maqlû and Šurpu tablets, written in cuneiform, contain what have been interpreted to depict medical and behavioral problems of OCD symptoms such as contamination, orderliness of objects, aggression, sex, and religion (Reynolds & Kinnier, 2012). According to Reynolds and Kinnier (2012), the word *ma"m"ıt(u)* seems to imply a compulsion to do or not to do a certain act as well as a fear or phobia of such action or inaction within a medical context. Some Šurpu tablets illustrated compulsive confessions of alleged sins, ritual offenses, unintended breaches of taboos, morality, and social order that may have offended the gods (Schwemer, 2011).

OCD as a Religious Problem

Numerous cases of OCD have been found in the well-documented annals of Christianity. OCD sufferers sought help from the clergy more than physicians due to beliefs that the disorder was caused by the devil, demons, or supernatural forces (Oldridge, 2019).

Around 600 A.D., John Climacus (579–649), abbot of St. Catherine Monastery in Sinai, seemed to understand the true nature of obsessions and suggested that "if you have blasphemous thoughts, do not think that you are to blame. God knows what is in our hearts and He knows that ideas of this kind come not from us. Those unclean and unspeakable thoughts come at us when we are praying, but, if we continue to pray to the end, they will retreat, for they do not struggle against those who resist them" (Climacus, 2012 [1605]).

Although illiterate, Margery Kempe (1373–1438) is known to have written the first English language autobiography, *The Book of Margery Kempe*. She dictated her spiritual journey to a local priest who wrote in her voice, "Our Lord withdrew from her all good thoughts . . . so now she had as many hours of foul thoughts and foul memories of lechery and all uncleanness. . . . she now horrible sights . . . of beholding men's members, and such other abominations. She saw (them) showing their bare members unto her. . . . When she should see the Sacrament, make her prayers, or do any other good deed, ever such cursedness was put into her mind" (Butler-Bowdon, 1944; Kempe & Butler-Bowdon, 1936). The account of her journey was fraught with sexual obsessions and scrupulous fears that she atoned for by compulsive self-denial and self-punishment.

In the fifteenth century, Antonius, born Antonio Pierozzi (1389–1459), the archbishop of Florence, believed that scrupulosity sometimes had a physical cause, and not necessarily a satanic one, and should be treated with "medicine or other physical remedies." Nonetheless, his advice for those trying to escape religious compulsions was to seek God's grace, study sacred Scripture, pray constantly, and put up a spirited resistance to the urge to compulsively confess (Collins, 1961).

Martin Luther (1483–1546), who founded the Protestant movement, also suffered from scrupulosity. The leader of the Reformation of the Catholic Church, which he considered corrupt and motivated by greed, he nailed a copy of his *95 Theses* to the door of the Wittenberg Castle church in 1517 to protest certain religious practices, one of which was selling indulgences. Indulgences transferred merits of the saints to people who could be absolved of lesser sins by paying a fee and doing good works. An example of a lesser sin was thinking lustful thoughts about someone who was not your spouse (Osborn, 2008).

Of his own scrupulosity, he said in verse three of his *Commentary of the Epistle to the Galatians* (1535), "When I was a monk I tried ever so hard to live up to the strict rules of my order. I used to make a list of my sins, and I was always on the way to confession, and whatever penances were enjoined upon me I performed religiously. In spite of it all, my conscience was always in a fever of doubt. The more I sought to help my poor stricken conscience the worse it got. The more I paid attention to the regulations the more I transgressed them" (Luther, 2012). It is unclear if Luther's religiosity was a product of obsessive perfectionistic black-and-white standards that left no gray area or an acceptance of the imperfect morality of human nature. Nonetheless, his theology resonated with a multitude who sectored off from the Roman Catholic Church.

St. Ignatius of Loyola (1491–1556) is another important religious figure worth mentioning in the history of OCD. Born as Íñigo López in Spain, he had an intense religious experience while recuperating from battle, which led to an extreme episode of scrupulosity. He wrote of his suffering, "After I have trodden a cross formed by two straws, or after I have thought, said, or done some other thing, there comes to me from 'without' a thought that I have sinned, and on the other hand it seems to me that I have not sinned; nevertheless I feel some uneasiness on the subject, inasmuch as I doubt and yet do not doubt" (Tek & Ulug, 2001). After applying his own innovative self-help technique of *agere contra* (do the opposite; what we now call *exposure and response prevention*), he overcame his fear and went on to establish the Jesuit order (Osborn, 2008).

Of course, William Shakespeare (1564–1616) fans are familiar with *Macbeth*, written in 1623. While sleepwalking, Lady Macbeth compulsively and symbolically tries to wash guilty blood off her hands:

Doctor: What is it she does now? Look how she rubs her hands.

Gentlewoman: It is an accustom'd action with her, to seem thus washing her hands. I have known her continue in this a quarter of an hour.

Lady Macbeth: Yet here's a spot.

Doctor: Hark, she speaks. I will set down what comes from her, to satisfy my remembrance the more strongly.

Lady Macbeth: Out, damn'd spot! out, I say! One; two: why, then 'tis time to do't. Hell is murky. Fie, my lord, fie, a soldier, and afeard? What need we fear who knows it, when none can call our pow'r to accompt? Yet who would have thought the old man to have had so much blood in him? (Shakespeare, Shilote, & Nkondo, 1982)

John Bunyan (1628–1688) was a British literary notable and preacher. After suffering with severe OCD, which he self-treated and recovered by reading Scripture, he wrote *Grace Abounding to the Chief of Sinners* (Bunyan, 2013) written in 1666 and *Pilgrim's Progress* (Bunyan, 1909), which was published in two parts in 1678 and 1684. In *Grace Abounding*, Bunyan (2013 [1666]) describes his obsessions:

> But it was neither my dislike of the thought, nor yet any desire and endeavour to resist it that in the least did shake or abate the continuation, or force and strength thereof; for it did always, in almost whatever I thought, intermix itself therewith in such sort that I could neither eat my food, stoop for a pin, chop a stick, or cast mine eye to look on this, or that, but still the temptation would come, sell Christ for this, or sell Christ for that; sell Him, sell Him. Sometimes it would run in my thoughts, not so little as a hundred times together, *Sell Him, sell Him, sell Him:* against which, I may say, for whole hours together, I have been forced to stand as continually leaning and forcing my spirit against it, lest haply, before I were aware, some wicked thought might arise in my heart, that might consent thereto; and sometimes the tempter would make me believe I had consented to it; but then I should be, as tortured upon a rack for whole days together.

As far as his scrupulosity, it is unusual that reading Scripture, the very source of his agony and distress, would also be the remedy.

Samuel Johnson (1709–1784) was a prolific writer of the arts as well lexicography. Along with OCD, Johnson is said to have also suffered with Tourette's syndrome. Johnson was said to "perform his gesticulations" at the threshold of a house or in doorways:

> It appeared to me some superstitious habit . . . to go out or in at a door or passage, by a certain number of steps from a certain point, or at least so as that either his right or left foot, (I am not certain which,) should constantly make the first actual movement when he came close to the door or passage. . . . I have . . . observed him suddenly stop, and then seem to count his steps with a deep earnestness; and when he had neglected or gone wrong in this sort of magical movement, I have seen him go back again, put himself in a proper posture to begin the ceremony, and, having gone through it, break from his abstraction, walk briskly on, and join his companion. (Boswell & Chapman, 1970)

Danish philosopher Søren Kierkegaard (1813–1855) also suffered from OCD. In 1848, he logged in his journal, "It is quite a particular form of spiritual tribulation when a man sins against his will, in the full sense of the word, haunted by the dread of sin; for example, when sinful thoughts come to him which he would more than willingly escape and does everything to avoid. . . . [In those cases] a man can truthfully say, I know that I did not occasion those evil thoughts, I know that I do everything I can to fight against them: consequently it is always against his will" (Kierkegaard & Dru, 1938).

OCD as a Disorder

Thinkers in the nineteenth century began to move away from thinking of OCD as a crisis of religion and toward the fields of philosophy, psychiatry, psychoanalysis, and science, due to prevailing developing ideas about rationalism (reason and experience) and positivism (experience based on proof). Societal attitudes and beliefs were shifting from the supernatural to the objective.

During this time, European psychiatrists used a variety of terms for the disorder. Some of these were *arithmomania* (compulsive counting), *mysophobia* (obsessive fear of contamination), *idée fixe* (focus on one thought), *délire partiel* (monomania/partial insanity), *délire emotif* (disease of the emotions), *folie avec conscience* (insanity with insight), *onomatomanie* (repeating obsession), *délire du toucher* (touching compulsions), and *grubelnsucht* (a ruminatory or questioning illness), and *zwangworstelfungen* (obsessional presentations; Berrios, 1996).

In 1877, Westphal's interpretation of the term *zwangsvorstellung* (compelled presentation or idea) formally operationalized the disorder as obsessive compulsive. He recognized the importance of including both thoughts and behaviors that were ego-dystonic in the nosology of OCD (Berrios, 1996).

The French physician J. E. D. Esquirol (1782–1840) authored the textbook *Des maladies mentales (Mental Maladies)* in 1838. He is said to have begun the "medicalization of madness" (Huertas, 2008). He described a patient's compulsive checking symptoms, saying that "such patients dissemble their condition, in presence of those who notice them, and have authority to decide on the question of their isolation; . . . [and] impose upon judicial magistrates in their legal capacity, when about to administer upon their persons or fortune" (Esquirol, 1965).

As far as treatments went, William Hammond (1828–1900) prescribed potassium, calcium, and sodium bromides to patients with OCD to help calm them down (Hammond, 1883). Henry Maudsley (1835–1918) and Pierre Janet (1859–1947) prescribed opium or morphine elixirs, on occasion adding low doses of arsenic (Janet & Raymond, 1903; Maudsley, 1895).

Janet and Sigmund Freud (1856–1939) included OCD in the diagnostic category psychasthenia, which also included phobias, fear, anxiety, and tics (Berrios, 1996). In his seminal work, *Les obsessions et la psychasthénie* (Janet & Raymond, 1903), Janet identified stages of psychasthenia that consisted of psychological and emotional deficits, problems with attention and concentration, and a breakdown in reality function. Janet claimed that obsessions and compulsions occurred in the deepest and primitive psychasthenic stage, characterized by a lack of psychological strength of will, difficulty directing attention, and nervous energy (Pitman, 1984, 1987).

Freud, father of psychoanalysis, conceptualized OCD as "maladaptive responses to conflicts between unacceptable, unconscious sexual or aggressive urges of the id (pleasure principle) and the drives and the demands of conscience and reality" (Freud & Bonaparte, 1954).

Some say that Freud might have been obsessed with sex since it was socially repressed during the Victorian Era (1837–1901). One of Freud's major contributions to the field of psychology was his five-stage theory of psychosexual development: oral, anal, phallic, latent, and genital. The theory is based on the construct that neurosis is the result of unconscious and dysfunctional responses to innate sexual fantasies and desires during childhood. Freud conceptualized the phallic stage for boys as the Oedipal complex, with the unconscious wish to kill the father in order to sleep with the mother. Girls suffered with the Electra complex by desiring their fathers and blaming their mothers for their not having a penis, known as penis envy (Freud, Strachey, Freud, Rothgeb, & Richards, 1953).

Freud argued that adult neurosis (functional mental disorder) often is rooted in childhood sexuality, and consequently he suggested that neurotic adult behaviors are manifestations of childhood sexual fantasy and desire. Freud insisted that his sexual theory applied to *all* mental illness.

Freud treated neuroses with psychoanalysis. The aim of psychoanalytic therapy is to release repressed emotions and experiences—that is, make the unconscious conscious. Treatment consisted of four to five visits a week of fifty minutes each session for several years. While the analyst sits behind the person's line of vision, the patient lies on a couch making free associations to his or her thoughts, as well as describing fantasies and dreams. The analyst then uses the material to formulate the cause of the unconscious conflicts and challenges the patient's defense mechanisms in order to bring the conflict into consciousness so that the patient can gain insight and resolve it. Modern views of treating OCD with psychoanalysis is that the treatment provides the opportunity for more obsessing without any symptom resolution.

Even Freud associated OCD with religion. His psychoanalytic theory on religion and OCD was based on his ideas of the id being in conflict with the superego (Kaplin et al., 2017). The patient was unconsciously responding to conflicts between sexual or aggressive id impulses and the demands of the ego conscience and experiences in reality. Issues of control between these forces led to ambivalence, which produced doubt, and to magical thinking, which manifested as superstitious compulsive acts. The ego had certain defense mechanisms: intellectualization and isolation (warding off the effects associated with the unacceptable ideas and impulses), undoing (carrying out compulsions to neutralize the offending ideas and impulses), and reaction formation (adopting character traits exactly opposite of the feared impulses; Thapaliya, 2017). The imperfect success of these defenses gave rise to OCD symptoms: anxiety, preoccupation with dirt or germs or moral questions, and fears of acting on unacceptable impulses (Epstein, 2006).

Freud said, "without as yet understanding the deeper connections, I described the obsessional neurosis as a distorted private religion and religion as a kind of universal obsessional neurosis" (Freud et al., 1953).

Asylums

In 1907, a case report was published by Dr. Nolan (1907) about an obsessional patient who asked to be admitted to the Downpatrick Asylum because she feared being responsible for causing harm to others. He believed that the calming environment of the asylum would have a curative effect. The patient had an obsessive fear that a pile of stones left along the road could cause a fatal accident, and she retraced her steps in order to check to see if any harm had been done. He stated that her doubts increased about the degree to which she might be responsible for others' well-being or death. When she was admitted to Downpatrick, she realized that she was not as badly off as the more acutely ill patients, accepted Dr. Nolan's treatment of tonics (generally, herbal concoctions), and was discharged after three months with some improvement.

Although the *Diagnostic and Statistical Manual* was published in 1953, OCD was not added to the *DSM* until the second edition in 1968 under the category Neurosis, along with anxiety neurosis and phobic neurosis (Vahabzadeh, Gillespie, & Ressler, 2015). OCD is now in the *DSM-V* under the new category Obsessive Compulsive and Related

Disorders (American Psychiatric Association, 2013). The recommendation to call it Obsessive Compulsive Spectrum Disorders was not upheld, but this term is commonly referred to in the research literature (Phillips et al., 2010).

The 1950s was also the era of deinstitutionalization when patients who been in state mental hospitals were transitioned out into the community, where they were to receive community-based mental health and housing services (Tuntiya, 2003). Since then, refinements in nosology, neuroanatomy, neurophysiology, pharmacology, learning theory, cognitive behavior therapy, and diagnostic imaging and technology have allowed us to reach a more therapeutically useful conceptualization of OCD. Although the causes of the disorder are still elusive, research in genetics, neurobiology, and brain structure is working toward identifying the etiology and pathogenesis of OCD.

History of Behavior Therapy

Viktor Frankl (1905–1997) is worth a quick mention as the founder of logotherapy, a precursor to behavior therapy. Frankl was an Austrian psychiatrist and a survivor of the Theresienstadt, Auschwitz, Kaufering, and Türkeim World War II concentration camps. The Nazis appointed Frankl head of the Rothschild Hospital, where he had secretly been keeping notes on his observations of humanity, and inhumanity, on scraps of paper he found in the camps. In 1946, he published a book in German based on his ideas and concepts that became the basis of logotherapy. This was translated into English in 1959, and in a revised and enlarged edition, it appeared as *The Doctor and the Soul: An Introduction to Logotherapy* (Frankl, 1965) in 1963. His other seminal work, *Man's Search for Meaning: The Classic Tribute to Hope from the Holocaust* (Frankl, 1963), originally titled *From Death-Camp to Existentialism*, was published in 1959.

In the meantime, as psychoanalysis seemed to be insufficient in treating OCD, treatment turned toward modifying behavior. Wolpe and Lazarus (1966) theorized that increasing adaptive behavior while extinguishing maladaptive phobic behaviors improved mental health. After the therapist conducts a behavioral analysis (or case formulation), the patient is taught relaxation techniques. The patient is then gradually exposed to the anxiety-producing stimulus through systematic desensitization (SD). This worked especially well for simple phobias (SP).

For example, Steven entered into therapy suffering from the common SP arachnophobia (fear of spiders). Wherever he went, he was preoccupied with scanning the environment for areas that might host spiders. Sometimes he would ask his partner to go ahead and let him know if it was safe. He was tired of being anxious and feeling disconnected from the people with whom he was socializing. He had anticipatory anxiety when going to unfamiliar places. Basements, attics, and dusty and cluttered areas might have cobwebs and caused "creepy" feelings.

Steven started seeing a behavior therapist who helped him overcome his fear through systematic desensitization. A spider was placed in a jar on the other side of the room and was gradually moved closer until he no longer felt afraid. Subsequently, the spider was taken out of the jar and moved closer to him until he felt ready to hold the spider himself. The process was slow and took a few months. Steven's determination enabled him to stick with the therapy, but other people might give up due to how tedious and prolonged SD can be. Unfortunately, SD had limited success in treating OCD (Foa, 2010).

An account by de Silva and Rachman (2004) related that around the same time that SD was being used, a London psychiatrist at Middlesex Hospital, Victor Meyer, experimented in treating two inpatients with severe OCD. One of them, who suffered with fears of disease and dirt, spent most of the day cleaning. The other patient was tortured by recurrent, disruptive blasphemous thoughts about sex. She had been treated with shock therapy, drugs, eleven years of psychoanalysis, and even psychosurgery, all to no avail.

Meyer decided to implement *apotrepic therapy*, now known as *exposure and response prevention* (ERP; Meyer, 1966). In this approach, patients would be put in the anxiety-provoking situations and ritualistic behaviors would be eliminated (de Silva & Rachman, 2004).

For the patient with contamination fears, Dr. Meyer and a nurse exposed her to objects that triggered her anxiety and prevented her from carrying out her cleaning rituals. They turned off the water in her room to prevent excessive hand washing and limited her access to cleaning agents. When the patient's urges to wash her hands decreased, she generalized their progress by conducting exposures to other triggering situations around the hospital (Wilson, 1992). Sometimes the therapist touched items perceived to be contaminated as a way of demonstrating normalized behavior and then encouraged the patients to do the same Once the patients were comfortable under the situations that were deemed to be most difficult, their supervision was progressively decreased. After four weeks, the patient's anxiety decreased, and she made further progress after eight weeks with a noticeable decrease in her cleaning behaviors.

Meyer's second patient's treatment consisted of exposing the patient to triggering items and developing imaginal scenes while she was prevented from performing any anxiety-reducing behaviors. After nine weeks of difficult and distressing intensive therapy, her OCD symptoms dropped to a manageable level. After having been hospitalized for extended amounts of time, even though both patients continued to have OCD symptoms, they were discharged home and were said to have regained normal lives.

After getting good results with his first few patients, Meyer used his apotrepic therapy on fifteen other OCD sufferers, ten of whom were reported to be "much improved or symptom free," and the other five patients were found to be "moderately improved" (Mavissakalian, Turner, & Michelson, 1985). Since this model showed success, outpatient therapists started using a modified version of it in their practices (Rachman et al., 1979; Rachman & Hodgson, 1980).

In the 1970s, researchers began to refine and rename Meyer's method into exposure and response prevention therapy, which remains the most effective psychological treatment of OCD (Clark, 2000). Since then, clinicians and researchers have expanded the field to attend to the cognitive and affective aspects of obsessive beliefs (Foa, 2010).

Established in 1986, the International Obsessive Compulsive Foundation's mission is to educate and increase public awareness about OCD. Their first success was a broadcast on the ABC news program *20/20* in 1987. "That opened the floodgates," said Jenny, who was involved with the foundation. "Thousands and thousands of people called [the foundation]. It was around the clock for about three weeks. People kept telling us over and over again, 'I thought I was alone'" (St. John Erickson, 1989). The report was followed by spots on talks shows such as Phil Donahue, Geraldo Rivera, Oprah Winfrey, and dozens of other TV talk shows, national magazines, and newspapers (Foundation). In 1989, Dr. Judith Rapoport published the book *The Boy Who Couldn't Stop Washing* which further launched public awareness of OCD with her 1991 appearance on the popular Phil Donahue TV talk show (Donahue, 1991).

Now known as the International OCD Foundation (IOCDF), the foundation has become a comprehensive resource for individual and family consumers. The website provides psychoeducational materials for all types of OCD and related disorders, national and international lists of therapists and support groups, community events, and programs. It sponsors local affiliates, performs outreach and advocacy, and hosts several social media platforms. The annual conference brings patients, families, clinicians, and researchers together under one roof to share knowledge and experiences. The annual One Million Steps Walk takes place in June all over the world.

The foundation publishes a monthly newsletter, has a training institute, and provides grants for innovative research. There is also the OCD Awareness Week in October. IOCDF formed a genetic collaboration in 2002 to consolidate global research efforts in identifying genetic causes of and treatments for OCD. According to its program director, the foundation has 3,500 members (Stephanie Cogen, email, 3/29/19). The foundation is tireless in its efforts to maximize all means of clinical expertise, communication, education, treatment, and research for the cause of alleviating suffering for all lives who are touched by OCD. The link to the website is https://iocdf.org.

The next chapter, "Theory and Research," will go into more detail about current theoretical concepts and targets of neurobiological research.

References

American Psychiatric Association. (2013). *Diagnostic and statistical manual of mental disorders* (5th ed.). Washington, DC: American Psychiatric Publishing.

Berrios, G. E. (1996). *The history of mental symptoms: Descriptive psychopathology since the nineteenth century*. Cambridge: Cambridge University Press.

Boswell, J., & Chapman, R. W. (1970). *Life of Johnson* (New ed.). London and New York: Oxford University Press.

Bunyan, J. (1909). *The pilgrim's progress*. New York: P. F. Collier and Son.

Bunyan, J. (2013 [1666]). *Grace abounding to the chief of sinners* (8th ed.). D. Price (Ed.). Retrieved from www.gutenberg.org

Butler-Bowdon, W. (Ed.). (1944). *The book of Margery Kempe: A modern version of the earliest known autobiography in English, A.D. 1436*. London: Devin-Adair Company.

Ciarrocchi, J. W. (1995). *The doubting disease: Help for scrupulosity and religious compulsions*. New York: Paulist.

Clark, D. A. (2000). Cognitive behavior therapy for obsessions and compulsions: New applications and emerging trends. *Journal of Contemporary Psychotherapy, 30*(2), 129–147. doi:10.1023/a:1026562628287

Climacus, J. (2012 [1605]). *Ladder of divine ascent* (4th ed.). Holy Transfiguration Monastery.

Collins, E. F. (1961). *The treatment of scrupulosity in the summa moralis of St. Antoninus: A historical-theological study* (Doctoral dissertation). Pontificia Universitas Gregoriana, Rome, Italy.

de Silva, P., & Rachman, S. (2004). *Obsessive-compulsive disorder: The facts* (3rd ed.). Oxford and New York: Oxford University Press.

Donahue, P. (Executive producer). (1991). Obsessive-compulsive disorder: The boy who couldn't stop washing with Judith Rapoport [Television series episode]. In *The Phil Donahue Show*. Chicago: CBS.

Epstein, T. (2006). *The unconscious life of the child with obsessive-compulsive disorder* (Master's thesis). University of the Witwatersrand, Johannesberg, South Africa.

Esquirol, E. (1965). *Mental maladies: Treatise on insanity* (E. K. Hunt, Trans.). Philadelphia: Lea & Blanchard.

Foa, E. B. (2010). Cognitive behavioral therapy of obsessive-compulsive disorder. *Dialogues in Clinical Neuroscience, 12*(2), 199–207. Retrieved from https://www.ncbi.nlm.nih.gov/pubmed/20623924

Foundation, I. O. History of the IOCDF. Retrieved from https://iocdf.org/our-history/

Frankl, V. E. (1963). *Man's search for meaning: The classic tribute to hope from the Holocaust*. Boston: Beacon.

Frankl, V. E. (1965). *The doctor and the soul, from psychotherapy to logotherapy* (2nd expanded ed.). New York: A. A. Knopf.

Freud, S., & Bonaparte, P. M. (1954). *The origins of psychoanalysis* (Vol. 216). London: Imago.

Freud, S., Strachey, J., Freud, A., Rothgeb, C. L., & Richards, A. (1953). *The standard edition of the complete psychological works of Sigmund Freud*. London: Hogarth Press.

Friedrich, P. (2015). Recurrent doubt: A brief story of OCD through its literary texts. In *The literary and linguistic construction of obsessive-compulsive disorder* (pp. 29–66). London: Palgrave Macmillan.

Hammond, W. A. (1883). *A treatise on insanity in its medical relations*. New York: Appleton.

The History of OCD. (2004). About OCD. Retrieved from https://www.ocduk.org/ocd/history-of-ocd/

Huertas, R. (2008). Between doctrine and clinical practice: Nosography and semiology in the work of Jean-Etienne-Dominique Esquirol (1772–1840). *History of Psychiatry, 19*(2), 123–140. doi:10.1177/0957154X07080659

Janet, P., & Raymond, F. (1903). *Les obsessions et la psychasthénie*. Paris: F. Alcan.

Kaplin, D., Giannone, D., Flavin, A., Hussein, L., Kanthan, S., Aw Young, S., . . . Mele, P. (2017). The religious and philosophical foundations of Freud's tripartite theory of personality. *Janus Head, 16*(1), 227–264.

Kempe, M., & Butler-Bowdon, W. (1936). *The book of Margery Kempe, 1436.* London: J. Cape.

Kierkegaard, S., & Dru, A. (1938). *The journals of Søren Kierkegaard.* London and New York: Oxford University Press.

Luther, M. (2012). *Commentary of the epistle to the Galatians.* CreateSpace Independent Publishing.

Maudsley, H. (1895). *The pathology of mind* (2nd ed.). New York: Appleton.

Mavissakalian, M., Turner, S. M., & Michelson, L. (Eds.). (1985). *Obsessive-compulsive disorder: Psychological and pharmacological treatment.* New York: Springer.

Meyer, V. (1966). Modification of expectations in cases with obsessional rituals. *Behaviour Research and Therapy, 4*(4), 273–280.

Nolan, M. J. (1907). Study of a case of melancholic folie raisonnante. *British Journal of Psychiatry, 53,* 615–626.

Oldridge, D. (2019). Demons of the mind: Satanic thoughts in seventeenth-century England. *Seventeenth Century,* 1–16.

Osborn, I. (2008). *Can Christianity cure obsessive-compulsive disorder?: A psychiatrist explores the role of faith in treatment.* Grand Rapids, MI: Brazos.

Phillips, K. A., Stein, D. J., Rauch, S. L., Hollander, E., Fallon, B. A., Barsky, A., . . . Leckman, J. (2010). Should an obsessive-compulsive spectrum grouping of disorders be included in DSM-V? *Depression and Anxiety, 27*(6), 528–555. doi:10.1002/da.20705

Pitman, R. K. (1984). Janet's obsessions and psychasthenia: A synopsis. *Psychiatric Quarterly, 56*(4), 291–314. Retrieved from https://www.ncbi.nlm.nih.gov/pubmed/6399751

Pitman, R. K. (1987). Pierre Janet on obsessive-compulsive disorder (1903): Review and commentary. *Archives of General Psychiatry, 44*(3), 226–232. Retrieved from https://www.ncbi.nlm.nih.gov/pubmed/3827518

Rachman, S., Cobb, J., Grey, S., McDonald, B., Mawson, D., Sartory, G., & Stern, R. (1979). The behavioural treatment of obsessional-compulsive disorders, with and without clomipramine. *Behavior Research and Therapy, 17*(5), 467–478. doi:10.1016/0005-7967(79)90063-9

Rachman, S., & Hodgson, R. J. (1980). *Obsessions and compulsions.* Upper Saddle River, NJ: Prentice Hall.

Reynolds, E. H., & Kinnier, W. J. V. (2012). Obsessive compulsive disorder and psychopathic behaviour in Babylon. *Journal of Neurology, Neurosurgery, and Psychiatry, 83*, 199–201.

Schwemer, D. (2011). Magic rituals: Conceptualization and performance. In K. Radner & E. Robson (Eds.), *The Oxford handbook of cuneiform culture* (pp. 418–446). Oxford: Oxford University Press.

Shakespeare, W. (2014). *Macbeth*. New York: Millenium Publications.

St. John Erickson, M. (1989). Inexplicable rituals. *Daily Press*. Retrieved from https://www.dailypress.com/news/dp-xpm-19890 601-1989-06-01-8905300261-story.html

Tek, C., & Ulug, B. (2001). Religiosity and religious obsessions in obsessive-compulsive disorder. *Psychiatry Research, 104*(2), 99–108. doi:S0165-1781(01)00310-9 [pii]

Thapaliya, S. (2017). The case of rat man: A psychoanalytic understanding of obsessive-compulsive disorder. *Journal of Mental Health and Human Behaviour, 22*(2), 132–135. doi:10.4103/jmhhb.jmhhb _22_17

Tuntiya, N. (2003). *The forgotten history: The deinstitutionalization movement in the mental health care system in the United States* (Master's thesis). University of South Florida. Retrieved from scholarcommons.usf.edu/etd/1496

Vahabzadeh, A., Gillespie, C. F., & Ressler, K. J. (2015). Fear-related anxiety disorders and post-traumatic stress disorder. In M. J. Zigmond, J. T. Coyle, & L. P. Rowland (Eds.), *Neurobiology of brain disorders: Biological basis of neurological and psychiatric disorders* (1st ed., pp. 612–621). Waltham, MA: Academic Press.

Wilson, P. H. (1992). *Principles and practice of relapse prevention*. New York: Guilford.

Wolpe, J., & Lazarus, A. A. (1966). *Behavior therapy techniques: A guide to the treatment of neuroses* (1st ed.). Oxford and New York: Pergamon.

CHAPTER 4

Theory and Research

In chapter 3, we reviewed Freud's theory that OCD acts as a defense against taboo thoughts and urges, especially related to the libido, in a discussion of how OCD was understood in the Victorian Age (Freud, Strachey, Freud, Rothgeb, & Richards, 1953). We also saw how behaviorally based empirical research developed into the evidence-based treatment of exposure and response prevention (Olatunji, Davis, Powers, & Smits, 2013). Several other etiological theories have been advanced since then, including learning and conditioning, cognition, neurobiology, genetics, and neuroevolution. Emotional/experiential appraisal and avoidance processes at work when OCD is activated have also been identified as important.

Psychological Research Methodology

Much of the behavioral and cognitive literature on OCD has been conducted in academic and community settings with nonclinical subjects for good practical reasons. It is more cost and time effective to achieve a critical mass of study subjects required for valid findings with an already established group.

Using analog subjects who are considered to represent the target population is a common design in experimental research (Hooley, Butcher, Nock, & Mineka, 2017). Since obsessive and compulsive symptoms occur in roughly 2–3 percent of the general population (Adam, Meinlschmidt, Gloster, & Lieb, 2012; de Bruijn, Beun, de Graaf, ten Have, &

Denys, 2010), analog samples are assumed to provide adequate data for analysis of the research question or hypothesis.

A study addressing the use of nonclinical subjects in correlational-designed research used, for example, to see if there is a relationship between superstition and OCD found support for the validity and generalizability of the data collected with such samples (Abramowitz et al., 2014). However, it is difficult to determine how findings from analog samples translate to clinical practice, and it is unclear if the studies are actually replicated (Reynolds & Streiner, 1998). The good news is that internet-based survey platforms provide access for researchers to recruit people with OCD for data that can be applied for clinical analysis and treatment (van Gelder, Bretveld, & Roeleveld, 2010).

Psychological Theories

Although there are many factors to consider for successful OCD treatment, identifying which ones are the most salient for each individual will provide the best plan for helping patients achieve normalized functioning.

Behavior

"Change the behavior; then the thoughts and feelings will follow" is a common refrain in behavioral treatment from OCD. This means that by when patients take the leap of faith, face obsessive fears, and allow the anxiety to run its natural course without trying to avoid the anxiety, the thoughts will subside, and, in turn, so will the emotions. When done properly, people get used to the feared situations in a normalized manner; then their thinking begins to resolve, and they understand that the emotions were only secondary to the obsessions. The effects of ERP result from exposure to the feared stimuli, causing an increase of physiology rates until they reach their peak, then naturally dropping off to baseline levels as long as urges to perform compulsive behaviors are resisted (Polman, Bouman, van Hout, de Jong, & den Boer, 2010). The process is known as *habituation*.

For example, George has hit-and-run obsessions and drives back to the area where he went over a bump. His anxiety high, he checks to make sure nothing happened until he can no longer stand being stuck checking. He feels guilty for leaving the "scene of the crime" and sometimes goes back to check again. When George follows his behavioral plan to drive over bumps and keep going, his anxiety begins to decrease;

he realizes how irrational his fear is, and he no longer feels guilty that he might be a negligent person.

Learning and Conditioning

Learning theory and classical conditioning explain how knowledge is received and processed through experience. A two-factor behavioral model of OCD consists of fear and avoidance of OCD triggers (Mowrer, 1960). When a person is in a triggering situation, the experience of fear teaches him or her to avoid that situation, even though there is no evidence of threat of harm (Solomon & Wynne, 1954). Through operant conditioning, avoidance behavior is negatively reinforced, since the desire not to experience anxiety takes priority over the functional aspects of being in those situations.

In chapter 3, we learned that Meyer's use of apotrepic therapy launched generations of empirical research on the behavioral theory of OCD. The research showed that patients' anxiety increased when facing obsessional stimuli and that the subsequent performance of compulsions decreased the anxiety (Rachman & Hodgson, 1980). Since practice of eliminating compulsions achieves habituation, it is critical that the therapist understand the compulsions' function in order not to assume what purpose they serve. Excessive showering for one person may serve as a decontamination ritual, while the drive behind this behavior for another may be the need to feel "right" or "complete." This distinction is crucial for designing the treatment plan that will effectively target the symptoms during ERP (Shafran, 2006).

For example, Sage visit a friend in the hospital, and she becomes highly anxious due to being in an environment of sick people. When Sage gets home, she goes into the shower to scrub off any microbes she worries are on her skin until she is convinced she has thoroughly washed them away. Her washing ritual results in sore, red, and raw skin. The high level of anxiety combined with the excessive behavioral response of thoroughly decontaminating herself prevent her from future visits to her sick friend, causing deep feelings of guilt.

Sage is conditioned to anticipate that going to a hospital is highly anxiety provoking, and her anxiety-reducing behaviors reinforce the idea that the hospital is a risky environment. She learns that avoidant behaviors, such as not going to the hospital, further prevent her OCD from being triggered. Sadly, the obsessional anxiety is never really extinguished, since the person consciously makes decisions about whether to face or avoid a feared situation that result in a life being controlled and limited by fear. Further, the triggering situation is not the source of the problem; the person still has OCD, which will find other ways of manifesting itself in situations that had been otherwise neutral (Rachman & Hodgson, 1980).

Cognitive (and Behavioral) Theory

Cognitive theory is based on how the mind learns, processes, and organizes information that creates beliefs (Dobson, 2010). Obsessions are said to be caused by catastrophic misinterpretations and appraisals that unwanted intrusive thoughts have some meaning (Rachman, 1998; Salkovskis, 1985). Similar to the theoretical behavioral model of OCD that behavioral change will effect changes thoughts and feelings (Baer, 1991), cognitive theory suggests that because thoughts precede emotions and behavior, the restructuring of distorted automatic negative thoughts will lead to changes in emotions and behavior (Beck, 1979; Ellis, 1962).

One line of questioning by cognitive theorists is why intrusive thoughts that are experienced by most people develop into obsessions in others. Although 90 percent of people experience intrusive thoughts of a similar content, only 2–3 percent develop clinically significant OCD symptoms (Krochmalik & Menzies, 2003). To reference examples of nonclinical intrusive thoughts, please refer back to table 1.1.

In cognitive theory development, researchers included the concept found in learning theory that negative experiences can lead to distorted beliefs about intrusive thoughts, in order to identify the cognitive mechanisms through which intrusive thoughts lead to obsessional anxiety and ritualizing (Salkovskis, Shafran, Rachman, & Freeston, 1999). The authors identified three main ideas: OCD is due to a dysfunction in cognitive processing; specific dysfunctional beliefs are causes of obsessions and compulsions; and poorer performance of neuropsychiatric executive functioning and memory may play a role in why intrusive thoughts become obsessions.

For example, Sandy is fearful that her intrusive thoughts of harm coming to her family will actually cause harm if she doesn't *do* something to prevent it, such as mentally ritualizing. Her ritual is conjuring an image of each family member being safe at school and work. She is unwilling to take the risk of shrugging off the intrusive thought because of a strong sense of responsibility to ensure that she has protected them. Here we can see that, again, Sandy does not feel she has superpowers to affect the outcome of reality, but she wants to avoid feeling responsible or guilty if something *did* happen.

Research has shown that the "importance of thoughts" and "need to control thoughts" domains respond better to treatment than others (Adams, Riemann, Wetterneck, & Cisler, 2012). Reviewing these domains with patients is helpful in conceptualizing what distorted beliefs may impact the quality of treatment.

Inhibitory Learning

Consideration has been given about what accounts for partial responses to ERP treatment and vulnerabilities for relapse. Even if there is a good initial course of ERP treatment, in certain cases, it may not be sufficient to generalize clinical gains beyond the specific settings in which the exposures were conducted. For example, Josh may have habituated to public bathrooms but became anxious when he joined a gym and started using the locker room. As a result, researchers began investigating the application of inhibitory learning theory for enhancing OCD treatment.

One basis of this theory is to inhibit the association of the current obsessive fear by combining various triggering elements within the same exposure session. The goal is for the patient to learn that the situation is safe no matter what conditions the feared situation presents (Arch & Abramowitz, 2015; Jacoby & Abramowitz, 2016). In Sage's case, while conducting the exposure in the hospital, having her use the hospital bathroom without washing her hands and then go home and cross-contaminate would have more of a synergistic effect. Another aspect of this method is learning that the emotions experienced during the exposure will also come and go (Craske, Treanor, Conway, Zbozinek, & Vervliet, 2014).

Eight strategies have been established under which inhibitory learning is accomplished. The first is challenging the patients' expectation of what they *think* is going to happen and what they *actually* experience in the feared situation (Craske et al., 2014). For example, someone with stabbing obsessions who has avoided using knives may overanticipate her level of fear about using one, but when she actually handles one and uses it long for a long-enough time, she will realize that she won't act on her feared thoughts.

The next strategy is to eliminate safety cues. A safety cue for someone with hit-and-run driving obsessions may be having a cell phone in the car, knowing that she can call someone if she gets triggered (Blakey & Abramowitz, 2016; Craske et al., 2014).

After that step, patients will benefit by exposure to their obsessive triggering in multiple contexts. When an expected feared outcome does not occur in the presence of multiple fear cues at the same time, the inhibitory learning process will be greater than when only one fear cue is present (Jacoby & Abramowitz, 2016). In the first example above, it will be more effective for the person to have all sharp knives out in the open while chopping vegetables alongside her roommate who is also cooking dinner.

Another helpful tool is affect labeling, which helps patients identify their emotions during the exposure rather than what they assume they are going to feel. Neuroscience has found an association between linguistics and inhibitory learning through the process of consciously identifying what feeling are being experienced in the moment. People may feel more guilt, anger, or sadness during an exposure session than anxiety (Craske et al., 2014).

The practice of exposure to varying levels of fear on the hierarchy, instead of in a linear manner, is yet another practice that can help develop a stronger tolerance to the obsessive trigger, since it may replicate the unpredictable nature of being triggered in real life (Knowles & Olatunji, 2019). Someone with moral perfectionism may agree to tell a "white lie" to the therapist, say a critical thought about someone they loved, and walk past someone and not hold the door while walking out, thus evoking Subjective Units of Distress Scale (SUDS) levels of sixty-five, ninety-five, and ninety, respectively.

Deepened extinction, another strategy, consists of entering into situations where the obsessive fear is anticipated to be triggered in order to confirm that there is a less likelihood or probability that it will occur (Craske, 2015). Someone with pedophilia obsessions would be able to go to a mall and go into toy stores, the children's section in department stores and a bookstore, and then visit the mall's play area all in one (perhaps prolonged) session.

Another cognitive process considered to help solidify treatment gains is reconsolidation. Reconsolidation involves retrieving already-stored conditioned fear or emotional memories while introducing new behavioral information (Craske et al., 2014). During that process, it is said that new learning is acquired and memories will be altered (Monfils, Cowansage, Klann, & LeDoux, 2009). Someone with emotional contamination may be triggered by seeing someone from high school who had a nosebleed in class and the memory of that incident will have now spread a fear of her town becoming contaminated. The person with OCD can reconsolidate the memory by approaching this person and having a normal conversation. The memory would already have been retrieved, but the normal interaction with the person would help neutralize the contamination fear and the related negative emotions.

Last is occasionally reinforcing extinction, which occurs when the feared obsessive consequence actually happens, contrary to the expectancy violation experience. A person with contamination fears may become sick after having used a public bathroom without washing his hands. Because he successfully challenged his fear through expectancy violations, inhibitory learning strengthened his ability to take this experience more in stride (Bouton, Woods, & Pineño, 2004).

Emotional Appraisal and Experiential Avoidance

Just as OCD sets off neurobiological false alarm signals that provoke a sense of threat in the absence of real danger, strong emotional reactions to obsessions are also set off as a result of how a person appraises them. Because of the distressing nature of obsessions, people appraise them as highly significant or threatening. Clark and colleagues (2003) consider such appraisals as the key cognitive process that leads to an escalation in the frequency and intensity of obsessive intrusive thoughts.

Some people are especially sensitive and reactive to their emotions. Most people would rather not have "negative emotions," such as sadness, guilt, disgust, anger, and shame, but they play a role in our humanity. The concept of emotional appraisal refers to the relationship people have to their emotions. Some people with anxiety have a sense of perceived threat that their emotions are too strong to manage (McCubbin & Sampson, 2006). Commonly appraised emotions in OCD are fear, guilt, physical and spiritual disgust, and NJREs (Power, 2006).

It would make sense, then, that rituals serve to facilitate emotional avoidance (Smith et al., 2012) and that people may use their OCD as a way of avoiding their problematic emotions (McCubbin & Sampson, 2006). According to Manos and colleagues (2010), compulsions function as attempts at emotional avoidance in which people try to control or reduce their obsessive thoughts as a means of not having the negative emotions associated with them.

Cognitively, the OCD-specific domain of inflated responsibility of thoughts is associated with emotional appraisal through thought action fusion (TAF), a belief that having a bad thought is as bad doing the action (Obsessive Compulsive Cognitions Working Group, 1997). Within TAF, there are two components. One is the moral TAF, which is the fear that having the thought has the same moral value as acting on it. The other is the likelihood TAF, which is the belief that having the thought will make it more likely to happen (Obsessive Compulsive Cognitions Working Group, 1997). When people with OCD fear that their thoughts may reflect badly on them morally or that they may increase the likelihood of causing harm to others, they perform overcompensating rituals, such as being overly nice, pleasing others, praying, or confessing the harming thought to the person.

For example, while Al is playing with his four-year-old niece, who adores him, he has the sudden thought "What's stopping me from wringing her neck?" Under normal circumstances, that thought might occur to someone, give a little pause, and then pass. For Al, though, it isn't an anxiety response that upsets him but his feelings of guilt, shame, and disgust for having the thought. As time goes on, he judges himself to be a threat to anyone considered vulnerable (e.g., children, elderly) and purposely avoids being around them, including his beloved niece. For Al, it does not help that he is someone who already avoids his emotions because of not being in touch with them or not knowing how to manage them. Now, not only does he avoid being around his niece, but he also wants to avoid anything that may precipitate those feelings.

The appraisal of disgust manifests itself in interesting ways with OCD. There can be a visceral reaction to rotting food or being around someone with a cold, not for fear of contamination but due to a situational reaction of disgust in the environment. There can also be a sense of self-disgust around religious or moral impurity. If someone is highly religious or has moral perfectionism, intrusive sexual or blasphemous thoughts can cause the person to feel he or she has violated a religious tenet or is morally reprehensible (Brakoulias et al., 2013).

Anger is especially difficult for OCD patients to tolerate, since it provokes a sense of threat and guilt. A study found that anger significantly correlated with OCD severity, leading to the conclusions that the suppression of anger may play an important role in the further understanding of OCD (Hart, 2010).

Experiential avoidance is characterized by an unwillingness to experience or be in contact with unpleasant internal experiences, for which efforts are made to escape (Hayes, Wilson, Gifford, Follette, & Strosahl, 1996). It differs from emotional avoidance in that the precipitant is situational, but it is similar in that the situations patients want to avoid evoke fear, emotions, thoughts, bodily sensations, and disgust.

Thought Suppression and Neutralizing

The act of trying *not* to have a thought *is* having the thought. Unwanted, upsetting thoughts are a universal experience, and people with OCD attribute irrational, negative meaning to these kinds of cognitions and are thus motivated to suppress them. These suppression attempts lead to the paradoxical effect of increasing, rather than decreasing, the frequency of the unwanted thought.

In 1994, Daniel Wegner published the book *White Bears and Other Unwanted Thoughts: Suppression, Obsession, and the Psychology of Mental Control.* Wegner and colleagues proposed that efforts to suppress unwanted thoughts involve two cognitive processes: a purposeful search for a distracting thought and an automatic search for the target suppressed thought (Wegner, Erber, & Zanakos, 1993). While people who do not want a certain thought try to think of something else, the mind still has an awareness of the unwanted cognition. Wegner ran a study in which subjects were asked to suppress thoughts about a white bear while they were thinking about other things. They were instructed to ring a bell whenever the thought of the bear appeared, which was more than once per minute. They were then asked to intentionally think of a white bear, and the results showed an increased frequency of the white bear thoughts during the suppression task. Because the automatic cognitive monitoring process searches for the target thought, it paradoxically increases the accessibility of that thought to consciousness (Wegner, Schneider, Carter, & White, 1987). Thus, by consciously trying to suppress thoughts of a white bear, the monitoring process searches for white bear thoughts, undermining suppression attempts.

The effect of the cognitive intention to suppress thoughts, especially with OCD, is that it leads to a rebound effect, where the thoughts increase (Tolin, Abramowitz, Przeworski, & Foa, 2002). Trying to avoid or suppress obsessions only serves to increase their frequency, intensity, and anxiety (Rachman, 1998; Salkovskis, Thorpe, Wahl, Wroe, & Forrester, 2003).

Another cognitive attempt to reduce the distressing and affectively heightened effects of obsessions is to neutralize them. Neutralizing is an intentional cognitive reaction in response to the way in which the person with OCD negatively interprets the content of an intrusive thought (Salkovskis et al., 2003).

A study was conducted where two subject groups listened to repeated recorded presentations of their intrusive thoughts. One group neutralized their obsessions by thinking of a self-reassuring thought for a brief amount of time, while the other group was instructed to use distraction by counting for the same brief amount of time. The authors found an initial decrease in anxiety for those who neutralized their obsessions compared to those using distraction. However, when the obsessional thought was reintroduced to the subjects who neutralized their obsessional thought a short while later, they experienced a greater increase in discomfort than did those who had distracted (Salkovskis et al., 2003).

From a neurostructural perspective, functional imaging research has proposed that the failure to suppress unwanted thoughts may be caused by increased glucose metabolism in the orbitofrontal cortex of the brain (Rubin, Villanueva-Meyer, Ananth, Trajmar, & Mena, 1992).

References

Abramowitz, J. S., Fabricant, L. E., Taylor, S., Deacon, B. J., McKay, D., & Storch, E. A. (2014). The relevance of analogue studies for understanding obsessions and compulsions. *Clinical Psychology Review, 34*(3), 206–217.

Adam, Y., Meinlschmidt, G., Gloster, A. T., & Lieb, R. (2012). Obsessive-compulsive disorder in the community: 12-month prevalence, comorbidity and impairment. *Social Psychiatry and Psychiatric Epidemiology, 47*(3), 339–349. doi:10.1007/s00127-010-0337-5

Adams, T. G., Riemann, B. C., Wetterneck, C. T., & Cisler, J. M. (2012). Obsessive beliefs predict cognitive behavior therapy outcome for obsessive compulsive disorder. *Cognitive Behaviour Therapy, 41*(3), 203–211. doi:10.1080/16506073.2011.621969

Arch, J., & Abramowitz, J. S. (2015). Exposure therapy for obsessive-compulsive disorder: An optimizing inhibitory learning approach. *Journal of Obsessive Compulsive and Related Disorders, 6*, 174–182.

Baer, L. (1991). *Getting control.* New York: Plume.

Beck, A. T. (1979). *Cognitive therapy of depression.* New York: Guilford.

Blakey, S. M., & Abramowitz, J. S. (2016). The effects of safety behaviors during exposure therapy for anxiety: Critical analysis from an inhibitory learning perspective. *Clinical Psychology Review, 49*, 1–15.

Bouton, M. E., Woods, A. M., & Pineño, O. (2004). Occasional reinforced trials during extinction can slow the rate of rapid reacquisition. *Learning and Motivation, 35*(4), 371–390. doi:10.1016/j.lmot.2004.05.001

Brakoulias, V., Starcevic, V., Berle, D., Milicevic, D., Moses, K., Hannan, A., . . . Martin, A. (2013). The characteristics of unacceptable/taboo thoughts in obsessive-compulsive disorder. *Comprehensive Psychiatry,* *54*(7), 750–757. doi:10.1016/j.comppsych.2013.02.005

Clark, D., Purdon, C., & Wang, A. (2003). The Meta-Cognitive Beliefs Questionnaire: Development of a measure of obsessional beliefs. *Behaviour Research and Therapy, 41*(6), 655–669.

Craske, M. G. (2015). Optimizing exposure therapy for anxiety disorders: An inhibitory learning and inhibitory regulation approach. *Verhaltenstherapie, 25*(2), 134–143. doi:10.1159/000381574

Craske, M. G., Treanor, M., Conway, C. C., Zbozinek, T., & Vervliet, B. (2014). Maximizing exposure therapy: An inhibitory learning approach. *Behavior Research and Therapy, 58*, 10–23. doi:10.1016/j .brat.2014.04.006

de Bruijn, C., Beun, S., de Graaf, R., ten Have, M., & Denys, D. (2010). Subthreshold symptoms and obsessive-compulsive disorder: Evaluating the diagnostic threshold. *Psychological Medicine, 40*(6), 989–997. doi:10.1017/s0033291709991012

Dobson, K. S. (2010). *Handbook of cognitive-behavioral therapies* (3rd ed.). New York: Guilford.

Ellis, A. (1962). *Reason and emotion in psychotherapy.* New York: L. Stuart.

Freud, S., Strachey, J., Freud, A., Rothgeb, C. L., & Richards, A. (1953). *The standard edition of the complete psychological works of Sigmund Freud.* London: Hogarth Press.

Hart, J. M. (2010). *Relationship between patient anger, experiential avoidance, initial levels of obsessive-compulsive and depressive symptoms, and response to intensive inpatient cognitive-behavioral treatment.* Fielding Graduate University, ProQuest Dissertations Publishing, Santa Barbara, CA.

Hayes, S. C., Wilson, K. G., Gifford, E. V., Follette, V. M., & Strosahl, K. (1996). Experiential avoidance and behavioral disorders: A functional dimensional approach to diagnosis and treatment. *Journal of Consulting and Clinical Psychology, 64*(6), 1152–1168.

Hooley, J. M., Butcher, J. N., Nock, M., & Mineka, S. (2017). *Abnormal psychology* (17th ed.). Boston: Pearson.

Jacoby, R. J., & Abramowitz, J. S. (2016). Inhibitory learning approaches to exposure therapy: A critical review and translation to obsessive-compulsive disorder. *Clinical Psychology Review, 49*, 28–40. doi:10.1016/j.cpr.2016.07.001

Knowles, K. A., & Olatunji, B. O. (2019). Enhancing inhibitory learning: The utility of variability in exposure. *Cognitive and Behavioral Practice, 26*(1), 186–200. doi:10.1016/j.cbpra.2017.12.001

Krochmalik, A., & Menzies, R. G. (2003). The classification and diagnosis of OCD. In R. G. Menzies & P de Silva (Eds.), *Obsessive compulsive disorder: Theory, research and treatment* (pp. 3–20). Chichester, UK: Wiley.

Manos, R., Cahill, S., Wetterneck, C., Conelea, C., Ross, A., & Riemann, B. (2010). The impact of experiential avoidance and obsessive beliefs on obsessive-compulsive symptoms in a severe clinical sample. *Journal of Anxiety Disorders, 24*(7), 700–708. doi:S0887-6185(10)00106-4 [pii] 10.1016/j.janxdis.2010.05.001

McCubbin, R. A., & Sampson, M. J. (2006). The relationship between obsessive-compulsive symptoms and appraisals of emotional states. *Journal of Anxiety Disorders, 20*(1), 42–57. doi:10.1016/j.janxdis.2004.11.008

Monfils, M. H., Cowansage, K. K., Klann, E., & LeDoux, J. E. (2009). Extinction-reconsolidation boundaries: Key to persistent attenuation of fear memories. *Science, 324*(5929), 951–955. doi:10.1126/science.1167975

Mowrer, O. H. (1960). *Learning theory and behavior.* New York: Wiley.

Obsessive Compulsive Cognitions Working Group. (1997). Cognitive assessment of obsessive-compulsive disorder. *Behaviour Research and Therapy, 35*(7), 667–681.

Olatunji, B. O., Davis, M. L., Powers, M. B., & Smits, J. A. J. (2013). Cognitive-behavioral therapy for obsessive-compulsive disorder: A meta-analysis of treatment outcome and moderators. *Journal of Psychiatric Research, 47*(1), 33–41. doi:10.1016/j.jpsychires.2012.08.020

Polman, A., Bouman, T. K., van Hout, W. J., de Jong, P. J., & den Boer, J. A. (2010). Processes of change in cognitive-behavioural treatment of obsessive-compulsive disorder: Current status and some future directions. *Clinical Psychology & Psychotherapy: An International Journal of Theory & Practice, 17*(1), 1–12.

Power, M. J. (2006). The structure of emotion: An empirical comparison of six models. *Cognition and Emotion, 20*(5), 694–713. doi:10.1080/02699930500367925

Rachman, S. (1998). A cognitive theory of obsessions. In E. Sanavio (Ed.), *Behavior and cognitive therapy today* (pp. 209–222). Oxford: Pergamon.

Rachman, S., & Hodgson, R. J. (1980). *Obsessions and compulsions.* Upper Saddle River, NJ: Prentice Hall.

Reynolds, S., & Streiner, D. (1998). Why we do not abstract analogue studies of treatment outcome and scale development. *Evidence Based Mental Health, 1*(4), 101–102. doi:10.1136/ebmh.1.4.101

Rubin, R., Villanueva-Meyer, J., Ananth, J., Trajmar, P., & Mena, I. (1992). Regional xenon 133 cerebral blood flow and cerebral technetium 99m hmpao uptake in unmedicated patients with obsessive-compulsive disorder and matched normal control subjects: Determination by high-resolution single-photon emission computed tomography. *Archives of General Psychiatry, 49,* 695–702. doi:10.1001/archpsyc.1992.01820090023004

Salkovskis, P. M. (1985). Obsessional-compulsive problems: A cognitive-behavioural analysis. *Behavior Research and Therapy, 23*(5), 571–583.

Salkovskis, P. M., Shafran, R., Rachman, S., & Freeston, M. H. (1999). Multiple pathways to inflated responsibility beliefs in obsessional problems: Possible origins and implications for therapy and research. *Behavior Research and Therapy, 37*(11), 1055–1072.

Salkovskis, P. M., Thorpe, S. J., Wahl, K., Wroe, A. L., & Forrester, E. (2003). Neutralizing increases discomfort associated with obsessional thoughts: An experimental study with obsessional patients. *Journal of Abnormal Psychology, 112*(4), 709–715. doi:10.1037/0021-843X.112.4.709

Shafran, R. (2006). Cognitive behavioral models of OCD. In J. S. Abramowitz & A. C. Houts (Eds.), *Concepts and controversies in obsessive compulsive disorder.* New York: Springer.

Smith, A. H., Wetterneck, C. T., Hart, J. M., Short, M. B., Björgvinsson, T., & Smith, A. H. (2012). Differences in obsessional beliefs and emotion appraisal in obsessive compulsive symptom presentation. *Journal of Obsessive-Compulsive and Related Disorders, 1*(1), 54–61.

Solomon, R. L., & Wynne, L. C. (1954). Traumatic avoidance learning: The principles of anxiety conservation and partial irreversibility. *Psychological Review, 61*(6), 353–385.

Tolin, D. F., Abramowitz, J. S., Przeworski, A., & Foa, E. B. (2002). Thought suppression in obsessive-compulsive disorder. *Behaviour Research and Therapy, 40*(11), 1255–1274.

van Gelder, M. M. H. J., Bretveld, R. W., & Roeleveld, N. (2010). Web-based questionnaires: The future in epidemiology? *American Journal of Epidemiology, 172*(11), 1292–1298. doi:10.1093/aje/kwq291

Wegner, D. M. (1994). *White bears and other unwanted thoughts: Suppression, obsession, and the psychology of mental control.* New York: Guildford.

Wegner, D. M., Erber, R., & Zanakos, S. (1993). Ironic processes in the mental control of mood and mood-related thought.

Journal of Personality and Social Psychology, 65(6), 1093–1104. doi:10.1037//0022-3514.65.6.1093

Wegner, D. M., Schneider, D. J., Carter, S. R., & White, T. L. (1987). Paradoxical effects of thought suppression. *Journal of Personality and Social Psychology, 53*(1), 5.

CHAPTER 5

Development and Causes

OCD is the result of a latent combination of neurobiological, genetic, behavioral, cognitive, and environmental factors. Research in OCD has identified neuroanatomy and structure, neurochemical and neurocircuit pathways in the brain's prefrontal cortex. Genetics also play a role in the transmission of the disorder. The onset of the disorder is usually precipitated by a particularly stressful psychosocial event, such as separation from home, unexpected life events, or illness (Taylor, 2011).

This chapter describes the interaction of all these systems, beginning with important fundamental neuroscientific knowledge based upon which the evolving research findings have been built. Even at this writing, new scientific discoveries are being made. The pace of OCD research is breakneck and will lead to better treatments.

Neuroanatomy and Structure of OCD

The prefrontal cortex (PFC) mediates a variety of cognitive functions, including response inhibition, planning, organizing, and verifying operations (Miller & Cohen, 2001). Executive functioning tasks take place in this area and orchestrates the selection, perception, and manipulation of important information, working memory, planning and organization, behavioral control, adaptation to changes, and decision-making. It also mediates motor, cognitive, and behavioral functions (Seo, Lee, & Averbeck, 2012; Tekin & Cummings, 2002). Its significance in OCD that future decisions are based on the outcome and reinforcement of learning through trial and error on the basis of reward or punishment

(Schönberg, Daw, Joel, & O'Doherty, 2007). Because compulsions provide initial relief, the sense of reward is reinforced and will be performed the next time the person encounters the triggering situation.

There are subsections in the PFC that have overlapping roles in the functioning of OCD. These sections will be described in order from the outer to inner structural regions of the brain. The section on neurocircuitry and neurotransmitters will explain how these areas comprise the OCD loop.

The orbitofrontal cortex (OFC), where judgment is based, processes affective and motivational functions (Rolls, 2000; Tekin & Cummings, 2002). The dorsolateral prefrontal cortex (DLPFC) is considered one of the more important areas of dysregulation in OCD, as it monitors motor and cognitive control, learning, memory, and planning (McGovern & Sheth, 2017; Miller & Cohen, 2001). The anterior cingulate cortex (ACC) manages cognitive, motor, emotional processing, response inhibition, and regulation of behavior based in the social context (Bush et al., 2002; Rolls, 2000). The striatum modulates motor, cognitive, and affective functions (Packard & Knowlton, 2002), and the thalamus is the sensory relay station and also monitors motor function (Gazzaniga, Ivry, & Mangun, 2014).

Other areas of OCD brain activity have also been found in the OCD network, namely the basal ganglia and the amygdala. The basal ganglia may represent the primary site of dysfunction in OCD (Rauch, Whalen, Curran, Shin, & Coffey, 2001). The basal ganglia functions are procedural sequencing, reward-based and habit learning, selection of behavioral control, habits, decision-making, cognition, and emotion (Haynes et al., 2018). Within this system, research has shown that neural communication errors from the basal ganglia to the frontal cortex occur through two pathways with opposing effects for the proper execution of movement (Li & Mody, 2016).

A lack of voluntary control over habits stored in the basal ganglia might lead to a reduced and ineffective regulation by prefrontal areas of habit learning and expression. Cognitive and behavioral therapy may produce changes in these areas by reprogramming pathological habits for appropriate ones (Dougherty et al., 2018). Abnormalities in the basal ganglia have been found to be associated with OCD severity and may determine whether patients respond to certain medications (Rosenberg & MacMillan, 2002).

The amygdala lies in the executive-functioning fear circuitry within the PFC and ACC and causes problems with safety learning (Apergis-Schoute et al., 2017). The role of the amygdala in OCD is said to be misinterpreting fear that then becomes conditioned and reinforced by compulsive or avoidant behaviors (Rauch, Shin, & Wright, 2003). Interesting findings have been made about which types of symptoms result from abnormalities in the amygdala's threat detection system. Variations in the amygdala within the frontal, striatal, and limbic regions may account for aggressive/checking and sexual/religious symptoms (Via et al., 2014).

Neurotransmitters and Neurocircuitry

This section describes what neurochemicals interact, create an imbalance, and result in a looped feedback neurocircuit. Neurotransmitters send chemical messages across the space between neurons, which is called the *synapse* (picture the Sistine Chapel where God is sending life to Adam without touching him). The feedback loop from the OFC, the ACC, DLPFC, the striatum, the thalamus, and then back to the OFC is referred to going forward as the *CSTC circuit* (Bokor & Anderson, 2014; Tang et al., 2016). Serotonin, dopamine, and glutamate have been identified as the neurotransmitters involved in sending signals that trigger obsessions and compulsive behaviors (Vaghi et al., 2017). Functional neuroimaging of the CSTC has shown impaired safety learning in people with OCD (Apergis-Schoute et al., 2017; Brennan & Rauch, 2017). Table 5.1 provides the putative neuroanatomical, neurofunctional, and neurochemical components of OCD.

Serotonin

Serotonin is a neurotransmitter active in a wide range of neurophysiological functions, such as regulating mood, cognitive and social behavior, sleep, circadian rhythms, temperature, sexual activity, and pain (Gross, Sasson, Chopra, & Zohar, 1998). Serotonin reuptake inhibitors (SRIs) have been prescribed for OCD since the tricyclic antidepressant drug clomipramine was discovered to reduce symptoms (Jenike, 1990). The serotonin transporter protein, 5HT, has been found to be lower in OCD patients in the prefrontal and thalamic cortical region of the brain, and to be higher in the caudate (Dougherty et al., 2018; Marazziti et al., 1997). Serotonin reuptake inhibitor medications and CBT have been shown to be effective in reducing caudate glucose metabolism and OCD symptoms, but there is no evidence that serotonin is the primary brain chemical involved in the disorder, as once believed (Dougherty et al., 2018).

Table 5.1   Neuroanatomy, Neurofunctions, and Neurochemicals of OCD

Anatomy	Function	Chemical
Prefrontal cortex	Response inhibition Planning Organizing Verifying	Dopamine
Orbitofrontal cortex	Judgment Affect Motivation	Serotonin Dopamine
Anterior cingulate cortex	Cognition Motor Emotional processing Response inhibition Behavioral regulation Error detection	Glutamate
Dorsolateral prefrontal cortex	Motor Cognitive Learning Memory Complex problem solving Plannning	Glutamate
Striatum	Motor Cognition Affect	Glutamate
Thalamus	Motor Sensory relay station	Serotonin Glutamate
Basal ganglia	Learning	Dopamine
Amygdala	Memory Decision-making Emotion appraisal Anxiety Fear Aggression	Dopamine Serotonin

Dopamine

Dopamine is a neurochemical that provides the motivation for reward in motor and habit-learning behavior (Huey et al., 2008). Dopamine is found to be lower in the basal ganglia and striatum of people with OCD (Olver et al., 2009; van der Wee et al., 2007). Too much dopamine results in excessive movement and is connected to excessive behaviors in the form of rituals (Saxena & Rauch, 2000). The antipsychotics olanzapine, Zyprexa (Koran, Ringold, & Elliott, 2000), and risperidone, Risperdal (Decloedt & Stein, 2010), as well as the antidepressant bupropion, Wellbutrin (Lambert, 2008), are common OCD medications used to augment the effects of the SSRIs.

Glutamate

Glutamate is the most abundant neurotransmitter in the brain (Pittenger, Bloch, & Williams, 2011). It regulates brain development by sorting large quantities of information to differentiate and eliminate nerve cells, as well as playing an important role in learning and memory (Zhou & Danbolt, 2014).

Research has attributed glutamate dysfunction within the CSTC circuit as playing a role in the pathophysiology of OCD, as shown in neuroimages produced by magnetic resonance spectroscopy (Dougherty et al., 2018; Gnanavel, Sharan, Khandelwal, Sharma, & Jagannathan, 2014). The identification of the gene SLC-A1A that carries glutamate has informed clinical OCD research trials with the medications riluzole, used for treating amyotrophic lateral sclerosis (Grant et al., 2016); memantine, used to treat moderate to severe confusion (dementia) related to Alzheimer's disease (Entezari et al., 2012); ketamine, an anesthetic (Rodriguez et al., 2015); and N-acetylcysteine, used as an antioxidant, for acetaminophen overdose, and to treat respiratory conditions (Couto & Moreira, 2018).

Brain Mass and Volume

Structural and functional images taken by functional magnetic resonance imaging (fMRI) with OCD patients have shown decreased gray matter volume in the bilateral cingulate cortex and bilateral striatum, where executive functions such as planning, performance monitoring, and short-term memory processing occur (Tang et al., 2016; van den Heuvel et al., 2005). Other fMRI results by Tang and colleagues (2016) found that patients with OCD had an overactivation of the right cerebellum and right parietal lobe and reduced activation of the left cingulate gyrus, putamen, and caudate nucleus. Interestingly, they also found that treatment with SSRIs seemed to correlate with improvement in brain structure, leading to symptom improvement.

Etiology

We have reviewed the interplay of the neurobiological pathways, structure, and neurofunctions of OCD. Research has also identified several etiological factors that help explain the cause of the disorder.

Genetics

The International Obsessive Compulsive Disorder Foundation Genetics Collaborative (IOCDF-GC) and the OCD Collaborative Genetics Association Studies (OCGAS) were established specifically for conducting genomic research (Genetics et al., 2018). Their research findings have been based on family and twin studies, genetic linage studies, candidate gene association, genome-wide studies, and genome sequencing studies (Purty, Nestadt, Samuels, & Viswanath, 2019). The data from a 1929–2005 review twin study reported that genetic factors accounted for heritability of 45–65 percent in early onset OCD (van Grootheest, Boomsma, Hettema, & Kendler, 2008). The most recent rate reported of OCD heritability was approximately 40 percent but may increase as research techniques advance (Taylor, 2016). While at this time no gene has been definitively confirmed, studies have found consistent markers that have the potential to be isolated with ongoing research. The genes of interest being studied in OCD are comprised of glutamate, serotonin, and dopamine.

Glutamate-related gene transporters are suspected of increasing the amount of glutamate in the brain and possibly lead to OCD symptoms (Zai & Richter, 2016). A specific marker under consideration is SLC1A1 (Stewart et al., 2013). This marker codes for the postsynaptic neuronal glutamate transporter located within the CSTC circuits (Dallaspezia, Mazza, Lorenzi, Benedetti, & Smeraldi, 2014), and is thought to be associated with early onset OCD (Purty et al., 2019). Others are SLITRK5 and DLGAP1 (Zai & Richter, 2016).

Serotonergic genes are under examination in OCD because of the treatment response of SSRI medications (Stewart et al., 2013). The gene receptors HTR1B and HTTLPR and the gene transporter HTTLPR have been studied as potential sequences in OCD (Pauls, Abramovitch, Rauch, & Geller, 2014; Purty et al., 2019; Zai & Richter, 2016). The marker MEF2BNB has also been considered to play a genetic role in OCD (den Braber et al., 2016).

The dopamine gene DRD4 has shown to be involved in the OCD symptom dimension of symmetry, and DRD3 is associated with early onset (Gasso et al., 2015).

As noted earlier, early onset OCD has been traced to family heritability in many cases (van Grootheest et al., 2008), and the course appears to be moderately stable across development due to genetic factors (Krebs, Waszczuk, Zavos, Bolton, & Eley, 2015; Krebs et al., 2015). A research question being investigated is whether neuroimaging measuring studies can identify genetic homogeneity in early OCD onset that carry distinct clinical patterns instead of relying on symptom type (Rosenberg & Hanna, 2000). These authors suggest that the diagnosis and treatment of OCD may be better informed if there are clinical distinctions between genetic transmission of the disorder and the onset being accounted for by other precipitating factors.

Symptom Dimensions

In a similar vein, research has been able to identify genetic components related to symptom dimensions controlled for by environmental factors. One genetic study, conducted on a large sample of female twins found a 36 percent genetic similarity on the obsessions, contamination, and checking symptoms dimensions (van Grootheest et al., 2008).

Another study found that the OCD dimensions of intrusive thoughts, contamination/cleaning, obsessive doubts, superstitions/rituals, and symmetry/hoarding were heritable (Katerberg et al., 2010). The authors found that the taboo and doubts factor and the contamination and symmetry/hoarding factor shared genetic influences and levels of severity.

Stressful Life Events

As stated at the beginning of the chapter, it appears empirically that OCD remains latent until precipitated by an important planned or unplanned change or stressful event (Taylor, 2011). The research, however, has not yet confirmed what the pathophysiological relationship between stress and OCD is, although stressful life events activate the same corticostriatal and limbic activity in the brain (Adams et al., 2018). Circular questions that are raised are whether a stressful or traumatic event is the triggering factor that interacts with the latent OCD, whether the event is a discrete cause of OCD symptoms, and whether there is an interaction between life events and genes (Goldberg et al., 2015). Academic, social, family dysfunction, loss of a loved one, and subjectively experienced challenges are a few examples of precipitating circumstances.

Having had one or more events was found to result in increased OCD severity, especially with obsessions, checking, and symmetry/

ordering, two of the four symptom dimensions that were specifically associated with the occurrence of traumatic life events. These results are generally supportive of how the form and content of specific OCD symptoms can be shaped by events in a patient's life (Cromer, Schmidt, & Murphy, 2007).

Problems with distress tolerance can also have an effect on how obsessions are experienced. Lower distress tolerance was predictive of more obsessions in people who were experiencing stressful life events (Macatee, Capron, Schmidt, & Cougle, 2013). Those who had a stressful life event prior to their first OCD episode were found to have a later onset, less family history of OCD, and contamination as a common symptom (Real et al., 2011).

At least one event preceded the onset of OCD in two hundred patients (60.8%), and this was significantly associated with female gender, abrupt onset of the disorder, and somatic obsessions (Rosso, Albert, Asinari, Bogetto, & Maina, 2012). These authors found three common traumatic events that consistently triggered specific OCD dimensions. Hospitalization of a family member, having a major personal physical illness, and experiencing loss of personally valuable object were associated with the symptom dimensions of symmetry obsessions, repeating, ordering/arranging, counting, and checking compulsions (Rosso et al., 2012).

Female Reproductive Events and OCD

Research has been conducted on the powerful effect hormones have on OCD. Studies have looked at whether changes in estrogen and progesterone increase women's OCD symptoms in the menstrual cycle, pre- and perinatal phases of pregnancy, and menopause (Lochner et al., 2004). Once again, serotonin, dopamine, and glutamate are found to play a role in worsening of OCD symptoms during these physiological events (Karpinski, Mattina, & Steiner, 2017). Karpinski and colleagues (2017) also reported being able to regulate these neurotransmitter systems by treating hormone levels pharmacologically with estrogen, progesterone, and oxytocin.

Premenstrual

Premenstrual syndrome (PMS) occurs typically a week before the onset of menstruation and for approximately 48 percent of women in an international study (Direkvand-Moghadam, Sayehmiri, Delpisheh, & Kaikhavandi, 2014). PMS causes emotional lability and physical discomfort in women (Ussher & Perz, 2013) and a worsening of OCD symptoms in 42 percent of female subjects in an outpatient study (Forray, Focseneanu, Pittman, McDougle, & Epperson, 2010; Williams & Koran, 1997). Another study found that the onset of OCD occurred during the same year of menarche, which is when the onset of menstruation begins (Labad et al., 2005).

Pregnancy

For some women, the onset of OCD may occur during pregnancy or childbirth, or it may worsen symptoms for those with active OCD (Forray et al., 2010). The estrogen hormones estradiol and progesterone have been found to increase dopamine over the course of pregnancy (Karpinski et al., 2017).

Research has reported an incidence rate of OCD onset and pregnancy in 1–13 percent of women (Fairbrother, Janssen, Antony, Tucker, & Young, 2016; Williams & Koran, 1997), and for women with preexisting OCD, 17–34 percent reported increase in severity (Forray et al., 2010; Williams & Koran, 1997). Interestingly, 22 percent of pregnant women with OCD experienced improvement in their symptoms, and 44–69 percent of women with preexisting OCD found no changes in severity (Forray et al., 2010; Williams & Koran, 1997).

Perinatal/Postpartum

The time after childbirth is expected to be filled with joy and bonding, but many women, 13 percent, are devasted by postpartum depression (Beck, 2001). Postpartum OCD onset occurs in 3 percent (Forray et al., 2010) and up to 21 percent (Buttolph & Holland, 1990; Williams & Koran, 1997) due to hormonal changes. Fluctuations in estrogen and progesterone levels that occur in the third trimester of pregnancy appear to alter serotonergic transmission, reuptake, and binding (Biegor, Reches, & Snyder, 1983). In women with OCD, 29–50 percent reported an increase in symptom severity after childbirth (Forray et al., 2010).

Evolutionary Biology

Evolutionary biology explains that when we become afraid or are in danger, our brain activates our precaution system, starting with the amygdala and setting off a surge of adrenalin that alerts our physiological functions of threat and presents us with an immediate decision to fight or flee (Adolphs, 2013). Whatever decision we make, our prefrontal cortex will remember that this particular situation should now be avoided.

With OCD, though, when the precaution mechanism is activated from an obsessive trigger, the same survival instincts are set in motion but in the absence of real threat or danger. There is only the *doubt* or the *feeling* of it. Further, the neurological basis of OCD provokes the feeling of imminent or potential danger even under ordinary, routine conditions for which there is no quantifiable evidence of threat, because there is none. Consider how basic survival needs transform into OCD symptoms. The need to be clean and neat turns into contamination obsessions that compel washing and cleaning rituals. The need to be safe results in avoidance and checking behaviors. Our awareness of death and the inability to know why seemingly random catastrophic events occur create existential fears of being able to know or have certainty about the future.

Every culture has a set of superstitious beliefs that create an illusion of having control of or preventing bad things from happening. OCD takes this concept further with scrupulosity (fear of offending God or disrupting the order of the universe) and moral perfectionism (perfect thoughts and behavior will prevent mistakes of harm). While hoarding is no longer considered an OCD subtype, we can see that it may be an outgrowth of nesting instincts.

Our evolved abilities to think ahead and consider how our actions may result in harm become overactive in the OCD imagination. Unfortunately, the adaptive ability to anticipate future needs or threats through our striatal-frontal brain circuits can create a life of catastrophic improbabilities (Brüne, 2006). People with OCD lose sight that just because an obsessive thought is provoked, it doesn't mean it has to be acted on.

References

Adams, T. G., Kelmendi, B., Brake, C. A., Gruner, P., Badour, C. L., & Pittenger, C. (2018). The role of stress in the pathogenesis and maintenance of obsessive-compulsive disorder. *Chronic Stress (Thousand Oaks), 2*. doi:10.1177/2470547018758043

Adolphs, R. (2013). The biology of fear. *Current Biology, 23*(2), R79–R93. doi:10.1016/j.cub.2012.11.055

Apergis-Schoute, A. M., Gillan, C. M., Fineberg, N. A., Fernandez-Egea, E., Sahakian, B. J., & Robbins, T. W. (2017). Neural basis of impaired safety signaling in obsessive compulsive disorder. *Proceedings of the National Academy of Science of the United States of America, 114*(12), 3216–3221. doi:10.1073/pnas.1609194114

Biegor, A., Reches, A., & Snyder, L. (1983). Serotonergic and noradrenergic hormones. *Life Sciences, 32,* 2015–2021.

Bokor, G., & Anderson, P. D. (2014). Obsessive-compulsive disorder. *Journal of Pharmacy Practice, 27*(2), 116–130. doi:10.1177/089719 0014521996

Brennan, B. P., & Rauch, S. L. (2017). Functional neuroimaging studies in obsessive-compulsive disorder: Overview and synthesis. In C. Pittenger (Ed.), *Obsessive-compulsive disorder: Phenomenology, pathophysiology, and treatment* (pp. 213–231). New York: Oxford University Press.

Brüne, M. (2006). The evolutionary psychology of obsessive-compulsive disorder: The role of cognitive metarepresentation. *Perspectives in Biology and Medicine, 49*(3), 317–329. doi:10.1353/pbm.2006.0037

Bush, G., Vogt, B. A., Holmes, J., Dale, A. M., Greve, D., Jenike, M. A., & Rosen, B. R. (2002). Dorsal anterior cingulate cortex: A role in reward-based decision making. *Proceedings of the National Academy of Science of the United States of America, 99*(1), 523–528. doi:10.1073/pnas.012470999

Buttolph, M. L., & Holland, A. D. (1990). Obsessive-compulsive disorders in pregnancy and childbirth. In M. Jenike, L. Baer, & W. Minichiello (Eds.), *Obsessive-compulsive disorders: Theory and management* (pp. 89–97). Chicago: Year Book Medical.

Couto, J. P., & Moreira, R. (2018). Oral N-acetylcysteine in the treatment of obsessive-compulsive disorder: A systematic review of the clinical evidence. *Progress in Neuro-Psychopharmacology and Biological Psychiatry, 86,* 245–254.

Cromer, K. R., Schmidt, N. B., & Murphy, D. L. (2007). An investigation of traumatic life events and obsessive-compulsive disorder. *Behavior Research and Therapy, 45*(7), 1683–1691. doi:10.1016/j .brat.2006.08.018

Dallaspezia, S., Mazza, M., Lorenzi, C., Benedetti, F., & Smeraldi, E. (2014). A single nucleotide polymorphism in SLC1A1 gene is associated with age of onset of obsessive-compulsive disorder. *European Psychiatry, 29*(5), 301–303. doi:10.1016/j.eurpsy.2014.02.006

Decloedt, E. H., & Stein, D. J. (2010). Current trends in drug treatment of obsessive-compulsive disorder. *Neuropsychiatric Disease and Treatment, 6,* 233–242.

den Braber, A., Zilhao, N. R., Fedko, I. O., Hottenga, J. J., Pool, R., Smit, D. J. A., . . . Boomsma, D. I. (2016). Obsessive-compulsive symptoms in a large population-based twin-family sample are predicted by clinically based polygenic scores and by genome-wide SNPs. *Translational Psychiatry, 6,* e731. doi:10.1038/tp.2015.223

Direkvand-Moghadam, A., Sayehmiri, K., Delpisheh, A., & Kaikhavandi, S. (2014). Epidemiology of premenstrual syndrome (PMS): A systematic review and meta-analysis study. *Journal of Clinical and Diagnostic Research, 8*(2), 106–109.

Dougherty, D. D., Brennan, B. P., Stewart, S. E., Wilhelm, S., Widge, A. S., & Rauch, S. L. (2018). Neuroscientifically informed formulation and treatment planning for patients with obsessive-compulsive disorder: A review. *JAMA Psychiatry, 75*(10), 1081–1087. doi:10.1001/jamapsychiatry.2018.0930

Entezari, N., Modabbernia, A., Najand, B., Askari, N., Tabrizi, M., Ashrafi, M., . . . Akhondzadeh, S. (2012). Memantine add-on in moderate to severe obsessive-compulsive disorder: Randomized double-blind placebo-controlled study. *Journal of Psychiatric Research, 47*(2), 175–180. doi:10.1016/j.jpsychires.2012.09.015

Fairbrother, N., Janssen, P., Antony, M. M., Tucker, E., & Young, A. H. (2016). Perinatal anxiety disorder prevalence and incidence. *Journal of Affective Disorders, 200*, 148–155.

Forray, A., Focseneanu, M., Pittman, B., McDougle, C. J., & Epperson, C. N. (2010). Onset and exacerbation of obsessive-compulsive disorder in pregnancy and the postpartum period. *Journal of Clinical Psychiatry, 71*(8), 1061–1068. doi:10.4088/JCP.09m05381blu

Gasso, P., Ortiz, A. E., Mas, S., Morer, A., Calvo, A., Bargallo, N., . . . Lazaro, L. (2015). Association between genetic variants related to glutamatergic, dopaminergic and neurodevelopment pathways and white matter microstructure in child and adolescent patients with obsessive-compulsive disorder. *Journal of Affective Disorders, 186*, 284–292. doi:10.1016/j.jad.2015.07.035

Gazzaniga, M. S., Ivry, R. B., & Mangun, G. R. (2014). *Cognitive neuroscience: The biology of the mind* (4th ed.). New York: W. W. Norton.

Genetics, I. O. C. D. F., Arnold, P. D., Askland, K. D., Barlassina, C., Bellodi, L., Bienvenu, O., . . . Burton, C. L. (2018). Revealing the complex genetic architecture of obsessive-compulsive disorder using meta-analysis. *Molecular Psychiatry, 23*(5), 1181.

Gnanavel, S., Sharan, P., Khandelwal, S., Sharma, U., & Jagannathan, N. R. (2014). Neurochemicals measured by 1 H-MR spectroscopy: Putative vulnerability biomarkers for obsessive compulsive disorder. *Magnetic Resonance Materials in Physics, Biology and Medicine, 27*(5), 407–417.

Goldberg, X., Soriano-Mas, C., Alonso, P., Segalàs, C., Real, E., López-Solà, C., . . . Cardoner, N. (2015). Predictive value of familiality, stressful life events and gender on the course of obsessive-compulsive

disorder. *Journal of Affective Disorders, 185,* 129–134. doi:10.1016/j
.jad.2015.06.047

Grant, J. E., Fineberg, N., van Ameringen, M., Cath, D., Visser, H.,
Carmi, L., . . . van Balkom, A. J. L. M. (2016). New treatment models for compulsive disorders. *European Neuropsychopharmacology,*
26(5), 877–884. doi:10.1016/j.euroneuro.2015.11.008

Gross, R., Sasson, Y., Chopra, M., & Zohar, J. (1998). Biological mod-
els of obsessive-compulsive disorder. In R. P. Swinson, M. M. Antony,
S. Rachman, & M. A. Richter (Eds.), *Obsessive-compulsive disorder:*
Theory, research, and treatment. New York: Guilford.

Haynes, W. I., Clair, A.-H., Fernandez-Vidal, S., Gholipour, B., Morgiève,
M., & Mallet, L. (2018). Altered anatomical connections of associa-
tive and limbic cortico-basal-ganglia circuits in obsessive-compulsive
disorder. *European Psychiatry, 51,* 1–8.

Huey, E. D., Zahn, R., Krueger, F., Moll, J., Kapogiannis, D., Wassermann,
E. M., & Grafman, J. (2008). A psychological and neuroanatomical
model of obsessive-compulsive disorder. *Journal of Neuropsychia-*
try and Clinical Neurosciences, 20(4), 390–408. doi:10.1176/appi
.neuropsych.20.4.390

Jenike, M. A. (1990). Treatment. In M. A. Jenike, L. Baer, & W. E. Minichiello (Eds.), *Obsessive compulsive disorder: Theory and manage-*
ment (pp. 249–282). Chicago: Year Book Medical.

Karpinski, M., Mattina, G. F., & Steiner, M. (2017). Effect of gonadal
hormones on neurotransmitters implicated in the pathophysiology of
obsessive-compulsive disorder: A critical review. *Neuroendocrinology,*
105(1), 1–16. doi:10.1159/000453664

Katerberg, H., Delucchi, K. L., Stewart, S. E., Lochner, C., Denys, D. A. J.
P., Stack, D. E., . . . Cath, D. C. (2010). Symptom dimensions in OCD:
Item-level factor analysis and heritability estimates. *Behavior Genet-*
ics, 40(4), 505–517. doi:10.1007/s10519-010-9339-z

Koran, L. M., Ringold, A. L., & Elliott, M. A. (2000). Olanzapine augmentation for treatment-resistant obsessive-compulsive disorder. *Jour-*
nal of Clinical Psychiatry, 61(7), 514–517. doi:10.4088/jcp.v61n0709

Krebs, G., Waszczuk, M. A., Zavos, H. M. S., Bolton, D., & Eley, T. C.
(2015). Genetic and environmental influences on obsessive-compulsive
behaviour across development: A longitudinal twin study. *Psychologi-*
cal Medicine, 45(7), 1539–1549. doi:10.1017/s0033291714002761

Labad, J., Menchón, J. M., Alonso, P., Segalàs, C., Jiménez, S., & Vallejo,
J. (2005). Female reproductive cycle and obsessive-compulsive disorder. *Journal of Clinical Psychiatry, 66*(4), 428–435. Retrieved from
https://www.ncbi.nlm.nih.gov/pubmed/15816784

Lambert, M. (2008). APA releases new guideline on treating obsessive-compulsive disorder. *American Family Physician, 1*(78), 131–135.

Li, B., & Mody, M. (2016). Cortico-striato-thalamo-cortical circuitry, working memory, and obsessive-compulsive disorder. *Frontiers in Psychiatry, 7,* 78. doi:10.3389/fpsyt.2016.00078

Lochner, C., Hemmings, S. M., Kinnear, C. J., Moolman-Smook, J. C., Corfield, V. A., Knowles, J. A., . . . Stein, D. J. (2004). Gender in obsessive-compulsive disorder: Clinical and genetic findings. *European Neuropsychopharmacology, 14*(2), 105–113. doi:10.1016/s0924-977x(03)00063-4

Macatee, R. J., Capron, D. W., Schmidt, N. B., & Cougle, J. R. (2013). An examination of low distress tolerance and life stressors as factors underlying obsessions. *Journal of Psychiatric Research, 47*(10), 1462–1468. doi:10.1016/j.jpsychires.2013.06.019

Marazziti, D., Pfanner, C., Palego, L., Gemignani, A., Milanfranchi, A., Ravagli, S., . . . Cassano, G. (1997). Changes in platelet markers of obsessive-compulsive patients during a double-blind trial of fluvoxamine versus clomipramine. *Pharmacopsychiatry, 30*(06), 245–249.

McGovern, R. A., & Sheth, S. A. (2017). Role of the dorsal anterior cingulate cortex in obsessive-compulsive disorder: Converging evidence from cognitive neuroscience and psychiatric neurosurgery. *Journal of Neurosurgery, 126*(1), 132–147. doi:10.3171/2016.1.Jns15601

Miller, E. K., & Cohen, J. D. (2001). An integrative theory of prefrontal cortex function. *Annual Review of Neuroscience, 24,* 167–202. doi:10.1146/annurev.neuro.24.1.167

Olver, J. S., O'Keefe, G., Jones, G. R., Burrows, G. D., Tochon-Danguy, H. J., Ackermann, U., . . . Norman, T. R. (2009). Dopamine D1 receptor binding in the striatum of patients with obsessive-compulsive disorder. *Journal of Affective Disorders, 114*(1–3), 321–326.

Packard, M. G., & Knowlton, B. J. (2002). Learning and memory functions of the basal ganglia. *Annual Review of Neuroscience, 25,* 563–593. doi:10.1146/annurev.neuro.25.112701.142937

Pauls, D. L., Abramovitch, A., Rauch, S. L., & Geller, D. A. (2014). Obsessive-compulsive disorder: An integrative genetic and neurobiological perspective. *Nature Reviews Neuroscience, 15*(6), 410–424. doi:10.1038/nrn3746

Pittenger, C., Bloch, M. H., & Williams, K. (2011). Glutamate abnormalities in obsessive compulsive disorder: Neurobiology, pathophysiology, and treatment. *Pharmacology & Therapy, 132*(3), 314–332. doi:10.1016/j.pharmthera.2011.09.006

Purty, A., Nestadt, G., Samuels, J. F., & Viswanath, B. (2019). Genetics of obsessive-compulsive disorder. *Indian Journal of Psychiatry, 61* (Suppl 1), S37–S42. doi:10.4103/psychiatry.IndianJPsychiatry_518_18

Rauch, S. L., Shin, L. M., & Wright, C. I. (2003). Neuroimaging studies of amygdala function in anxiety disorders. *Annals of the New York Academy of Sciences, 985*(1), 389–410.

Rauch, S. L., Whalen, P. J., Curran, T., Shin, L. M., & Coffey, B. (2001). Probing striatothalamic function in obsessive-compulsive disorder and Tourette syndrome using neuroimaging methods. *Advances in Neurology, 85,* 207–224.

Real, E., Labad, J., Alonso, P., Segalàs, C., Jiménez-Murcia, S., Bueno, B., . . . Menchón, J. M. (2011). Stressful life events at onset of obsessive-compulsive disorder are associated with a distinct clinical pattern. *Depression and Anxiety, 28*(5), 367–376. doi:10.1002/da.20792

Rodriguez, C. I., Kegeles, L. S., Levinson, A., Ogden, R. T., Mao, X., Milak, M. S., . . . Simpson, H. B. (2015). In vivo effects of ketamine on glutamate-glutamine and gamma-aminobutyric acid in obsessive-compulsive disorder: Proof of concept. *Psychiatry Research, 233*(2), 141–147. doi:10.1016/j.pscychresns.2015.06.001

Rolls, E. T. (2000). The orbitofrontal cortex and reward. *Cerebral Cortex, 10*(3), 284–294. doi:10.1093/cercor/10.3.284

Rosenberg, D. R., & MacMillan, S. (2002). Imaging and neurocircuitry of OCD. In K. L. David, D. Charney, J. T. Coyle, & C. Nemeroff (Eds.), *Neuropsychopharmacology. The Fifth Generation of Progress,* 1621–1646.

Rosso, G., Albert, U., Asinari, G. F., Bogetto, F., & Maina, G. (2012). Stressful life events and obsessive-compulsive disorder: Clinical features and symptom dimensions. *Psychiatry Research, 197*(3), 259–264. doi:10.1016/j.psychres.2011.10.005

Saxena, S., & Rauch, S. L. (2000). Functional neuroimaging and the neuroanatomy of obsessive-compulsive disorder. *Psychiatric Clinics of North America, 23*(3), 563–586.

Schönberg, T., Daw, N. D., Joel, D., & O'Doherty, J. P. (2007). Reinforcement learning signals in the human striatum distinguish learners from nonlearners during reward-based decision making. *Journal of Neuroscience, 27*(47), 12860–12867. doi:10.1523/jneurosci.2496-07.2007

Seo, M., Lee, E., & Averbeck, B. B. (2012). Action selection and action value in frontal-striatal circuits. *Neuron, 74*(5), 947–960. doi:10.1016/j.neuron.2012.03.037

Stewart, S. E., Yu, D., Scharf, J. M., Neale, B. M., Fagerness, J. A., Mathews, C. A., . . . Pauls, D. L. (2013). Genome-wide association study of obsessive-compulsive disorder. *Molecular Psychiatry, 18*(7), 788–798. doi:10.1038/mp.2012.85

Tang, W., Zhu, Q., Gong, X., Zhu, C., Wang, Y., & Chen, S. (2016). Cortico-striato-thalamo-cortical circuit abnormalities in obsessive-compulsive disorder: A voxel-based morphometric and fMRI study of the whole brain. *Behavioural Brain Research, 313*, 17–22. doi:10.1016 /j.bbr.2016.07.004

Taylor, S. (2011). Early versus late onset obsessive-compulsive disorder: Evidence for distinct subtypes. *Psychological Review, 31*(7), 1083–1100.

Taylor, S. (2016). Disorder-specific genetic factors in obsessive-compulsive disorder: A comprehensive meta-analysis. *American Journal of Medical Genetics Part B: Neuropsychiatric Genetics, 171B*(3), 325–332. doi:10.1002/ajmg.b.32407

Tekin, S., & Cummings, J. L. (2002). Frontal-subcortical neuronal circuits and clinical neuropsychiatry: An update. *Journal of Psychosomatic Research, 53*(2), 647–654. doi:10.1016/S0022-3999(02)00428-2

Ussher, J. M., & Perz, J. (2013). PMS as a process of negotiation: Women's experience and management of premenstrual distress. *Psychology & Health, 28*(8), 909–927. doi:10.1080/08870446.2013.765004

Vaghi, M. M., Vértes, P. E., Kitzbichler, M. G., Apergis-Schoute, A. M., van der Flier, F. E., Fineberg, N. A., . . . Robbins, T. W. (2017). Specific frontostriatal circuits for impaired cognitive flexibility and goal-directed planning in obsessive-compulsive disorder: Evidence from resting-state functional connectivity. *Biological Psychiatry, 81*(8), 708–717. doi:10.1016/j.biopsych.2016.08.009

van den Heuvel, O. A., Veltman, D. J., Groenewegen, H. J., Cath, D. C., van Balkom, A. J. L. M., van Hartskamp, J., . . . van Dyck, R. (2005). Frontal-striatal dysfunction during planning in obsessive-compulsive disorder. *JAMA Psychiatry, 62*(3), 301–309. doi:10.1001/archpsyc .62.3.301

van der Wee, N. J., Ramsey, N. F., van Megen, H. J., Denys, D., Westenberg, H. G., & Kahn, R. S. (2007). Spatial working memory in obsessive-compulsive disorder improves with clinical response: A functional MRI study. *European Neuropsychopharmacology, 17*(1), 16–23.

van Grootheest, D. S., Boomsma, D. I., Hettema, J. M., & Kendler, K. S. (2008). Heritability of obsessive-compulsive symptom dimensions.

American Journal of Medical Genetics Part B: Neuropsychiatric Genetics, 147B(4), 473–478.

Via, E., Cardoner, N., Pujol, J., Alonso, P., Lopez-Sola, M., Real, E., . . . Menchon, J. M. (2014). Amygdala activation and symptom dimensions in obsessive-compulsive disorder. *British Journal of Psychiatry, 204*(1), 61–68.

Williams, K. E., & Koran, L. M. (1997). Obsessive-compulsive disorder in pregnancy, the puerperium, and the premenstruum. *Journal of Clinical Psychiatry, 58*(7), 330–334; quiz 335–336. doi:10.4088/jcp .v58n0709

Zai, G. A. K., Kennedy, J. L, & Richter, M. P. A. (2016). *Genetics of obsessive-compulsive disorder: From phenotypes to pharmacogenetics* (Doctoral dissertation). University of Toronto, Canada.

Zhou, Y., & Danbolt, N. C. (2014). Glutamate as a neurotransmitter in the healthy brain. *Journal of Neural Transmission (Vienna), 121*(8), 799–817. doi:10.1007/s00702-014-1180-8

CHAPTER 6

Effects and Costs

The burden of OCD doesn't only impact individual sufferers; it also touch the lives of those with whom they are connected, such as family, friends, coworkers, and people in the community. When measuring the effects and costs of OCD from an epidemiological standpoint, important factors include mortality, comorbidity, disability, and effects on the quality of life, as well as the cost of interventions and their clinical effectiveness (Fineberg et al., 2019). Socioeconomically, the cost of OCD is significant. Some people with mild OCD can hide their symptoms, or for them, the symptoms are triggered only in specific situations and can be coped with fairly well. Those in the moderate-to-severe range have more trouble managing their symptoms, and they interfere with functioning. Either way, the symptoms can be managed to maximize the best level of well-being.

Successful identification, diagnosis, and treatment of OCD can help reduce the overall burden the disorder has on the personal, societal, and global domains of life. This chapter outlines the various components that contribute to the impact OCD has on the microscopic and macroscopic levels of life.

Quality of Life

According to Jacoby, quality of life (QOL) refers to subjective well-being, including enjoyment and satisfaction with various life activities, while functional impairment consists of measurable difficulty in engaging in activities (e.g., work, social, leisure activities) due to psychological symptoms (Jacoby, Leonard, Riemann, & Abramowitz, 2014).

Quality of life is also measured by connection to social networks, personal happiness and enjoyment, reliability, ability to work and keep social commitments, and participation in life activities (Asnaani et al., 2017). It also consists of people's perception of their position in life within the context of their culture, value system, goals, expectations, standards, psychological and physical health, social connectedness, and overall concerns about well-being (Hou, Yen, Huang, Wang, & Yeh, 2010; Theofilou, 2013).

OCD exacts a price on the quality of life not only of individual sufferers but also of the people in their lives. The quality of life for people with high-moderate to extreme clinical levels of OCD often begins to erode and take a toll on almost all domains of life (Velloso et al., 2018). One study found that for people with severe OCD, relationships and social functioning were the domains most impacted by OCD, while managing the household was the most common problematic area for those in the moderate range (Ruscio, Stein, Chiu, & Kessler, 2010). The effect of OCD on relationships is more fully addressed in chapter 9.

Behaviors, Barriers, and Delays in OCD Diagnosis and Treatment

Duration of Untreated Illness (DUI)

The duration of untreated illness, defined as the time elapsing between the onset of a disorder and the beginning of the first pharmacological treatment, has been increasingly investigated as a predictor of outcome and course across different psychiatric disorders (Dell'Osso, Buoli, Hollander, & Altamura, 2010). DUI appears to be among the predictors of treatment outcome and to have a significant impact on the course of illness for untreated individuals (Dell'Osso et al., 2010; Erzegovesi et al., 2001).

Study results have confirmed that patients with OCD have had a long DUI, due to factors such as severity, secrecy, poor insight, parental and cultural attitudes, and lack of access to psychiatric services (Belloch, Del Valle, Morillo, Carrió, & Cabedo, 2009; Torres et al., 2017). Families with children who have OCD may not take it seriously or may not know where to find help (Goodwin, Koenen, Hellman, Guardino, & Struening, 2002; Stengler-Wenzke, Trosbach, Dietrich, & Angermeyer, 2004).

Unfortunately, OCD has one of the longest durations of untreated illness among psychiatric disorders. The delay from the time of symptom onset to entering treatment can run from eight to seventeen years (García-Soriano, Rufer, Delsignore, & Weidt, 2014; Grabe et al., 2001), and when professional help was consulted, it took, on average, two years before the diagnosis was made (Skoog & Skoog, 1999). Studies have reported that 38–90 percent of OCD sufferers do not even enter into treatment (Goodwin et al., 2002; Sagayadevan et al., 2018). On average, patients with OCD seek therapeutic help when the disorder has become chronic (Skoog & Skoog, 1999).

Some reasons patients have given for the delay are believing that OCD symptoms were just a part of life, experiencing symptoms that waxed and waned over time, and believing they that could or should overcome the symptoms on their own (Poyraz et al., 2015). Those who did seek treatment stated that being supported by others to seek help, hearing about others' experiences of OCD, and having confidence in their health provider provided motivation toward getting help (Robinson, Rose, & Salkovskis, 2017). In one study, half of the subjects interviewed stated that they considered the problem to be temporary (Belloch et al., 2009). In other studies, fluctuation in symptoms, belief that they did not have an illness or that they could take care of it on their own, and experiencing low distress levels were others reasons provided for not seeking help (Erzegovesi et al., 2001; Poyraz et al., 2015). Level of insight also seems to influence whether OCD help was pursued. Those with poor insight into their symptoms would not appear to see the need for treatment, while those with good insight showed a pattern of getting help (Erzegovesi et al., 2001; García-Soriano et al., 2014).

Intervention programs designed to identify early onset OCD are likely to increase referrals to effective treatment and decrease the costs and consequences associated with untreated illness. In addition, educative public health programs aimed at promoting early OCD diagnosis should be disseminated to general practitioners and consideration should be given to translating scientific knowledge into information easily available for the general population, thus increasing the recognition of OCD by the lay public and primary care clinicians (Dell'Osso et al., 2010).

Symptoms of OCD are typically portrayed as washing, cleaning, checking, and arranging. When people's symptoms don't conform to those specific types, they often don't realize that they have a treatable problem and may delay seeking help until their lives become unmanageable. Earlier intervention will result in preventing disruptions in educational, vocational, financial, emotional, relational, social, and general well-being.

Help-Seeking Settings

Where sufferers go for help plays an important role in determining how or whether an OCD diagnosis is made. Lack of awareness on the part of the individual and those from whom they seek help that the struggle stems from a psychiatric problem may contribute to OCD, and it is often left undiagnosed or mistaken for other kinds of psychological problems.

Medical

Uncertainty about where to seek help often leads people to turn to their medical practitioner, especially in males (Doherty & Kartalova-O'Doherty, 2010; Harris et al., 2016). General practitioners, primary care physicians, and pediatricians may not be aware of their patients' suffering (Vuong, Gellatly, Lovell, & Bee, 2016). In addition to lack of patient disclosure of symptoms, OCD may go undiagnosed due to the unlikelihood of physicians screening for it. A very seasoned pediatrician developed a grant-funded website dedicated to addressing and disseminating information about children's emotional issues. He included a page depicting a case of a child with OCD that he had missed diagnosing. The child's parents wrote about their experience, and an OCD expert provided tips on how to recognize the signs of early onset OCD (https://www.cehl.org).

Further, a misdiagnosis may be made because of lack of patient and physician awareness about the nature of the problem, especially since OCD symptoms manifest in so many different forms. Glazier and colleagues (2015) conducted an online survey of physicians from five major medical hospitals, and the results showed that more than half misdiagnosed OCD and, thus, the patients were not referred for treatment.

The most common misdiagnoses made by medical professionals were attention-deficit/hyperactivity disorder, another anxiety disorder, an autism spectrum disorder, depression, or a psychotic disorder (Fenske & Petersen, 2015; Grant, 2014). Altogether, the lost opportunities to make timely and appropriate referrals for treatment cost precious time, decrease quality of life, and lengthen the duration of OCD episodes (Vuong et al., 2016).

Patient fear of the reaction by health professionals contributed to delay in being clinically diagnosed and referred to treatment, especially for sexual and violent obsessions (Robinson et al., 2017). This fear was actually validated in a study of clinicians who responded to vignettes of a friend disclosing certain types of obsessions. The clinicians' attitudes revealed a greater likelihood of social rejection by those with contamination, harming, and sexual obsessions than those with other types of obsessions (Steinberg & Wetterneck, 2017).

People with intrusive harming obsessions reported being afraid of criminalization, being considered a danger, or being judged insane if they disclosed having sexual or violent obsessions (Robinson et al., 2017; Torres et al., 2006; Vuong et al., 2016). People with intrusive thoughts about harming children were reported to disclose their thoughts after reaching a crisis point, not because they realized they had OCD but because they were afraid that they were capable of acting on them and wanted to ensure that children were safe (Vuong et al., 2016).

One study found that most of the 201 African American participants in a focus group reported that they contacted physicians, ministers, and hospitals when experiencing emotional distress. Only 9 percent said that they consulted psychologists, psychiatrists, or community mental health facilities (Thompson, Bazile, & Akbar, 2004). Hispanics and other minorities were also found less likely to visit a specialist in mental health (Gallo, Marino, Ford, & Anthony, 1995).

Clinicians with a good level of awareness, kindness, and understanding can be very important to those seeking help. Validation, sensitivity, and support of patients' experiences leading up to seeking help can help create a safe and trusting environment for effective treatment.

Pastoral/Clergy

People in distress often go to their clergy for support and guidance. For people with OCD, it is unclear if parishioners seek pastoral counseling because they don't know that they have OCD or because they feel guilty or believe they are being punished for something bad or sinful they did, or both. They may have feelings of distrust toward mental health treaters or shame about having mental health challenges due to negative perceptions or stigmatization within their community. Clergy may also be consulted when there is a lack of access to mental health care, when there is a problem with affordability of care, or when people simply do not know where else to turn.

Indeed, one study confirmed that clergy continue to be contacted in higher proportions by people with psychological problems than psychiatrists or general medical doctors (Farrell & Goebert, 2008). Wang and colleagues (2003) reported that nearly one-quarter of those seeking help from clergy have the most seriously impairing mental disorders and yet only seek help from their clergy.

Clergy Efficacy/Preparedness

In a study conducted in an urban African American faith community, ministers reported that people seeking pastoral counseling came by referral from health professionals or were self-referred or that the ministers sought out people they perceived to be struggling (Young, Griffith, & Williams, 2003). The authors also reported that some ministers frequently made referrals to a social worker, hospital emergency services, or a community mental health center. A minority of ministers made direct referrals to pastoral counselors, psychiatrists, psychologists, and institutional chaplains (Young et al., 2003).

A study of Protestants examined how prepared clergy felt to recognize and manage mental health issues within their congregations. The majority of subjects felt they had insufficient training or knowledge about how to recognize mental illness. When a referral was recommended, some clergy felt it was important that the professional share the same religious faith as the parishioner (Farrell & Goebert, 2008).

It is essential that clergy be aware of the OCD scrupulosity and moral subtypes, since people who suffer with these symptoms may not be aware that they are actually experiencing symptoms of a disorder. These types of symptoms are often mistaken as problems of faith, morality, or spirituality due to the content of the obsessions (Shapiro, 2014). People with OCD who have blasphemous, violent, or sexual obsessions may confess them to clergy, who might interpret them as sins to be atoned for or give advice that may be carried out as OCD rituals and not in the spirit of healthy faith practice. When this occurs, sufferers often end up feeling worse about themselves, inadequate, unworthy, and discouraged when the clerical advice did not work.

Positive religious attitudes were found to predict follow-up on the advice given by clergy (Kovess-Masfety et al., 2017). As such, training and collaboration with mental health professionals can better ensure that the most appropriate interventions are delivered (Oppenheimer, Flannelly, & Weaver, 2004). Likewise, clinicians' understanding of patients' religious and faith beliefs may provide more validating support (Farrell & Goebert, 2008).

Psychosocial, Demographic, and Clinical Factors

Race/Ethnicity/Culture/Class/Socioeconomics

Help-seeking behaviors in racial and ethnic minority communities have been examined, and there are several barriers that interfere with utilizing mental health services. For example, the cost of treatment, geographic limitations of access to services, lack of mental health literacy, and cultural differences in health beliefs are some reasons for disparities, inequalities, and underrepresentation in clinical health care settings (Gallo et al., 1995).

One study compared barriers that parents from different ethnic groups face when trying to access specialized OCD services for their children. Several common barriers included a lack of knowledge of OCD, lack of resources, mistrust in the mental health system, previous negative experiences, lack of time and financial challenges, inconvenient location of services, and bullying. Barriers identified by parents from the ethnic minority groups but not by white parents largely consisted of perceived or real attitudes within their communities. Stigma, discrimination, negative attitudes, mistrust of the health care system, and different beliefs about mental health issues were experienced as external factors, while shame and denial were internal experiences of parents that interfered with getting help.

Another study examined reasons for help-seeking avoidance within an African American community. Along with responses similar to those found in the study cited above, others were affordability, impersonal quality of service, lack of cultural understanding and sensitivity, and fear of being stereotyped by the health care clinicians (Thompson et al., 2004).

An international home-based study was conducted that examined the role religious advisors play in mental health care according to disorder severity, sociodemographics, religious involvement, and country income groups. Of the 101,258 people in ten high-income, six upper-middle income, and five low/lower-middle-income countries, 12 percent were found to use religious services. In the low- to lower-middle-income population, it was as much as 30 percent, while 20 percent in some upper-middle-income countries reported their preference in seeking religious resources for help. Attending religious services at least once a week was a strong predictor of religious provider usage, especially when they needed comfort through difficult times (Kovess-Masfety et al., 2017).

Age of Onset

The consequences of early onset and undiagnosed OCD may include disruption in stages of psychosocial development and impact on the potential future success of sufferers. Symptoms can disrupt academics, acquisition of normative social skills, learning future vocational options/opportunities, and possible future earnings, and they can contribute to depression and affect marital/relationship status, familial relatedness, and the overall quality of the life cycle, depending on how much time was lost before getting help (Wang et al., 2012; Watson, 2007).

In general, OCD in childhood or adolescence may hinder normative developmental behaviors that affect social and personal functioning (Fontenelle, Mendlowicz, & Versiani, 2006). Additionally, diagnosing and treating OCD at early ages may have long-term benefits by preventing neurostructural changes as times goes on (Rotge et al., 2009). Unfortunately, there was a longer delay in seeking help for those with early onset of the disorder than those with later onset (Gallo et al., 1995).

Family accommodation of symptoms, such as performing rituals for the child or allowing the household to function around the OCD, may account for a longer duration of untreated illness (Albert et al., 2017). Consequences of these behaviors, other than sustaining or worsening the OCD episode, can result in the breakdown of family relationships and negatively impact the quality of life of those who are directly affected (Peris et al., 2008). Family accommodation is explored more in depth in chapter 9.

Altogether, the lost opportunities to make timely and appropriate referrals for treatment cost precious time, decrease quality of life, and lengthen the duration of OCD episodes.

Psychosocial Functioning and Impact of Symptom Types

Some types of symptoms have been found to affect treatment-seeking behaviors and social activities. On one hand, study findings showed that people with aggressive, harming, and sexual obsessions were compelled to seek treatment because of their high levels of distress (García-Soriano et al., 2014). On the other hand, other studies reported that people with these symptoms avoided seeking help out of fear of what the symptoms might mean about them, fear that the thoughts would be mistaken as posing a danger or threat to others, or shame about just having the thoughts in the first place (Robinson et al., 2017).

Contamination fears and checking behaviors have been found to create more emotional problems, interfere with social functioning, and contribute to poorer physical health (Albert, Maina, Bogetto, Chiarle, & Mataix-Cols, 2010). Contamination, symmetry, and overresponsibility for harm were symptoms identified to interfere with fulfillment of duties and responsibilities in the various roles people play, such as participation in household functioning, enjoyment of leisure activities, social relationships, and physical health (Schwartzman et al., 2017). Generally, people

Table 6.1   Role Interference

	Moderate/Severe %	Severe %
Home management	70	75
Work	37	80
Relationships	44	80
Social life	37	80
Any domain	74	87

Source: Ruscio et al. (2010).

with OCD were more likely to have periods of unemployment or to be underemployed, earn less money, have less participation in social activities, and be unmarried (Sahoo, Sethy, & Ram, 2017).

Table 6.1 shows the different levels of impairment between moderate/severe to severe OCD in home management, work, relationships, social life, and any unspecified domain.

Emotions

Clearly, OCD has an emotional impact on sufferers. One's level of self-esteem, sense of personal identity, level of maturity, range of innate emotional sensitivity, and sense of self-security are characteristics that can contribute to how the sufferer emotionally internalizes having OCD (Abdulkadir et al., 2016). Family, social, and cultural attitudes about mental illness are external cues for how patients may also internalize how they feel about having the disorder. As a result, many OCD sufferers hide their symptoms out of embarrassment, shame, or fear of stigma (García-Soriano et al., 2014).

Sometimes OCD serves as emotional avoidance. One study found the inability to recognize and deal with emotions in 20–40 percent of patients with OCD (De Berardis et al., 2005). OCD may also play a distracting role in people who have experienced a difficult event in their past. A person with OCD may feel overwhelmed when emotions, somatic symptoms, memories, or situations of the event emerge during exposure therapy (Hayes, Wilson, Gifford, Follette, & Strosahl, 1996). Keeping "busy" by performing rituals is an effective way of avoiding the emotions, but it unfortunately maintains the OCD status quo. The literature on the phenomenon is sparse, although it is empirically recognized by experienced OCD treaters that the need to face and experience emotions is a cause of some resistance when patients become stuck in treatment. Patients can become unexpectedly emotionally overwhelmed when their symptoms improve and the protective layer of the OCD starts to peel away (Prasko et al., 2016).

Embarrassment

People with contamination obsessions who perform overt cleaning and washing rituals may avoid being in public and attending social events. Uncertainty about what contaminant might be on anything they touch could trigger urges to wash or clean their hands or perform avoidant behaviors that might look odd to others. Engaging in activities such as playing/attending sports games, going to the mall, being around large crowds of people (i.e., going to concerts or movies, going downtown, taking public transportation), eating out, using public bathrooms, or being in a potentially contaminating situation can cause high levels of anxiety and ruin any sense of enjoyment or pleasure (Schwartzman et al., 2017).

People with overt checking rituals also experience embarrassment by being out in public. Obsessions about the fear of causing harm can complicate tasks such as parking cars, paying for purchases, walking by people (especially children and elders who are perceived to be more vulnerable), and going out to eat (fear of stabbing someone with the knife). People also become embarrassed when their checking or repeating behaviors are performed in public or in situations where they become obvious to others (Weingarden & Renshaw, 2015). Some people may deny that others are observing their rituals, such as checking and repeating, but they are actually noticeable (Brooks, 2011).

Shame

Shame is damaging in interpersonal relationships and motivates social withdrawal (Tangney & Dearing, 2002). It is strongly linked with depression and suicide, and it can be a barrier to treatment (Hastings, Northman, & Tangney, 2000). Shame was found to be stronger predictor of lower quality of life than OCD severity (Singh, Wetterneck, Williams, & Knott, 2016).

Shame about having a mental disorder and feeling the need to hide it are a common reaction for people, as family and social stigma continues to prevail in our culture (Belloch et al., 2009; García-Soriano et al., 2014; Weingarden & Renshaw, 2015). With OCD, it is very difficult for people with fear-of-causing-harm obsessions to cope with the emotional distress they experience. People often feel shame about the content of the obsessions, overidentify with their symptoms, and have trouble finding the motivation to seek help and support (Wheaton, Kellie, & Aditi Sarda, 2016). They often worry about causing shame to their families by admitting that they have a mental disorder, fear that the family may react by trivializing the disorder, and can even have trouble admitting to themselves they have a problem (Stengler-Wenzke et al., 2004; Torres et al., 2007).

Harming obsessions are not the only thoughts that cause shame in people with OCD. Contamination obsessions can cause internal feelings of being impure and shameful. People worry that they are passing this contamination quality along to whatever they touch and to the people who touch those things (Cougle, Lee, Horowitz, Wolitzky-Taylor, & Telch, 2008). These authors also found that higher contamination severity caused some to feel shame from an internal sense of being dirty (Cougle et al., 2008). Fears of contaminating others can also cause health consequences, because of excessive and time-consuming hand washing, cleaning, and checking rituals that can lead to dermatological problems, dental damage, and other hygiene problems (Albert et al., 2010).

Guilt

Healthy guilt serves a purpose. In evolutionary term, prosocial emotions, such as empathy and reciprocal altruism, teach us that when we have done something wrong to another, we must make amends (Trivers, 1971). But just like anything else, OCD turns people's sense of conscience and values against them.

Guilt underlies almost all OCD subtypes and symptoms (Shapiro & Stewart, 2011). A common dialectic for those in treatment is, "If my rituals are protecting the ones I love, giving them up means I am selfish, no longer care about what happens to my loved ones, and I neglected to do whatever I could to prevent harm, but the only way I will get my symptoms under control is if I stop ritualizing." People feel they are trading the safety of others for their own benefit.

Fifteen common themes were identified in a study of guilt in OCD. These consisted of the following:

1. Forbidden thoughts, feelings, and behaviors
2. Hyperresponsibility/omnipotence
3. Conflicts between internal standards and external behaviors

4. Rituals alleviating existing guilt
5. Fear of guilt as a motivating factor in rituals
6. Inadequate justification
7. Being a bad mother/wife
8. Being a bad daughter/son
9. Being a bad friend
10. Interpersonal isolation/alienation
11. Perceived failing of the self
12. Waste
13. Difficulty coping with guilt
14. Clinical improvement and the loss of conscientiousness
15. Emergent reparation (Savoie, 1996)

Obsessive guilt can also be a factor driven by perfectionism and needing to feel "right" (Mancini, Gangemi, Perdighe, & Marini, 2008). Being able to tolerate the uncertainty of having done something wrong or being "bad" can be especially challenging for most people with OCD who go so far out of their way to avoid causing grief to someone.

Stigma

Stigma has been mentioned throughout the chapter as a treatment-interfering emotion in OCD. Not only are people afraid of social stigma about having a disorder, but often they stigmatize themselves and become further demoralized (Belloch et al., 2009; García-Soriano et al., 2014). Another way stigma presents in OCD (and other mental health issues) is the sense of wanting to be normal and fit in. Some people may believe that they are personally flawed because of how they've allowed the OCD to overtake their lives (Murphy & Perera-Delcourt, 2014).

Psychoanalytic theory may have had a role in contributing to the stigmatization of OCD. The psychoanalytic formulation of OCD was that it manifested from repressed sexual or aggressive impulses. These impulses were said to be controlled by the unconscious defense mechanisms of *undoing* and *reaction formation* that served to neutralize the thoughts; in this concept, behaving in the opposite manner to the urges would ensure that they were not acted on (Freud et al., 1953). Emotional consequences of this theory and practice might be feelings of shame and guilt for having normal urges, feeling that they needed repressing in order to live as a morally acceptable person. The topic of stigma is addressed more fully in chapter 10.

Suicidality and Depression

Suicide is contemplated, attempted, or committed by a substantial amount of people with OCD. While early studies found the suicide rate of people with OCD to be rarer compared to other mental health problems (Alonso et al., 2010; Goodwin, Guze, & Robins, 1969; Koran, Thienemann, & Davenport, 1996), recent studies have reported higher incidences (Maina, Salvi, Tiezzi, Albert, & Bogetto, 2007), and it is likely these results are underestimated (Kamath, Reddy, & Kandavel, 2007). It is clear that OCD causes deep suffering that can be a hidden and fatal problem.

Mortality

One report found that 2 percent of all *completed* suicides in the United States, thirty-one thousand, could be attributed to OCD (DuPont, Rice, Shiraki, & Rowland, 1995). Others found the rates of completed suicides to be up to 15 percent (Alonso et al., 2010; Dell'Osso et al., 2010; Fernandez de la Cruz et al., 2017; Maina et al., 2007). A previous suicide attempt was the strongest predictor of committing suicide, and a higher risk of suicide was found in those with a comorbid personality or substance use disorder (Fernandez de la Cruz et al., 2017). International prevalence studies examining the rates of those with OCD considering suicide in the United States, Australia, Brazil, India, Italy, Japan, South Africa, and Spain was 6–36 percent (Alonso et al., 2010; Angelakis, Gooding, Tarrier, & Panagioti, 2015; Brakoulias et al., 2017; Torres et al., 2011).

Suicide attempts were made by 11–59 percent of people with OCD (Brakoulias et al., 2017; Kamath et al., 2007; Torres et al., 2011). As mentioned in the section on emotions, a portion of people with OCD in a severe episode have difficulty experiencing or managing strong emotions, and a suicide attempt may be one way of expressing their deep psychological and emotional pain A suicidal act may, therefore, be a way of expressing an intolerable psychological pain (Albert, De Ronchi, Maina, & Pompili, 2018).

Comorbid depression has been a confirmed predictor of suicidal behavior in OCD (Chaudhary, Kumar, & Mishra, 2016). The Epidemiological Catchment Area (ECA) study found that 32 percent of OCD patients were diagnosed with concurrent comorbid major depressive disorder (MDD) (Regier et al., 1988). The Canadian National Collaborative Group found the rate of lifetime comorbidity of OCD and

MDD to be 60 percent (Weissman et al., 1994). Upward of 75 percent of OCD patients presenting to clinics are experiencing significant primary or secondary depression (Masellis, Rector, & Richter, 2003). It is unclear which of these studies reported rates of depression secondary to having OCD (i.e., the depressive symptoms remit once the OCD is treated), although from analyzing the ECA data, researchers stated that the depression was secondary for most of the study participants (Rasmussen & Eisen, 1989).

There is hardly any discrimination in risk of suicide and OCD symptoms types. Aggressive, philosophical, existential, odd or superstitious obsessions, sexual, religious, cleanliness/contamination, symmetry, ordering, and repeating rituals were associated with severe depression and risk of suicide (Alonso et al., 2010; Chaudhary et al., 2016; Hong et al., 2004; Kamath et al., 2007). Specific risk of suicide rates by symptom types were cleanliness and contamination (57%), religious obsessions (45%), sexual obsessions (33%), repeating rituals (31%), and other obsessions such as need to touch and ask for reassurance (26%; Chaudhary et al., 2016; Kamath et al., 2007) and symmetry/ordering (Alonso et al., 2010).

Clinicians should be aware that suicidal thoughts can be obsessions (Wetterneck, Williams, Tellawi, & Bruce, 2016). People may be afraid that they will act on their thoughts but are not depressed and have no wish to be dead. The thoughts are ego-dystonic, while genuine suicidality is a result of severe depression, planning, and an intent to follow through with the plan. Once the function of the obsessions is understood, these thoughts are treated the same as any other OCD symptom.

Socioeconomic Costs to Society

Reports on the socioeconomic costs of OCD mostly date back to the 1990s and will be assumed to approximate current trends. The World Health Organization identified OCD as the tenth leading cause of disability out of all health conditions in the world (Murray & Lopez, 1996). DuPont and colleagues (1995) provided the following economic statistics from the Epidemiological Catchment Area study of the burden of OCD on society: the total estimated costs of OCD were $8.4 billion, which was 6 percent of the estimated costs of all mental illnesses combined for that year; the estimated 1990 direct costs of OCD to the U.S. economy were $2.1 billion; and the indirect cost, such as lost productivity, was $6.2 billion They also reported that OCD accounted for 6 percent of the

1990 estimated cost of all mental illness based on lost expected future earnings adjusted by age, sex, and expenses incurred by hiring others to perform household and related tasks. Contributing costs, unrelated to treatment, were unemployment, disability, and public assistance (Leon, Portera, & Weissman, 1995).

Levels of Care

The expense of a course of treatment for OCD or per episode or over a lifetime can depend on the level of care required. Patients with sub-clinical or mild range of OCD severity typically do well with weekly outpatient therapy, which is the least costly. People with low severity also experience less disruption in their daily routines, such as work and general functioning.

Others' lives can become so functionally impaired that residential or inpatient level of care becomes necessary, contributing to overall burden of having and treating the disorder. All told, the effect and costs of OCD have been found to be significant.

Ancillary Services

Direct Costs

Although inpatient hospitalization for OCD sufferers is generally not the rule, it does incur an economic burden on society. A 1990 study reported the total costs of OCD were estimated to be $8.4 billion, 6 percent of the estimated costs of all mental illnesses combined for that year of $147.8 billion (DuPont et al., 1995). This study also assessed the indirect costs of OCD, such as lost productivity of individuals suffering from or dying from the disorder, and estimated them at $6.2 billion.

DuPont (1995) reported the breakdown direct costs of OCD as $756 million for specialist institutions, federal and county private psychiatric hospitals, residential treatment, correction facilities, and mental health centers; $120 million on short-stay hospital care; $95 million for physicians; $120 million for professional services such as psychologists and social workers; $791 million for nursing homes; $53 million for medications; and $199 million for net private health insurance. Indirect costs, such as lost days of work or reduced productivity, were $6 billion, and lost earning potential due to suicide was $26 million. Based on these data, the annual direct cost per person with OCD is $820, and the indirect cost is $1,870.

The most recent Epidemiologic Catchment Area study for OCD by the National Institute of Mental Health was also conducted in 1990. The report revealed that of the two hundred forty-eight thousand study participants, 7 percent had at least one inpatient admission. Of those admissions, 36 percent were to general hospitals, 3 percent were to state and county mental hospitals, 10 percent were to residential support units, 11 percent were to private mental hospitals, 21 percent were to Veteran's Affairs hospital psychiatric units, 14 percent were to alcohol and drug treatment, and 1 percent were to nursing homes (Regier et al., 1993).

A consumer-based study was conducted by mailing a questionnaire to members of the Obsessive Compulsive Foundation. There were 710 (27%) members who responded and who were most likely a self-selected sample, having had experienced hospitalization due to OCD. Of those, 25 percent had an inpatient stay, 50 percent had more than one admission, and 10 percent had more than five admissions. The study also calculated that the economic cost per hospitalization was $12,000, and the lifetime hospitalization cost was determined to be $5 billion (Hollander, 1997).

Indirect Costs

High social costs of OCD are also reflected in the high rates of unemployment, disability, and public assistance (Leon et al., 1995). Family members suffer as well for indirect out-of-pocket expenses, such as cleaning and hygiene supplies, hot water bills from long showers, throwing out clothing perceived to be contaminated, and gas spent on going back to locations due to driving hit-and-run obsessions (Singer, 2018). Other social consequences of OCD involve patients' symptoms causing household disruption, disharmony, anger, resentment about demands to participate in rituals, burnout from the burden of dependency, having restricted access to rooms or living space due to the need for control over the household environment, problems with taking holidays and vacations, and interference with work obligations (Boisseau, Schwartzman, & Rasmussen, 2017; Torres et al., 2017).

Needless to say, better dissemination of information about OCD to service professionals, early diagnosis and treatment, and reduction in duration of untreated illness will contribute to lessening the economic burden OCD has on society. Improving access to health care utilization in a timely manner will help minimize how OCD impacts patients and their families' level of reduced productivity and earnings (Greist et al., 2003).

References

Abdulkadir, M., Tischfield, J. A., King, R. A., Fernandez, T. V., Brown, L. W., Cheon, K. A., . . . Dietrich, A. (2016). Pre- and perinatal complications in relation to Tourette syndrome and co-occurring obsessive-compulsive disorder and attention-deficit/hyperactivity disorder. *Journal of Psychiatric Research, 82,* 126–135. doi:10.1016/j.jpsychires.2016.07.017

Albert, U., Baffa, A., & Maina, G. (2017). Family accommodation in adult obsessive-compulsive disorder. *Psychological Research and Behavior Management, 10,* 293–304.

Albert, U., De Ronchi, D., Maina, G., & Pompili, M. (2018). Suicide risk in obsessive-compulsive disorder and exploration of risk factors: A systematic review. *Current Neuropharmacology, 17*(8), 681–696. doi: 10.2174/1570159x16666180620155941

Albert, U., Maina, G., Bogetto, F., Chiarle, A., & Mataix-Cols, D. (2010). Clinical predictors of health-related quality of life in obsessive-compulsive disorder. *Comprehensive Psychiatry, 51*(2), 193–200. doi:10.1016/j.comppsych.2009.03.004

Alonso, P., Segalas, C., Real, E., Pertusa, A., Labad, J., Jiménez-Murcia, S., . . . Menchón, J. (2010). Suicide in patients treated for obsessive-compulsive disorder: A prospective follow-up study. *Journal of Affective Disorders, 124*(3), 300–308.

Angelakis, I., Gooding, P., Tarrier, N., & Panagioti, M. (2015). Suicidality in obsessive compulsive disorder (OCD): A systematic review and meta-analysis. *Clinical Psychology Review, 39,* 1–15.

Asnaani, A., Kaczkurkin, A. N., Alpert, E., McLean, C. P., Simpson, H. B., & Foa, E. B. (2017). The effect of treatment on quality of life and functioning in OCD. *Comprehensive Psychiatry, 73,* 7–14. doi:10.1016/j.comppsych.2016.10.004

Belloch, A., Del Valle, G., Morillo, C., Carrió, C., & Cabedo, E. (2009). To seek advice or not to seek advice about the problem: The help-seeking dilemma for obsessive-compulsive disorder. *Social Psychiatry and Psychiatric Epidemiology, 44*(4), 257–264. doi:10.1007/s00127-008-0423-0

Boisseau, C. L., Schwartzman, C. M., & Rasmussen, S. A. (2017). Quality of life and psychosocial functioning in OCD. In C. Pittenger (Ed.), *Obsessive-compulsive disorder: Phenomenology, pathophysiology, and treatment* (pp. 57–64). New York: Oxford University Press.

Brakoulias, V., Starcevic, V., Belloch, A., Brown, C., Ferrao, Y. A., Fontenelle, L. F., . . . Viswasam, K. (2017). Comorbidity, age of onset and suicidality in obsessive-compulsive disorder (OCD): An international collaboration. *Comprehensive Psychiatry, 76,* 79–86. doi:10.1016/j .comppsych.2017.04.002

Brooks, C. F. (2011). Social performance and secret ritual: Battling against obsessive-compulsive disorder. *Qualitative Health Research, 21*(2), 249–261.

Chaudhary, R. K., Kumar, P., & Mishra, B. P. (2016). Depression and risk of suicide in patients with obsessive-compulsive disorder: A hospital-based study. *Industrial Psychiatry Journal, 25*(2), 166–170. doi:10.4103/ipj.ipj_63_16

Cougle, J., Lee, H., Horowitz, J., Wolitzky-Taylor, K., & Telch, M. (2008). An exploration of the relationship between mental pollution and OCD symptoms. *Journal of Behavior Therapy and Experimental Psychiatry, 39*(3), 340–353. doi:S0005-7916(07)00052-3 [pii]10.1016/j .jbtep.2007.08.007

De Berardis, D., Campanella, D., Gambi, F., Sepede, G., Salini, G., Carano, A., . . . Ferro, F. M. (2005). Insight and alexithymia in adult outpatients with obsessive-compulsive disorder. *European Archives of Psychiatry and Clinical Neuroscience, 255*(5), 350–358. doi:10.1007 /s00406-005-0573-y

Dell'Osso, B., Buoli, M., Hollander, E., & Altamura, A. C. (2010). Duration of untreated illness as a predictor of treatment response and remission in obsessive-compulsive disorder. *World Journal of Biological Psychiatry, 11*(1), 59–65. doi:10.3109/15622970903418544

Doherty, T. D., & Kartalova-O'Doherty, Y. (2010). Gender and self-reported mental health problems: Predictors of help seeking from a general practitioner. *British Journal of Health Psychology, 15*(Pt 1), 213–228. doi:10.1348/135910709X457423

DuPont, R. L., Rice, D. P., Shiraki, S., & Rowland, C. R. (1995). Economic costs of obsessive-compulsive disorder. *Medical Interface, 8*(4), 102–109. Retrieved from https://www.ncbi.nlm.nih.gov/pubmed /10141765

Erzegovesi, S., Cavellini, M. C., Cavedini, P., Diaferia, G., Locatelli, M., & Bellodi, L. (2001). Clinical predictors of drug response in obsessive compulsive disorder. *Journal of Clinical Psychopharmacology, 21,* 272–275.

Farrell, J. L., & Goebert, D. A. (2008). Collaboration between psychiatrists and clergy in recognizing and treating serious mental illness. *Psychiatric Services, 59*(4), 437–440. doi:10.1176/ps.2008.59.4.437

Fenske, J. N., & Petersen, K. (2015). Obsessive-compulsive disorder: Diagnosis and management. *American Family Physician, 92*(10),

896–903. Retrieved from https://www.ncbi.nlm.nih.gov/pubmed/265 54283

Fernandez de la Cruz, L., Rydell, M., Runeson, B., D'Onofrio, B. M., Brander, G., Ruck, C., . . . Mataix-Cols, D. (2017). Suicide in obsessive-compulsive disorder: A population-based study of 36,788 Swedish patients. *Molecular Psychiatry, 22*(11), 1626–1632. doi:10 .1038/mp.2016.115

Fineberg, N. A., Dell'Osso, B., Albert, U., Maina, G., Geller, D., Carmi, L., . . . Zohar, J. (2019). Early intervention for obsessive compulsive disorder: An expert consensus statement. *European Neuropsychopharmacology, 13*(51), 1–17. doi:10.1016/j.euroneuro.2019.02.002

Fontenelle, L. F., Mendlowicz, M. V., & Versiani, M. (2006). The descriptive epidemiology of obsessive-compulsive disorder. *Progress in Neuro-Psychopharmacology & Biological Psychiatry, 30*(3), 327–337. doi:10.1016/j.pnpbp.2005.11.001

Freud, S., Strachey, J., Freud, A., Rothgeb, C. L., & Richards, A. (1953). *The standard edition of the complete psychological works of Sigmund Freud.* London: Hogarth Press.

Gallo, J. J., Marino, S., Ford, D., & Anthony, J. C. (1995). Filters on the pathway to mental health care, II. Sociodemographic factors. *Psychological Medicine, 25*(6), 1149–1160.

García-Soriano, G., Rufer, M., Delsignore, A., & Weidt, S. (2014). Factors associated with non-treatment or delayed treatment seeking in OCD sufferers: A review of the literature. *Psychiatry Research, 220* (1–2), 1–10. doi:10.1016/j.psychres.2014.07.009

Glazier, K., Swing, M., & McGinn, L. K. (2015). Half of obsessive-compulsive disorder cases misdiagnosed: Vignette-based survey of primary care physicians. *Journal of Clinical Psychiatry, 76*(6), e761–767. doi:10.4088/JCP.14m09110

Goodwin, D., Guze, S. B., & Robins, E. (1969). Follow-up studies in obsessional neurosis. *JAMA Psychiatry, 20*(2), 182–187. doi:10.1001 /archpsyc.1969.01740140054006

Goodwin, R., Koenen, K. C., Hellman, F., Guardino, M., & Struening, E. (2002). Help seeking and access to mental health treatment for obsessive-compulsive disorder. *Acta Psychiatrica Scandinavica, 106*(2), 143–149. doi:10.1034/j.1600-0447.2002.01221.x

Grabe, H. J., Meyer, C., Hapke, U., Rumpf, H.-J., Freyberger, H. J., Dilling, H., & John, U. (2001). Lifetime-comorbidity of obsessive-compulsive disorder and subclinical obsessive-compulsive disorder in northern Germany. *European Archives of Psychiatry and Clinical Neuroscience, 251*(3), 130–135. doi:10.1007/s004060170047

Grant, J. E. (2014). Clinical practice: Obsessive-compulsive disorder. *New England Journal of Medicine, 14*(371), 646–653. doi: 10.1056 /NEJMcp1402176

Greist, J. H., Bandelow, B., Hollander, E., Marazziti, D., Montgomery, S. A., Nutt, D. J., . . . Zohar, J. (2003). WCA recommendations for the long-term treatment of obsessive-compulsive disorder in adults. *CNS Spectrums, 8*(8 Suppl 1), 7–16.

Harris, M. G., Baxter, A. J., Reavley, N., Diminic, S., Pirkis, J., & Whiteford, H. A. (2016). Gender-related patterns and determinants of recent help-seeking for past-year affective, anxiety and substance use disorders: Findings from a national epidemiological survey. *Epidemiology and Psychiatric Sciences, 25*(6), 548–561. doi:10.1017 /S2045796015000876

Hastings, M. E., Northman, L. M., & Tangney, J. (2000). Shame, Guilt, and Suicide. In T. Joiner & D. Rudd (Eds.), *Suicide science: Expanding the boundaries,* 67–79. New York: Springer Press.

Hayes, S. C., Wilson, K. G., Gifford, E. V., Follette, V. M., & Strosahl, K. (1996). Experiential avoidance and behavioral disorders: A functional dimensional approach to diagnosis and treatment. *Journal of Consulting and Clinical Psychology, 64*(6), 1152.

Hollander, E. (1997). Obsessive-compulsive disorder: The hidden epidemic. *Journal of Clinical Psychiatry, 58*(Suppl 12), 3–6. Retrieved from https://www.ncbi.nlm.nih.gov/pubmed/9393389

Hong, J. P., Samuels, J., Bienvenu, O. J., III, Cannistraro, P., Grados, M., Riddle, M. A., . . . Nestadt, G. (2004). Clinical correlates of recurrent major depression in obsessive-compulsive disorder. *Depression and Anxiety, 20*(2), 86–91. doi:10.1002/da.20024

Hou, S.-Y., Yen, C.-F., Huang, M.-F., Wang, P.-W., & Yeh, Y.-C. (2010). Quality of life and its correlates in patients with obsessive-compulsive disorder. *Kaohsiung Journal of Medical Sciences, 26,* 397–407.

Jacoby, R. J., Leonard, R. C., Riemann, B. C., & Abramowitz, J. S. (2014). Predictors of quality of life and functional impairment in obsessive-compulsive disorder. *Comprehensive Psychiatry, 55*(5), 1195–1202. doi:10.1016/j.comppsych.2014.03.011

Kamath, P., Reddy, Y. C., & Kandavel, T. (2007). Suicidal behavior in obsessive-compulsive disorder. *Journal of Clinical Psychiatry, 68*(11), 1741–1750.

Koran, L. M., Thienemann, M. L., & Davenport, R. (1996). Quality of life for patients with obsessive-compulsive disorder. *American Journal of Psychiatry, 153*(6), 783–788. doi:10.1176/ajp.153.6.783

Kovess-Masfety, V., Evans-Lacko, S., Williams, D., Andrade, L. H., Benjet, C., Ten Have, M., . . . Gureje, O. (2017). The role of religious advisors in mental health care in the World Mental Health surveys. *Social Psychiatry and Psychiatric Epidemiology, 52*(3), 353–367. doi:10.1007/s00127-016-1290-8

Leon, A. C., Portera, L., & Weissman, M. M. (1995). The social costs of anxiety disorders. *British Journal of Psychiatry Supplement* (27), 19–22. Retrieved from https://www.ncbi.nlm.nih.gov/pubmed/7794589

Maina, G., Salvi, V., Tiezzi, M. N., Albert, U., & Bogetto, F. (2007). Is OCD at risk for suicide?: A case-control study. *Clinical Neuropsychiatry, 3*, 117–121.

Mancini, F., Gangemi, A., Perdighe, C., & Marini, C. (2008). Not just right experience: Is it influenced by feelings of guilt? *Journal of Behavior Therapy and Experimental Psychiatry, 39*(2), 162–176. doi: 10.1016/j.jbtep.2007.02.002.

Masellis, M., Rector, N. A., & Richter, M. A. (2003). Quality of life in OCD: Differential impact of obsessions, compulsions, and depression comorbidity. *Canadian Journal of Psychiatry, 48*(2), 72–77.

Murphy, H., & Perera-Delcourt, R. (2014). "Learning to live with OCD is a little mantra I often repeat": Understanding the lived experience of obsessive-compulsive disorder (OCD) in the contemporary therapeutic context. *Psychology and Psychotherapy, 87*(1), 111–125. doi:10.1111/j.2044-8341.2012.02076.x

Murray, C. J., & Lopez, A. D. (1996). The global burden of disease: A comprehensive assessment of mortality and disability from diseases, injuries, and risk factors in 1990 and projected to 2020. Cambridge, MA: Harvard University Press.

Oppenheimer, J. E., Flannelly, K. J., & Weaver, A. J. (2004). A comparative analysis of the psychological literature on collaboration between clergy and mental-health professionals—perspectives from secular and religious journals: 1970–1999. *Pastoral Psychology, 53*(2), 153–162.

Peris, T. S., Bergman, R. L., Langley, A., Chang, S., McCracken, J. T., & Piacentini, J. (2008). Correlates of accommodation of pediatric obsessive-compulsive disorder: Parent, child, and family characteristics. *Journal of the American Academy of Child and Adolescent Psychiatry, 47*(10), 1173–1181. doi:10.1097/CHI.0b013e3181825a91

Poyraz, C. A., Turan, ş., Sağlam, N. G., Batun, G., Yassa, A., & Duran, A. (2015). Factors associated with the duration of untreated illness among patients with obsessive compulsive disorder. *Comprehensive Psychiatry, 58*, 88–93. doi:10.1016/j.comppsych.2014.12.019

Prasko, J., Hruby, R., Ociskova, M., Holubova, M., Latalova, K., Marackova, M., . . . Vyskocilova, J. (2016). Unmet needs of the patients with obsessive-compulsive disorder. *Neuroendocrinology Letters, 37*(5), 373–382.

Rasmussen, S. A., & Eisen, J. L. (1989). Clinical features and phenomenology of obsessive compulsive disorder. *Psychiatric Annals, 19*(2), 67–73.

Regier, D. A., Boyd, J. H., Burke, J. D., Jr., Rae, D. S., Myers, J. K., Kramer, M., . . . Locke, B. Z. (1988). One-month prevalence of mental disorders in the United States. Based on five epidemiologic catchment area sites. *Archives of General Psychiatry, 45*(11), 977–986.

Regier, D. A., Narrow, W., Rae, D., Manderscheid, R., Locke, B., & Goodwin, F. (1993). The de facto US mental and addictive disorders service system: Epidemiologic catchment area prospective 1-year prevalence rates of disorders and services. *Archives of General Psychiatry, 50*, 85–94.

Robinson, K. J., Rose, D., & Salkovskis, P. M. (2017). Seeking help for obsessive compulsive disorder (OCD): A qualitative study of the enablers and barriers conducted by a researcher with personal experience of OCD. *Psychology and Psychotherapy, 90*(2), 193–211. doi:10.1111/papt.12090

Rotge, J. Y., Guehl, D., Dilharreguy, B., Tignol, J., Bioulac, B., Allard, M., . . . Aouizerate, B. (2009). Meta-analysis of brain volume changes in obsessive-compulsive disorder. *Biological Psychiatry, 65*(1), 75–83. doi:10.1016/j.biopsych.2008.06.019

Ruscio, A. M., Stein, D. J., Chiu, W. T., & Kessler, R. C. (2010). The epidemiology of obsessive-compulsive disorder in the National Comorbidity Survey Replication. *Molecular Psychiatry, 15*(1), 53–63. Retrieved from http://dx.doi.org/10.1038/mp.2008.94

Sagayadevan, V., Lee, S. P., Ong, C., Abdin, E., Chong, S. A., & Subramaniam, M. (2018). Quality of life across mental disorders in psychiatric outpatients. *Annals of the Academy of Medicine Singapore, 47*(7), 243–252. Retrieved from https://www.ncbi.nlm.nih.gov/pubmed/30120432

Sahoo, P., Sethy, R. R., & Ram, D. (2017). Functional impairment and quality of life in patients with obsessive compulsive disorder. *Indian Journal of Psychological Medicine, 39*(6), 760–765. doi:10.4103/IJPSYM.IJPSYM_53_17

Savoie, D. (1996). A phenomenological investigation of the role of guilt in obsessive-compulsive disorder. *Journal of Phenomenological Psychology, 27*(2), 193–218.

Schwartzman, C. M., Boisseau, C. L., Sibrava, N. J., Mancebo, M. C., Eisen, J. L., & Rasmussen, S. A. (2017). Symptom subtype and quality of life in obsessive-compulsive disorder. *Psychiatry Research, 249,* 307–310. doi:10.1016/j.psychres.2017.01.025

Shapiro, L. J. (2014). Understanding OCD: Skills to control the conscience and outsmart obsessive compulsive disorder. Santa Barbara, CA: Praeger.

Shapiro, L. J., & Stewart, S. E. (2011). Pathological guilt: A persistent yet overlooked factor in obsessive compulsive disorder. *Annals of Clinical Psychiatry, 23*(1), 63–70.

Singer, J. (2018). The cost of OCD—And yes, I'm talking about money. PsychCentral. Retrieved from https://psychcentral.com/blog/the-cost-of-ocd-and-yes-im-talking-about-money/

Singh, S., Wetterneck, C. T., Williams, M. T., & Knott, L. E. (2016). The role of shame and symptom severity on quality of life in obsessive-compulsive and related disorders. *Journal of Obsessive-Compulsive and Related Disorders, 11,* 49–55. doi:https://doi.org/10.1016/j.jocrd.2016.08.004

Skoog, G., & Skoog, I. (1999). A 40-year follow-up of patients with obsessive-compulsive disorder [see comments]. *Archives of General Psychiatry, 56*(2), 121–127. Retrieved from https://www.ncbi.nlm.nih.gov/pubmed/10025435

Steinberg, D. S., & Wetterneck, C. T. (2017). OCD taboo thoughts and stigmatizing attitudes in clinicians. *Community Mental Health Journal, 53*(3), 275–280. doi:10.1007/s10597-016-0055-x

Stengler-Wenzke, K., Trosbach, J., Dietrich, S., & Angermeyer, M. C. (2004). Experience of stigmatization by relatives of patients with obsessive compulsive disorder. *Archives of Psychiatric Nursing, 18*(3), 88–96. Retrieved from https://www.ncbi.nlm.nih.gov/pubmed/15199536

Tangney, J. P., & Dearing, R. L. (2002). *Shame and guilt.* New York: Guilford.

Theofilou, P. (2013). Quality of life: Definition and measurement. *Europe's Journal of Psychology, 9,* 150–162.

Thompson, V. L. S., Bazile, A., & Akbar, M. (2004). African Americans' perceptions of psychotherapy and psychotherapists. *Professional Psychology: Research and Practice, 35*(1), 19.

Torres, A. R., Fontanelle, L. F., Shavitt, R. G., Hoexter, M. Q., Pittenger, C., & Miguel, E. C. (2017). Epidemiology, comorbidity, and burden of OCD. In C. Pittenger (Ed.), *Obsessive-compulsive disorder: Phenomenology, pathophysiology, and treatment* (1st ed., pp. 35–46). New York: Oxford University Press.

Torres, A. R., Prince, M. J., Bebbington, P. E., Bhugra, D., Brugha, T. S., Farrell, M., . . . Singleton, N. (2006). Obsessive-compulsive disorder: Prevalence, comorbidity, impact, and help-seeking in the British National Psychiatric Morbidity Survey of 2000. *American Journal of Psychiatry, 163*(11), 1978–1985.

Torres, A. R., Prince, M. J., Bebbington, P. E., Bhugra, D. K., Brugha, T. S., Farrell, M., . . . Singleton, N. (2007). Treatment seeking by individuals with obsessive-compulsive disorder from the British Psychiatric Morbidity Survey of 2000. *Psychiatric Services, 58*(7), 977–982. doi:10.1176/ps.2007.58.7.977

Torres, A. R., Ramos-Cerqueira, A. T., Ferrao, Y. A., Fontenelle, L. F., do Rosario, M. C., & Miguel, E. C. (2011). Suicidality in obsessive-compulsive disorder: Prevalence and relation to symptom dimensions and comorbid conditions. *Journal of Clinical Psychiatry, 72*(1), 17–26; quiz 119–120. doi:10.4088/JCP.09m05651blu

Trivers, R. L. (1971). The evolution of reciprocal altruism. *Quarterly Review of Biology, 46, 35–57.*

Velloso, P., Piccinato, C., Ferrão, Y., Perin, E. A., Cesar, R., Fontenelle, L. F., . . . do Rosário, M. C. (2018). Clinical predictors of quality of life in a large sample of adult obsessive-compulsive disorder outpatients. *Comprehensive Psychiatry, 86,* 82–90. doi:10.1016/j.comppsych.2018.07.007

Vuong, T. M., Gellatly, J., Lovell, K., & Bee, P. (2016). The experiences of help-seeking in people with obsessive compulsive disorder: An internet study. *Cognitive Behaviour Therapist, 9.*

Wang, P. S., Berglund, P. A., & Kessler, R. C. (2003). Patterns and correlates of contacting clergy for mental disorders in the United States. *Health Services Research, 38*(2), 647–673. doi: 10.1111/1475-6773.00138

Wang, X., Cui, D., Wang, Z., Fan, Q., Xu, H., Qiu, J., . . . Xiao, Z. (2012). Cross-sectional comparison of the clinical characteristics of adults with early-onset and late-onset obsessive compulsive disorder. *Journal of Affective Disorders, 136*(3), 498–504. doi:10.1016/j.jad.2011.11.001

Watson, H. J. (2007). *Clinical and research developments in the treatment of paediatric obsessive-compulsive disorder* (Doctoral dissertation). Curtin University, Bentley and Perth, Australia.

Weingarden, H., & Renshaw, K. D. (2015). Shame in the obsessive compulsive related disorders: A conceptual review. *Journal of Affective Disorders, 171,* 74–84. doi:10.1016/j.jad.2014.09.010

Weissman, M., Bland, R., Canino, G., Greenwald, S., Hwu, H., Lee, C., . . . Wickramaratne, P. (1994). The cross national epidemiology of obsessive compulsive disorder: The Cross National Collaborative Group. *Journal of Clinical Psychiatry, 55* (Suppl), 5–10.

Wetterneck, C. T., Williams, M. T., Tellawi, G., & Bruce, S. L. (2016). Treatment of suicide obsessions in obsessive-compulsive disorder with comorbid major depressive disorder. In E. A. Storch & A. B. Lewin (Eds.), *Clinical handbook of obsessive-compulsive and related disorders: A case-based approach to treating pediatric and adult populations* (pp. 431–445). Cham, Switzerland: Springer.

Wheaton, M. G., Kellie, L. S., & Aditi Sarda, M. (2016). Self-concealment in obsessive-compulsive disorder: Associations with symptom dimensions, help seeking attitudes, and treatment expectancy. *Journal of Obsessive-Compulsive and Related Disorders, 11*, 43–48. doi:http://dx.doi.org/10.1016/j.jocrd.2016.08.002

Young, J. L., Griffith, E. E. H., & Williams, D. R. (2003). The integral role of pastoral counseling by African-American clergy in community mental health. *Psychiatric Services, 54*(5), 688–692. doi:10.1176/appi.ps.54.5.688

CHAPTER 7

Assessment and Treatment

A thorough assessment of OCD symptoms is worth doing in order to ensure that the treatment plan effectively targets overt and covert symptoms. It is essential to know the patient's feared consequences of not ritualizing so that the exposure specifically targets them. One person's fear about being contaminated might be causing others to become sick, while another's could be becoming sick herself. Patients can fill out assessment measures ahead of time in order to have more time for treatment planning in the therapy session. There are several other important psychological considerations to have in mind during the assessment process.

Issues to Consider during OCD Assessment

Psychological Factors

Even though OCD symptoms are ego-dystonic and do not fit within a sufferer's value system, individuals with OCD are self-judgmental, self-critical, and self-stigmatizing. They experience shame and feelings of guilt because they believe that the content of their negative intrusive thoughts, images, or impulses reflects unacceptable aspects of their character (Shapiro, 2014). In turn, they associate the performance of rituals as demonstrations of morality, virtue, and caring, which only reinforces the cycle of OCD.

The dichotomous nature of OCD sets up all/nothing, good/bad, right/wrong, and black/white psychological binds, or no-win situations, because sight is lost about the gray area. Patients do not identify with their obsessions yet experience them as real and distressing. This typically results in distress and doubts about the valued aspects of self-identity. Dialects and self-ambivalence are other ways of understanding the OCD paradox. A dialectic is being able to hold two differing concepts at the same time (Chapman, 2006), and self-ambivalence reflects a person's experience of having dichotomous and conflicting beliefs about self-worth, virtue, and value that impairs the sense of lovability and social acceptance (Bhar, Kyrios, & Hordern, 2015).

Awareness of certain personality traits may be useful, since they have been found to be positively related to certain OCD symptom dimensions. Obsessive compulsive personality disorder was described in chapter 3, but subclinical obsessive-compulsive personality traits, such as ordering and checking, may have an affective-motivational underpinning that may undermine the treatment process (Ecker, Kupfer, & Gönner, 2014). A study of OCD patients with comorbid cluster C personality disorders (anxious and fearful) reported that responsibility for harm, injury, or bad luck symptoms were significantly greater than other OCD symptom dimensions (Bulli, Melli, Cavalletti, Stopani, & Carraresi, 2016).

Post-Traumatic Stress Disorder/Trauma

It has been suggested that OCD and post-traumatic stress disorder (PTSD) lie on the same anxiety-fear continuum, based on the recurrent and intrusive thoughts experienced in both disorders (Gershuny, Baer, Radomsky, Wilson, & Jenike, 2003). OCD prevalence in people with traumatic life events was reported to be 30–82 percent (Cromer, Schmidt, & Murphy, 2007). It is unclear why the range is so broad.

Successful treatment outcome in patients with PTSD and contamination OCD may rely on the readiness or willingness to disclose the traumatic event during the assessment process (Dykshoorn, 2014). It has been found that treating one disorder may result in precipitating the other. Clinicians should provide psychoeducation about the role OCD may have served in protecting the patient from (re)experiencing the effect of PTSD or trauma (Gershuny et al., 2003).

Another important characteristic common to both disorders is the psychological and physiological disgust response in the face of traumatic and OCD triggers. Traumatic physical abuse may manifest as an OCD self-contamination symptom, compelling the person to perform excessive hand washing, showering, cleaning, or avoidant behaviors in order to feel emotionally clean (Badour, Bown, Adams, Bunaciu, & Feldner, 2012).

Cross-Cultural Factors

Every culture has its own norms for social order that may seem different but serve the same purpose. Eating with hands or making direct eye contact might be considered rude in one culture but a way of life in another. Making direct eye contact may be considered aggressive in one society or a way of making a connection somewhere else.

Similarly, the nature of obsessions and compulsions appear to have consistent themes regardless of geography, but they manifest according to local cultural or religious norms (Clark & Inozu, 2014; Esfahani, Motaghipour, Kamkari, Zahiredin, & Janbozorgi, 2012). People from different cultures and religions may have the same metaphysical fears (fear of offending and being cursed by God, not being sincere enough in practicing their faith) and similar symbolic elements of ritual practice (prayer, fasting, etc.), but they may be carried out differently according to the religious and cultural traditions of the group.

For example, the use of water is a common element in purification. Oestigaard (2017) describes the following uses of water. Muslims use it for purification prior to their five daily prayers. Hindus wash their hands and feet prior to entering the place of worship. Jews have a ritualized hand wash before meals that that is performed three times, as well as a monthly ritual purification bath (mikveh) women undergo after their menses, and Catholics dip their fingers in holy font water and make the sign of the cross on themselves prior to sitting in the pews (2017). It is easy to see how people with religious scrupulosity and contamination OCD use water excessively to purify and decontaminate their souls.

Superstitious beliefs serve a similar purpose in that, like religion, people seek metaphysical answers to events that seem random or try to placate supernatural forces to prevent negative events beyond human control (Shapiro, 2014). These irrational cultural superstitious beliefs and practices are magnified by OCD and are transformed into more rigid rules and behaviors. Examples include seeing the "unlucky" number thirteen and then performing an undoing ritual such as adding the unlucky numbers one and three together, which becomes a "lucky" number four. The person then might count in multiples of fours until the bad luck feeling goes away. The childhood superstition of "step on a crack and break your mother's back" can cause someone to look down while walking in order to avoid stepping on them, then go back to where the triggering crack was, and walk around it until the bad luck feeling had been undone.

Family History

We often assume that a person has had a normal baseline to use as a reference to life before OCD. However, early onset OCD may preclude normal development (Derisley, 2008), or being raised by a parent with untreated OCD may condition ritualistic behaviors in children by normalizing OCD rules in the home environment (Chacon et al., 2018).

Studies show that the rates of OCD and subthreshold obsessive compulsive disorder were significantly greater among the relatives of the patients with OCD at 7–16 percent (Nestadt et al., 2000; Skriner et al., 2016). Further, family history of OCD was associated with greater severity and a longer duration of illness (Arumugham et al., 2014).

Motivation

Because behavior therapy for OCD requires patients to confront their feared situations without ritualizing, readiness for change should be addressed in order to get a sense of how compliant the patient will be in treatment. Consider the following issues while assessing patients' motivation:

- What measurable goals does the patient have that he or she is willing to work hard to achieve?
- Is the patient presenting in treatment for him or herself or for the sake of a loved one? Some patients are pressured by those affected by the OCD, and their insight and motivation may likely be very limited or nonexistent. If patients are motivated by others, see if there are specific symptoms they are willing to work on for the sake of their relationships rather than convincing them that they are the source of the problem.
- Does the patient use emotional avoidance as a coping strategy? Some people get caught up in their symptoms as a way of distracting themselves from difficult emotions or problems.

Insight

Insight is the extent to which someone believes the intrusive thoughts or obsessions to be unreasonable. Insight is considered neither absent nor present, but is based on a range (Markova & Berrios, 1992). Figure 7.1 displays the range and types of insight. For the most part, sufferers know that the behaviors or mental rituals are not associated in a rational way with what they are designed to "fix" and are clearly excessive. They do not expect other people to react to the obsessive trigger in the same manner.

For example, people drive over bumps in the road without much realization or thought, but when Stan drives over a bump, he experiences a surge of anxiety because he thinks he might have hit someone with his car. As a result, he feels compelled to drive back to where he thinks the bump was to make sure nothing happened. The problem with OCD is that a nonevent can't be verified or proven, and the person is left with obsessive uncertainty and symptoms of physiological distress. People with poor insight are considered to have overvalued ideas, meaning that they have a stronger belief that their obsessions are more real or true than people with better insight.

Rational	Worry	Rumination	Obsession	Overvalued Ideas	Delusion

$\longrightarrow$

Figure 7.1   Range of Insight

Rational thoughts are realistic, and the majority of people would agree with your belief about the possibility and probability of a particular outcome. If the sky is dark and overcast, we likely all agree that rain is coming. We might not know how much or for how long, but we know that we should take an umbrella if we don't want to get wet.

Worry thoughts are normal, insightful, and controllable, but they can be somewhat preoccupying. Some people believe that a state of worry means they are on top of things in a somewhat superstitious way: "If I think about all the worst-case scenarios, then I'll be prepared." In getting ready for public speaking, people might try to anticipate what could go wrong as a way to be ready for that eventuality. There is nothing wrong with that strategy until the worrying interferes with their confidence and they start to psych themselves out.

Ruminations are more intense than worry thoughts; they are preoccupying and interfere with one's ability to concentrate or focus. Persistent worry thoughts and ruminations about "real life" concerns (money, health, making good judgments and decisions) may be indicative of generalized anxiety disorder (GAD). Other symptoms of GAD might include fatigue, irritability, problems falling or staying asleep, sleep that is often restless and unsatisfying, restlessness, and often becoming startled very easily. Physical problems may consist of muscle tension, shakiness, headaches, and digestive problems. Ruminations can cause paralysis in decision-making, as the anxiety begins to override the ability to make the "right" decision. A good course of cognitive behavior therapy will help reduce these symptoms.

Obsessions are always-negative and often-taboo thoughts that spike anxiety and cannot be controlled. People with OCD and excellent insight will say that they know the thoughts are irrational and that they need not be pushed away. Someone with good insight believes this about 80–95 percent. Fair insight means the person believes that the thoughts are realistic and are less flexible to change. The person is less willing to take the rational risk by doing the opposite of the obsession, which is what exposure therapy entails.

Overvalued ideation (OVI) is poor insight. People can agree that how you describe the excessiveness of their beliefs make sense but cannot do this on their own; "patients who were extremely certain that their feared consequences would occur evidenced poorer outcome [with exposure/response therapy] than patients with mild or moderate certainty, despite the reduction of such certainty at post-test" (Foa, Abramowitz, Franklin, & Kozak, 1999). A high-functioning attorney with whom I have worked for many years will not forego excessive checking in his practice because he fears uncertainty will or can lead to catastrophic outcomes for his clients. His work takes three times longer than his colleagues, and he is always behind. The intention of therapy is not to cause carelessness but to encourage patients to accept that perfection is an ideal, not a goal. Achieving that "right" feeling is transitory and does not actually produce a better product.

Magical ideation is an irrational belief that things unrelated to each other have a cause and effect relationship (Rosengren & French, 2013). It predicts OCD symptom dimensions of contamination concerns and cleaning/washing compulsions; unacceptable violent, religious, and sexual obsessions and related compulsions; and symmetry obsessions and ordering compulsions (Spears, 2014). Almost all obsessions could be understood in this way, but some obsessions make more sense than others. A person with contamination obsessions knows that germs are spread through airborne particles or touching surfaces and that hand washing helps prevent transmitting illness. On the other hand, someone with magical ideation may believe that seeing the color red, which represents blood, requires hand washing because of the association that person makes between the color and the feared consequence of contamination.

Patients with delusional beliefs have zero insight and fully believe that they are realistic. Common delusions are believing that a cabal is after you because you have special information or power, or that you are the messiah God sent to save the world. One might wonder, though, if we would recognize a messiah or prescribe medication for that individual.

Willingness to Accept Negative Internal
Experiences and Emotions

Willingness is a clinical marker of acceptance in engaging in distressing tasks. In OCD treatment, adhering to assigned exposures is associated with improved outcomes despite the presence of unpleasant and unwanted thoughts, emotions, and bodily sensations (Wheaton et al., 2016). Data shows that more willingness right before and during the exposure session as well as a willingness to engage in future exposures were associated with faster symptom reduction during six weeks of residential-level exposure therapy for adults with severe OCD.

Ways of addressing willingness prior to beginning treatment are the following:

- Providing psychoeducation about how behavioral treatment for OCD requires fully facing the obsessive fear without deliberate avoidance or neutralizing behaviors, both mentally and physically
- Asking how willing the person is to experience high levels of distress during treatment in order to experience symptom relief later

Patients may not actually know ahead of time, so it might be helpful to ask how they have managed challenging situations aside from their OCD. Since most people have undergone difficulties or feared situations, learning how they managed them can provide useful data about their ability to withstand levels of distress. An example might be how they persevered through personal challenges, so consider asking if they persevered through learning a sport, musical instrument, socializing, and so on. Many people with OCD are triggered by negative experiences, such as bad or unpleasant feelings, anger, sadness, and fear (Li, Bai, & Wang, 2013). Individuals with OCD engaging in exposure therapy may benefit from being coached to accept rather than control negative internal experiences. For OCD, this often involves reminding patients why experiencing uncomfortable internal experiences during the specific exposure at hand will lead to a life more worth living (Reid et al., 2017).

During the assessment, it is helpful to determine whether the triggering situation has an emotional component. Many people with OCD are triggered by negative emotions (e.g., anger, sadness, loneliness) but don't necessarily realize it. People who are in an OCD episode may want to push their negative emotions away, just like they do for anxiety. If patients believe that experiencing negative emotions is an indication that they are bad, wrong, disordered, or defective, then they will engage in emotion control, suppression, and avoidance strategies to manage their affective state.

Helpful questions to assess negative internal experiences include the following:

- Does the patient believe that his or her inability to control or eliminate negative internal experiences is a sign of weakness?
- Have attempts to control a negative internal experience only made it worse?
- Does a negative internal experience indicate a sign of personal problems?
- Can the patient accept that negative internal experiences are an inevitable part of being alive?

Cognitive Belief Domains Specific to OCD

The Obsessive Compulsive Cognitions Working Group identified six cognitive domains specific to OCD (Obsessive Compulsive Cognitions Working Group, 1997): overimportance of thoughts, importance of controlling thoughts, perfectionism, inflated responsibility, overestimation of threat, and intolerance for uncertainty.

Research has found that certain domains respond better to treatment than others (Adams, Riemann, Wetterneck, & Cisler, 2012). Changes in obsessive beliefs broadly, and changes in the importance of and control of thoughts specifically, were positively related to overall symptom reduction in OCD (Adams, Riemann, Wetterneck, & Cisler, 2012). Familiarizing the patient with these domains is helpful in conceptualizing distorted beliefs. The clinician should assess the rigidity or flexibility of the person's thinking and then provide psychoeducation about why and how the beliefs are beyond the norm. For example, having an obsession about dropping the baby doesn't mean that the patient is more likely to do so, and he is no more responsible for the thought than other parents who have the same thought, only more fleetingly.

Overimportance of thoughts involves the belief that every thought, image, or impulse means something very important and must be attended to. People with OCD believe that thoughts and actions are synonymous and that their feared consequences should be prevented. Some people with exaggerated intrusive "bad" thoughts believe that they have sinned if they have an inappropriate sexual thought. A Catholic person with such thoughts might pursue confession and penance, but doing so would not be effective.

Importance of controlling thoughts reflects the belief that it is possible and obligatory to have complete control over intrusive thoughts, images, and impulses. An OCD sufferer might think, "I must be weak or really believe these thoughts if I have them. To be a good person, I must find a way to avoid having them." No one has the ability to block thoughts completely, and the effort made to resist thoughts only makes them stronger.

Perfectionism is a common concern for people with OCD for several reasons. Some people with OCD have polarized beliefs. Perfection becomes the only acceptable standard and value. Imperfect results are considered failures and are wrong or bad. Others think themselves "lazy" or to have fallen short of their own or others' expectations. Some are driven to seek perfection simply as a matter of achieving that "just right" feeling.

Inflated responsibility is another problematic cognitive domain. This belief triggers an exaggerated sense that the feared obsessive consequences should be prevented, even though there is no actual or imminent danger of their occurrence. Depending on the content of the obsessions, some sufferers may experience this as a moral imperative. Common negative thoughts that everyone has are experienced as moral failures that provoke a disproportionate amount of guilt. There is almost always a moral double standard, in that the person with OCD does not attribute responsibility to others who have the same thoughts.

Overestimation of threat results from obsessive fear. People with OCD tend to overestimate levels of threat because of the anxiety they experience in triggering situations. Because certainty cannot be achieved, their default belief becomes "better to be safe than sorry."

Intolerance of uncertainty in OCD is similar to perfectionism, heightened fear, threat of risk, and the need to control thoughts. Individuals with OCD believe that every effort should be made to stop them from making mistakes, causing harm, and creating negative consequences from "bad" thoughts. Their goal is to feel "right" by being certain, so that they are effective for the next task at hand. The obsessive cognition may appear as the thought "Not being sure increases the possibility that something bad could happen. I will keep checking until I am sure that I left no stone unturned to prevent harm."

OCD Assessment

It may take several sessions with a new patient to fully develop a good assessment of symptoms and a functional analysis of the reasons he or she is seeking treatment. Both of these components are essential to developing an effective treatment plan.

Assessment Tools

Chapter 1 explained how to diagnose OCD and patients' symptoms. The Y-BOCS (Goodman et al., 1989) has been considered the gold standard of measuring symptom severity. It was designed to be administered by a clinician, but most often it is used as a self-rating tool. Many OCD treaters take a weekly rating, while other use it as a pre- and postmeasure. The Y-BOCS short version is a ten-item scale, including five questions about obsessions: how much time the person spends on obsessions, how much impairment or distress the patient experiences, the level of interference in daily life, how much effort the person makes in trying to control the thoughts, and how much resistance and control the person actually has over these thoughts. It is followed by five similar questions about compulsions (e.g., time spent, distress, interference, impairment, resistance). Each item is rated from zero (no symptoms) to four (extreme symptoms), with a total possible score ranging from zero to forty. The clinical severity cutoff scores are provided in table 7.1 for reference when using the scale.

The Y-BOCS has been translated into several languages and adapted to be culturally sensitive. Some of these are Italian (Melli, Avallone, et al., 2015), Spanish (Vega-Dienstmaier et al., 2001), Thai (Hiranyatheb et al., 2015), Japanese (Nakajima et al., 1995), Chinese (Peng, Yang, Miao, Jing, & Chan, 2011), Brazilian Portuguese (de Souza et al., 2007), Dutch (Arrindell, de Vlaming, Eisenhardt, van Berkum, & Kwee, 2002), French (Mollard, Cottraux, & Bouvard, 1989), Icelandic (Ólafsson, Ragnar P., Snorrason, & Smári, 2010), German (Weck, Gropalis, Neng, & Witthoft, 2013), and Persian (Esfahani et al., 2012).

The Yale-Brown Obsessive Compulsive Symptom Checklist classifies symptom types and is designed in a yes-or-no format. Researchers began to wonder if the results of the checklist captured the fuller clinical

Table 7.1 Y-BOCS Symptom Severity

Score	Level of Impairment
0–7	Subclinical
8–15	Mild
16–23	Moderate
24–31	Severe
32–40	Extreme

Source: Goodman et al. (1989).

picture, since it asks patients to report on the specific symptoms rather than symptoms that commonly cluster together.

The Dimensional Obsessive Compulsive Scale (DOCS) was created to reexamine how OCD is expressed, from research that identified four dimensions more fully reflecting patients' clinical experience. The endorsement of several symptom types tended to be perceived to indicate higher severity, while having symptoms that were not listed led to an inaccurate lower level of severity (Eilertsen et al., 2017).

The four dimensions are contamination obsessions and washing/cleaning compulsions; obsessions about responsibility for causing harm or making mistakes and checking compulsions; obsessions about order and symmetry and ordering/arranging compulsions, and repugnant obsessional thoughts concerning sex, religion, and violence, along with mental compulsive rituals and other covert neutralizing strategies (Abramowitz et al., 2010). Scores on each of the four subscales range from zero (no symptoms) to twenty (extreme). When all the subscale scores are summed, the highest possible total score is eighty. They also reflect distinct patterns of comorbidity, genetic transmission, neural substrates, and treatment response (Mataix-Cols, Rosario-Campos, & Leckman, 2005).

The DOCS has been translated into Hungarian (Harsanyi, Csigo, Demeter, Nemeth, & Racsmany, 2009), Italian (Melli, Chiorri, et al., 2015), Spanish, (López-Solà et al., 2014), Icelandic (Ólafsson et al., 2013), and Korean (Kim et al., 2013). For the Chinese translation by Dr. Jianping Wang and colleagues, and the French translation by Dr. Serge Larouche, visit https://www.unc.edu/~jonabram/DOCS_download.html.

Instincts and the Sociocultural Role of Ritual

Every culture has norms for social order that vary from place to place, and every culture has people with OCD (Ayuso-Mateos, 2002). Evolutionary biology explains how our precaution system detects imminent or actual threat and how behaviors developed to respond to them (Boyer & Liénard, 2006). During an OCD trigger, the precaution mechanism (fight or flight) is set off in the absence of actual threat or danger due to obsessive doubt and a not-right-feeling (Lienard & Boyer, 2008).

Functional and social ritual behaviors practiced within a cultural group seem to foster cooperation and help set expectations needed for maintaining social order (Port, 2000). The role of cooperative relationships (mating, group, family, kinship, and affiliation to the larger community) meets the essential preservation needs for procreation, producing food, and defending against threat. Further, certain specialized behaviors were adapted to maintain safety, sustenance, and well-being for the benefit of the group, such as checking, washing, counting, needing to confess, hoarding/nesting, and skills requiring precision (Polimeni, Reiss, & Sareen, 2005).

An interesting study was conducted in the furthest corners of the world by the World Health Organization. The study found universal themes that were consistent across cultures. Beliefs about the significance of specific numbers and colors; need for specified prayers or incantations; special attention to thresholds, pollution and purification; disgust about bodily secretions; concern with illness; separating or mixing items; setting boundaries; and important ways of making special transitions. Consistent behaviors were touching, tapping, or rubbing; ways of creating order or meaning; concern about symmetry or exactness; ordering or arranging things; concern with rules or morality; and telling/asking, and confessing (Ayuso-Mateos, 2002).

Cultural or social rituals are often practiced in repetition, which may become compulsive behaviors in those predisposed to OCD. Verbal rituals, such as making repetitious nonsense sounds, repeating special words, repeating prayers or incantations, and repeating the steps of a certain ritual, can become an excessive expression of cultural practices (Ayuso-Mateos, 2002).

The symptom dimensions of contamination/cleaning, hoarding, symmetry/ordering, taboo thoughts/mental compulsions, and doubt/checking are commonplace in Western samples (Bloch, Landeros-Weisenberger, Rosario, Pittenger, & Leckman, 2008); however, cultural diversity within Western samples has historically been scant (Williams, Powers, Yun, & Foa, 2010). Hispanic and Latin American subjects appear to have more contamination and aggression than other cultural identities (Washington, Norton, & Temple, 2008). Clinical samples in Indian studies identified contamination and pathological doubt to be more primary than other symptom dimensions (Jaisoorya et al., 2017). In East Asian samples, symptom of contamination and symmetry were most prominent; Japanese patients were more concerned with contamination, while Chinese patients had more of a need for symmetry (Liu, J., Cui, & Fang, 2008). The findings suggest that there are elements of symptom dimension that generalize to certain regions and religious groups across the world (Williams, Chapman, Simms, & Tellawi, 2017).

There are many common and idiosyncratic factors involved in OCD. Getting a sense of what purpose the rituals serve and what influences may have contributed to how they developed is a good strategy for understanding the relationship between the thoughts and behaviors.

Case Study: Avi

Assessment

Avi was a law student under tremendous stress. He currently worried about plagiarism and was falling behind in his work, due to the amount of cross-checking he did between his sources and his writing. When he made a point or a legal opinion, he was unsure if he's using something he already heard or if he might be using someone else's words. After all, he was fighting against committing the kinds of ethical issues he wanted to protect as an attorney.

When he was in high school, he had difficulty getting to school on time. Before leaving the house, he made sure the items in his room were perfectly lined up. Avi was shy, but as he gained confidence by excelling in his academics, he tried out for the debate team and eventually became captain. His teammates loved him because of how much preparation he did for each competition. He took piano lessons since first grade, and after finishing his homework, he practiced until his parents told him to stop. His parents, teachers at school, debate coach, and his piano teacher all praised him for his work. Because of his diligence in these areas, he made few friends and was a bit socially behind. He did, however, participate in community service.

Avi went on to a prestigious college and then law school, where academics were more challenging. He had heard that sometimes people pay others to do their work and didn't understand how they could trust not getting caught. This played on his conscience even though he knew he would never resort to that kind of behavior. In fact, he was getting good grades, but he often went without sleep in order to finish papers or study for exams. During study groups, Avi asked clarifying questions that caused frustration with the other students. At times, he would request a meeting with his professors to make sure that he understood the assignments in spite of details being clearly explained in the syllabus. He had trouble managing time because he tried to attend to every demand to his utmost ability and became overwhelmed.

On night, Avi was working on a paper and was suddenly afraid that he might be plagiarizing material he was including in his work. He went back to the articles he was using but didn't find any verbatim sentences. This was a long and tedious process, but he felt some relief when he was done. Then he had the doubting thought "But what if I am stealing the *ideas* I am using?" This brought on more anxiety and checking that interfered with meeting the paper's deadline. He contacted his professor and told her what happened. She referred him to the university's student mental health clinic.

After his intake interview, he was told that he likely suffered from OCD, due to his excessive concern about stealing and his checking behaviors. The intake counselor also pointed out the pattern of OCD traits he had over the course of his development (i.e., need for order, perfectionism, putting academics before social/leisure activities). The clinician explained to Avi that the level of academic stress he was experiencing most likely precipitated this first full-blown OCD episode. Avi stated that he had always been anxious and thought it was just normal and that he had always found a way to get by. Avi felt doubly stigmatized about having a mental disorder that, if disclosed, could discourage his being hired at a firm or getting clients in private practice. He also wondered if he could actually graduate from law school, given the level of detail involved in studying law. He didn't know if he would be supported by the university, if disclosing became necessary, given the culture of stigma and the level of competition among his peers.

Since OCD is covered by the Americans With Disabilities Act (1973), he qualified for academic accommodation. Avi had to decide whether to take advantage of this support without knowing if there would be ramifications in the future. Avi's options were to power through like he always had, disclose to the university that he had OCD and ask for accommodation so he could keep up, or take a medical leave of absence to focus solely on treatment and symptom control. Avi decided to see a psychiatrist for medication and continue with his studies.

Avi was referred to a psychiatrist, who prescribed an antidepressant medication and informed Avi that it might take up to a month before it began to work. The psychiatrist also told Avi the potential side effects and informed him that just taking medication without getting into treatment might or might not provide him with a stabilized recovery. At that point, Avi agreed to enter into behavior therapy, and he was provided a referral. In a way, Avi was lucky that he had access to such excellent resources in a city with so many teaching hospitals.

Using the Y-BOCS symptom checklist, Warren, Avi's behavior therapist, assessed his current and past symptoms as perfectionism/not-just-right-experiences, some moral perfectionism, symmetry/exactness, and the obsessive need to know/be sure. Warren explained to Avi what perfectionism and NJREs were and gave several examples going back to childhood from the history he had collected.

Avi was trying to accept that his high standards in schoolwork, piano playing, and preparing for debates and his avoidance of socializing were driven by his anxiety of failing, disappointing others, and needing to feel right about many unimportant things that came up every day. He knew that he worked harder than most people and was rewarded with praise and honors for his excellence. Sadly, the people reinforcing his behaviors did not know that the extent of time he put into his projects and the high level of anxiety he experienced doing them were signs of OCD. He realized why piano playing had become to feel like a chore and had stopped being enjoyable. When Warren helped him connect his behaviors to the disorder, Avi expressed relief at understanding the source of the pressure to perform and the high baseline anxiety he had been used to. He now learned that he might not have to live under such pressure for the rest of his life, even though he wasn't sure how well he would do with his studies and career.

Treatment

After getting to know Avi from few sessions, Warren and Avi began creating a treatment plan consisting of the situations that provoked Avi's obsessions and compulsions and the level of anxiety associated with each one rated in hierarchical form. An abbreviated version of Avi's treatment plan highlighting his symptoms and the spirit of suggested exposure tasks will be provided following the section in this chapter that describes the components of ERP in table 7.2.

Accurate assessment and diagnosis are the essential first steps toward effective treatment planning. Treatment planning needs to be customized for each individual's needs. Drawing on information gathered from the assessment, the clinician and patient can then build an effective treatment plan.

Typically, medication and/or behavior therapy are the recommended treatments for OCD. Combining and complying with both of these modalities will provide the best conditions for treatment success (Hirschtritt, Bloch, & Mathews, 2017). It is important for clinicians to recognize that compulsions are sometimes maintained as habits and that, when asked, the patient may not remember the impetus behind the behavior, meaning that it can be more easily stopped. On the other hand, the behaviors may now be so ingrained into the patient's daily routine that subtle (or not so subtle) resistance to treatment may occur as the therapist and patient get close to actually disrupting the patient's rituals or compulsions. Addressing and validating this ambivalence will be important for establishing a trusting therapeutic relationship. Setting reasonable goals and pace of treatment interventions may help counter resistance.

Table 7.2 Avi's Treatment Plan (Abbreviated)

Situation	SUDS Level	Fear	Ritual	Exposure
Attending a study group	6	Saying ideas/giving opinions in case they were "stolen" Negative reaction by others	Avoids attending May attend but does not say anything	First study group, it's okay to stay as long as possible and just listen. Do not ask any questions, but it's okay to make a comment if you resist not reviewing it or seeking reassurance after the meeting is over. Resist checking websites
Attending social events/ leisure	6	Falling behind Being too distracted from getting work done Wasting time	Mentally reviews his work Leaves early Checks the time Spends waking time on studies Spends time outside of class at the library Avoids being home so as not to be distracted	Initially, ask someone to go for coffee and stay focused on the conversation. Resist checking the time or talking about law. Join a club on campus. Stay for at least a half hour at the first meeting and talk to people. Stay the entire time in the next meeting. Resist asking reassurance questions. Ask people about themselves and listen.
Reading for class	7	Having more information to "steal"	Reads slowly/checks to make sure he "knows" what not to plagiarize	Start with setting timer for twenty minutes and read with a blocker as a barrier from going back to reread. Increase study time without checking back.

172

Speaking in a study group	7	Will says somebody else's ideas Not saying perfectly what he means and be misunderstood	Seeks reassurance from others that what he said made sense and was clear	Make at least one comment or ask a question unrelated to plagiarism, etc., then increase level of participation and interaction by asking questions or expressing own thoughts. Resist asking for reassurance or mentally reviewing what you said. Do not prepare ahead of time what you are going to say.
Speaking in class	7	Will says somebody else's ideas Not saying perfectly what he means and be misunderstood	Seeks reassurance from others that what he said made sense and was clear	Ask one question or make one statement without further attention to it. Sit with the uncertainty about what you said. Resist mentally reviewing to check what you said and the responses you got.
Writing a paper	8	Plagiarizing Getting caught and reported Getting a poor grade	Rewords excessively Checks excessively from sources to his text	Ask colleague if he wants to sit and work together (no asking, clarifying, or reassurance questions). Pace yourself and manage your time per normal productivity. Resist perfectionism (finding "right" words, getting stuck on grammar, semantics, etc.). When stuck, get up and take a walk and then resume your work.

(continued)

Table 7.2 (Continued)

Situation	SUDS Level	Fear	Ritual	Exposure
Studying for an exam	9	Learning material that he'll use by mistake. Getting caught by professor and being reported	Rereads and checks excessively	Set time limits for studying. Okay to attend the study group and focus on material. Only use the material you have unless it is clear and absolute that you need to look something up. Okay to study with others to reduce isolation, obsessing, and checking.
Handing in a paper	9	Getting caught plagiarizing. Failing. Being expelled	Repeatedly checks the copy before and after turning it in. Rereads his copy to find any mistakes or use of material too close to the original. Seeks reassurance from professor by asking if it was received. Explains he may have borrowed some ideas	After having closed the document, send as attachment without looking, checking, delaying, asking for clarification, or an extension.
Taking an exam	10	Getting caught plagiarizing. Failing/not maintaining GPA. Being expelled	Checks. Chooses words excessively. Mentally reviews the text	Get a good night's sleep, eat breakfast, get some physical exercise. Be mindful of the time. Read/write fluidly and complete responses according to what you actually know without second-guessing. Do not ask to reschedule. Resist perfectionism in order to fully finish the exam. Once handed in, resist asking to look at it/check it.

Some manifestations of resistance or ambivalence may appear as the patient distracting the therapist by talking about issues not related to treatment goals, avoiding the topics associated with behavioral, minimizing the impact of compulsive behaviors, or considering dropping out of treatment. Cognitive behavioral augmenting modalities can be helpful for treatment interfering or other complicating psychosocial factors. These will be provided after the medication section.

Behavioral and Psychosocial Treatments

Exposure and Response Prevention

Exposure and response prevention is the gold-standard psychological treatment for OCD. The effectiveness of ERP treatment has been reliably studied over time, and as a result, recent research has focused on methods to improve patients' residual and difficult-to-treat symptoms. It has been shown to be at least, if not more, effective than medication alone (Franklin & Foa, 2011). Exposure involves the patient engaging in the distress-provoking situation, while response prevention consists of the patient resisting all ritualistic urges in the exposure situation. With willingness, practice, and consistency, the patient experiences increasingly lower level of distress in the face of the obsessive fear.

This process, called habituation, is similar to when we wade into cold water but stay in it until we get used to it and swim comfortably (Abramowitz, 2006). As stated, creating a foundation of mutual trust will be one of the most powerful tools when patients are undergoing exposure work so that they can be encouraged to stay in their triggering situation despite the high level of distress. When not used as providing reassurance, the therapist can help the patient keep in mind that the exposure is not inherently risky or problematic (i.e., having germy hands) and that obsessive doubt is the predominant problem. The goal of treatment is to help individuals learn how to tolerate uncertainty and discomfort. Therapists model courage by not allowing their own or the patient's distress or anxiety levels to interfere with following through on the exposure tasks. Intense distress or anxiety is temporary, especially if the patient is willing to tolerate it. The distress will eventually taper off on its own. Supporting patients to take the leap of faith will result in symptom reduction and resolution.

Exposure to the distressing event can be conducted in a gradual or flooding manner. Conducting the exposure at a gradual pace enables the patient to experience a moderate-enough anxiety level to manage on a daily basis. The advantage is decreasing the risk of treatment dropout; however, it will prolong the overall course of treatment. If patients have hit-and-run driving obsessions, they may be willing to drive down their street without checking, then drive home. Gradually the exposure will become more challenging as they drive around the neighborhood, into the center of town, around schools, and then on the highway.

Flooding, or implosion, consists of patients facing the most triggering situation at maximum intensity for up to an hour until they are no longer capable of experiencing further fear (Boulougouris & Marks, 1969). Some patients opt for just getting it over with. While difficult, this method produces sudden gains by the rapid and stable habituation of anxiety within the first few exposure sessions (Buchholz, Abramowitz, Blakey, Reuman, & Twohig, 2019).

Another consideration is the frequency of exposure sessions. Spaced sessions are spread out over a broader range of time (weekly or biweekly), while massed sessions are multiple times a week. Spaced sessions require diligent daily between-session practice, while some patients opt for massed exposures as a way to maintain the level of exposure intensity with the aid of the therapist, also requiring practice between sessions. Research findings report that although massed sessions result in quicker extinction learning, spaced sessions produce more resilient extinction learning at follow-up (Cain, Blouin, & Barad, 2003). Whether more or less frequent sessions are held is decided empirically. Patients with more severe or interfering symptoms may initially meet more frequently during the initial phase of treatment and then transition to spaced sessions once their functioning is more stabilized.

In Warren's work with Avi, he helped foster an attitude of being willing to fail, in the spirit of accepting that mistakes are normal, and increasing Avi's cognitive flexibility. If Avi could approach his work with a sense of "What do I have to lose" or "What's the worst that can happen?" he could be freer and feel better about doing his most reasonable best. Avi could learn that his rituals wouldn't serve the intended purpose of protecting his moral scruples around cheating or plagiarizing.

Although Avi had other OCD symptoms, this hierarchy focused on the salient aspects of symptoms that were interfering with his studies. Once these symptoms were under better control, his therapist recommended that he address the others in order to have a full course of treatment and extinguish rituals that could lead to relapse. In the end, Avi decided to go into mental health law.

Tips on Effective Behavioral Coaching

ERP is simple but not easy. People intentionally put themselves in distressing situations and stay there without making any purposeful efforts to reduce or avoid their anxiety. ERP is collaborative, and ultimately the patient takes responsibility for treatment decisions.

Behavioral coaches can be a family member, friend, or supervised paraprofessional. Good behavioral coaches are respectful, able to manage their own emotions and anxiety, supportive, interested, self-confident, and challenging. Coaches are ineffective when they provide reassurance; are permissive, overly empathetic, or sensitive to the patient's distress/anxiety; are overcontrolling; or appear anxious.

When a family member is enlisted as a behavioral coach, he or she should be someone who is encouraging and patient, stays unemotionally reactive during the ERP process, does not try to push the individual with OCD into doing tasks to which he or she has not agreed, is not critical, and does not try to use logic for challenging the obsessions.

The following are coaching guidelines for successful exposure practices:

- Try to make yourself as invisible as possible so as not to distract from the exposure.
- Periodically ask about the patient's distress or anxiety level and urges to ritualize during exposure, using SUDS (0 = no distress, 10 = panic attack).
- If a drop in SUDS is observed, ask the patient if the drop was due to habituation, distraction, ritualizing, or something else.
- If an increase in SUDS is noted, keep the patient focused on the exposure task by asking what he or she is thinking about, but don't do too much cognitive or emotional processing.
- Whenever possible, end the exposure when the patient has habituated to the feared situation. Successful habituation is indicated by the report of a SUDS level of six or below for that obsessive trigger and no performance of rituals.
- Before moving on to the next exposure, the patient should have habituated to the current one to ensure that situation is at a stable and normalized level.
- Keep talking or answering of questions to a minimum. The patient may seem confused or want reassurance that what he or she is doing is safe.
- If the patient reports low anxiety, ask if he or she has been thinking about other things and stopped focusing on the exposure task due to

avoidance. Together you can recite the feared consequences in order to stay connected to the exposure.

- If the exposure is verbal (e.g., reading trigger words or scenarios aloud) and the patient seems detached and is speaking too slowly, too quickly, too quietly, or too loudly, ask the person to adjust his or her behavior according to what would be considered a normal manner. This goes for body language as well.
- If the patient is having a hard time getting started, you may model normalized behavior, such as touching a faucet or modeling a hand wash, and then have the patient perform the task. This should be a one-time intervention. However, it is important to sense whether this would provide reassurance, since the patient may think that you would not perform an unsafe behavior.
- Exposures should not go further than what the person can replicate on his or her own without ritualizing.
- Exposures should never consist of something you would never do yourself. This is the best way to ensure the task is within the normal risk level. If the exposure is within the norm and you are uncomfortable with the exposure task, the patient will likely pick up on your discomfort (i.e., not hand washing after bathroom use). You may not like the exposure task but should be able to demonstrate as much flexibility as the patient is being asked to do.
- Do not be put off by the patient's need to express a lot of emotion (e.g., crying, moaning, frustration). This expression is part of the therapeutic process, since it is likely that he or she has been ritualizing to avoid these feelings. Emotional habituation will happen as the patient lets the emotions run their course. However, you may need to use judgment at times to ensure that the patient does not become emotionally averse to returning to the task at the next opportunity.
- Avoid engaging in well-intentioned soothing, comforting, or reassuring. This gives the patient the message that he or she should be upset in the feared situation. Cheerleading and validating the patient by saying, "You are working really hard right now. I can see you're upset but hang in there," is an appropriate way of providing support.

Consistency and duration of the exposures are the two conditions most conducive to successful habituation (Telch, Cobb, & Lancaster, 2014). As such, patients should agree to follow through with conducting the exposure task every day on their own. It is helpful for patients to track their daily exposure practices by describing what they did, how long they did it, and what their SUDS level were and to report any unexpected challenges that may have occurred. This is helpful data for monitoring patients' progress through the course of treatment.

Imaginal Exposures

When in vivo exposure is not able to be conducted (e.g., fear of burning a house down, violent/sexual obsessions, fear of going to hell), imaginal exposure is an effective way for patients to face their fears (Foa, 2010). Sometimes imaginal exposure is conducted to prepare patients who feel too anxious about direct contact with the exposure trigger so that they experience some kind of habituation first.

The following are instructions for how to effectively help the person connect to obsessive fears in imagination (Tompkins, 2016).

The first step is to decide what obsessive fear to develop into the imaginal exposure. The triggering situation should consist of a specific situation so that the details are focused and specific. There may be other triggering aspects to the chosen exposure scenario, but those can be addressed in subsequent imaginal ERPs. Directions should be given about describing the scene with a vivid movie-like script and images that match the details of the triggering situation. The idea is to describe it in a way that evokes the emotions and physiological responses the obsession creates and to make a direction connection to it. It should not be rushed, so it may take more than one session to complete. The idea is to make it include all the qualities of the triggering situation so that the maximum anxiety and habituation is allowed to occur.

Just like with in vivo ERPs, all rituals, in this case mental, should be blocked. For example, if a patient is worried about hitting someone with her car, she should describe how the whole episode unfolds. Details about the accident, gory details, and the feared life consequences from trial to prison are to be included. Again, taking the time to imagine the details will have a better effect on habituation. If the person reassures herself by saying, "That would never happen to me," she should get back to the obsession that the accident happened and continue.

Some people may want to audio record the script and listen to it repeatedly, while others may prefer to write scripts by hand or type them. The benefit to the latter is that when patients rewrite the scripts, they experience another exposure, which is more cognitively active than listening to the same unchanging recording. In session, the patient can read the script aloud to the therapist, which is an even more cognitively and affectively deliberate process. The therapist can ask for more details in parts of the scene where there may have been some intentional or unintentional avoidance on the patient's part.

Patients will likely be distressed at what the therapist might think of them and seek reassurance that they are not a monster, especially if the scripts involve pedophilia obsessions. The therapist can validate how difficult it must be for patients to make themselves so vulnerable and support how brave and motivated they are toward recovery.

Biological Treatments

Medication

The most effective medications in the treatment of OCD are serotonin reuptake inhibitors (Dougherty et al., 2018). However, one disadvantage of relying solely on medication is that it takes as long as four to six weeks to see if the person responds. If the patient does not respond to the medication, another medication will be tried for another four to six weeks, and so on.

There appears to be a trend in people with somatic OCD where they avoid taking medication due to fears of side effects. Others may refuse to take medications because of contamination fears. Some individuals reject medication due to a sense of moral failure, in that they are not trying hard enough and would be "cheating" by relying on an artificial way of taking the edge off of their anxiety or becoming falsely dependent by taking medication. If this is the case, continued assessment of the person's progress in behavior therapy will determine whether this becomes a clinical issue. If the patient remains stuck with no change or symptom reduction, the clinician should address the obsessive beliefs about the role of medication and recommend having an evaluation with a psychiatrist.

Table 7.3 provides a list of various medications that are commonly prescribed to treat OCD.

Medication Augmentations

Several studies have identified second-line medications that help augment the effects of SSRIs when OCD symptoms persist (Pittenger & Bloch, 2014; Pittenger, Bloch, & Williams, 2011). Along with serotonin, the neurotransmitter glutamate has been found to have an important

Table 7.3   First-Line Prescribed Medication for OCD

Medication	Dose (Mg Per Day)
Selective Serotonin Reuptake Inhibitors	
Fluvoxamine (Luvox)	150–300
Sertraline (Zoloft)	50–200
Citalopram (Celexa)	20–80
Escitalopram (Lexapro)	10–40
Fluoxetine (Prozac)	20–80
Paroxetine (Paxil)	20–60[a]
Serotonin Reuptake Inhibitor	
Clomipramine (Anafranil)	Up to 300[b]
Serotonin Norepinephrine Reuptake Inhibitors	
Venlafaxine (Effexor)	Up to 225
Duloxetine (Cymbalta)	Up to 120[c]

Source: [a]Bloch, McGuire, Landeros-Weisenberger, Leckman, and Pittenger (2009)
[b]DeVeaugh-Geiss, Landau, and Katz (1989)
[c]Sansone and Sansone (2011)

role in OCD and is shown to successfully augment the effect of first-line prescribed medications for OCD and related disorders (Oliver et al., 2015). The glutamate supplemental medications for OCD are provided in table 7.4.

Neurotherapeutic Interventions

Transcranial Magnetic Stimulation (TMS)   - *ALT*

Transcranial magnetic stimulation is becoming more widely used as a noninvasive alternative treatment for OCD. First used in 1985 for treatment of depression, it was approved by the FDA in 2018 for OCD after promising results in experimental research (Pallanti, Marras, Salerno, Makris, & Hollander, 2016).

In TMS, the patient wears a cap of coils that send short pulses of magnetic energy to stimulate nerve cells on the left side of the frontal cortex. As TMS magnetic fields move into the brain, they produce very small electrical currents that activate cells that help normalize functional connectivity and serotonin and dopamine levels (Dubin, 2017). The

Table 7.4   Glutamate Supplements for OCD Augmentation

Medication	Dose
N-Acetyl Cysteine (NAC)	3,000 mg/day (Kariuki-Nyuthe, Gomez-Mancilla, & Stein, 2014; Oliver et al., 2015)
D-Cycloserine	Up to 50 mg/day (Mataix-Cols et al., 2017)
Memantine (Namenda)	Up to 10 mg/day (Bakhla, Verma, Soren, Sarkhel, & Chaudhury, 2013)
Lamotrigine (Lamictal)	Up to 150 mg/day (Hussain et al., 2015)
Riluzole (Rilutek)	05 mg bid (Pittenger et al., 2015)
Ketamine (Ketalar)	0.5 mg/kg IV forty minutes (Rodriguez et al., 2013)

typical initial treatment course consists of five treatments per week over a period of four to six weeks, for an average of twenty to thirty total treatments. Each treatment session lasts about one hour. For a more detailed description, visit http://www.butler.org/programs/outpatient /transcranial-magnetic-stimulation.cfm.

Studies reported TMS reductions in OCD severity (Li & Mody, 2016). Dunlop and colleagues (2016) found that 50 percent of the patients in their study responded to the treatment. Over half of the patients who did not respond to medication treatment and who were treated with TMS experienced a 25 percent reduction in their Y-BOCS scores (Pallanti et al., 2016). Denys and colleagues (2010) also found a decrease of 24 percent in Y-BOCS scores in the outcome of their study of sixteen treatment-refractory patients who received TMS.

Deep Brain Stimulation (DBS)

Some individuals diagnosed with OCD who do not seem to respond to medication treatment can be also successfully treated with deep brain stimulation. DBS is an invasive but reversible treatment that inserts an electrode into the nucleus accumbens located in the basal ganglia part of the brain. The electrode is attached to a pulse generator unit implanted into the chest (Tarsy, Vitek, Starr, & Okun, 2008). Since the pulse generator runs on batteries, it is important that the battery level be checked when patients are experiencing an increase in symptoms as well as the frequency of the electrical current to ensure that the level is optimal for the patient (Hitti, Vaughan, Ramayya, McShane, & Baltuch, 2018).

DBS has been found to release dopamine in the striata and effectively decrease symptoms in responders (Figee et al., 2014). A meta-analysis of thirty-one studies found that the global percentage drop in Y-BOCS scores of eighty-three participants was estimated at 45 percent, especially for those with sexual and religious obsessions and older age of onset (Alonso et al., 2015). Another meta-analysis that included twenty studies, found that sixty-two patients who underwent DBS had a 40 percent decrease in YBOCS score (Pepper, Hariz, & Zrinzo, 2015). A long-term study of six to nine years conducted with six individuals who underwent DBS found that participants maintained symptom reduction from post-treatment to follow-up (Fayad et al., 2016).

DBS is not indicated until medication and behavior therapy trials have been conducted. While it may seem like an unpleasant option, it is considered a blessing by those who experience symptom relief.

Psychosurgery

Surgical procedures have alleviated psychiatric symptoms for treatment refractory individuals since the 1930s, if not sooner (Faria, 2013). Since more innovative techniques have been developed over the past few decades, these interventions are less commonly recommended. For those who consider this option, there is a thorough screening process, and patients must meet several criteria, including symptom severity, chronicity, disability, and failure in all other treatment modalities.

After the patient applies for surgery, a multidisciplinary team consisting of psychiatrists, neurosurgeons, and other specialists involved in patient care reviews the case to confirm that adequate conventional treatment has been ineffective. The surgery must only be performed to restore function and relieve suffering, and patients must demonstrate the ability to make rational decisions (Shah, Pesiridou, Baltuch, Malone, & O'Reardon, 2008). The reports of success offer hope to those that have not benefitted from traditional interventions, and even a modest improvement can make a difference in the quality of life for patients with very severe and incapacitating OCD.

Bilateral Anterior Capsulotomy

Bilateral anterior internal capsulotomy creates bilateral lesions in the brain guided by a three-dimensional image of an MRI scan taken prior to the procedure (Banks et al., 2015). In one study of thirty-seven patients, five-year postoperative results showed a decrease of more than

50 percent in twenty-seven of the subjects, a decrease of 20–50 percent in six subjects, and a decrease by less than 20 percent in four subjects (Liu, Zhong, & Wang, 2017). The mean Y-BOCS severity scores of seven OCD patients before having the psychosurgery was thirty-three (out of forty), and at twelve-month follow-up, it was twenty-one, achieving an overall efficacy rate of 29–71 percent (Zhang, Wang, & Wei, 2013).

Dorsal Anterior Cingulotomy

Another psychosurgery available is a dorsal anterior cingulotomy. It is performed by severing the anterior cingulate cortex and the cingulum bundle (Nijensohn & Goodrich, 2014). A study of sixty-four patients who underwent this procedure reported that over half experienced a full response, as measured by a more than 35 percent decrease in Y-BOCS scores, and 7 percent were partial responders (Sheth, 2013). At the five-year follow-up, 47 percent had a full response, and 22 percent were partial responders. In addition, depression scores decreased by 17 percent (Sheth, 2013).

Another study reported a mean change in Y-BOCS scores from baseline to twelve months of 36 percent. At the twelve-month follow-up, a 35 percent or higher improvement rate of Y-BOCS scores was achieved (Kim et al., 2003). Banks and colleagues (2015) reported a response rate of 45–75 percent following the surgery. This response rate is significant considering that these patients had been refractory to conventional therapy for years or even decades.

Other Treatment Delivery Models

Home- and Community-Based Treatment

In severe cases in which a person is hospitalized for OCD, staff can be enlisted to assist him or her with a few exposure tasks. A therapeutic milieu that provides the needed support for recovery may include structure and services, such as medication, individual and group therapies, contact with other patients, and leisure activities. However, the majority of those with OCD will be receiving treatment in outpatient settings.

Ideally, exposures should be conducted in vivo, or right in the triggering situation. Some triggers can be replicated in the office, such as contamination exposures, but often they occur at the person's home or out in the community. Someone with pedophilia obsessions who conduct exposures at a community park, at the mall, toy stores, and so on will have a more effective experience than if the exposures were talked about in the office, done in imagination, or assigned as homework.

Outpatient therapists can find ERPs challenging to conduct due to time constraints and limited access to triggering situations within the standard fifty-minute session. Insurance providers are making allowances for prolonged service time and have added billing codes for sessions that are longer than forty-five minutes (https://pimsyehr.com/resources/coding-billing/cpt-code-changes/437-com-cdb-cpt-pcc-2016-cpt-code-changes-for-mental-behavioral-health).

Surprisingly, little research has been conducted on home-based in vivo treatment for OCD. The two existing research studies found differing results. One study found that 64 percent of the sample benefitted from exposures that were conducted in their homes where they were most triggered (Rosqvist et al., 2001). The other study reported that no differences were found between home-based and office-based treatment and that the outcome in both settings provided significant results (Rowa et al., 2007). It is unclear if the research methodology accounted for the differing outcomes.

Computer- and Electronic-Based Applications

Advances in technology have made it possible to conduct mental health treatment remotely. This is important for people who live in geographical areas where there is no access to treaters who specialize in OCD or for people who have difficulties with mobility.

Initially developed as a telephone-based treatment program (now internet-based), BT Steps provided a structured sequence of self-help behavioral exercises that has guided the format of more recent electronic application interventions (Baer & Greist, 1997). A study of eighty-seven participants with moderate OCD significant were randomly assigned to twelve weeks of treatment with either BT Steps alone, BT Steps with nontherapist coaching, or BT Steps with CBT therapist coaching. Each modality provided clinically significant reduction in symptoms; 48 percent of the patients stated that they preferred the computer method, 33 percent preferred meeting in person with a therapist, and 19 percent had no preference of delivery type (Kobak, Greist, Jacobi, Levy-Mack, & Greist, 2015).

Several studies have shown promising results for delivering treatment electronically. A meta-analysis of eighteen studies with a total of 823 individuals with OCD concluded that remote delivery of treatment resulted in a meaningful reduction of symptoms (Wootton, Dear, Johnston, Terides, & Titov, 2013). A study provided OCD patients with sixteen to eighteen twice-weekly, ninety-minute sessions by videoconference, between-session phone supports, and an additional maintenance session after two weeks. Significant improvements were made by patients using this treatment protocol in their OCD symptoms (Goetter et al., 2013).

Text messaging has also become a convenient option for some therapists who are comfortable giving out their phone number. Since this is a more recent delivery of care, the research being conducted is not yet available in the literature. One study did report a preference to therapy provided in an office setting, but no significant difference in treatment results was found between technology- or therapist-delivered therapies (Dèttore, Pozza, & Andersson, 2015).

Electronic consumer-based-treatment mobile-phone applications (apps) have become available as either self-help or therapist-assisted programs. Apps are being used to assess and track symptoms as well as to provide systemized treatment (Van Ameringen, Turna, Khalesi, Pullia, & Patterson, 2017). The advantages of using phone apps is that they are always available, are user-friendly, and can provide direct real-time feedback and data to the individual and therapist. Since this treatment modality is new as of this writing, there is a lack of empirical evidence to support how effective it is (Van Ameringen et al., 2017). The International OCD Foundation has listed several that have been reviewed for quality control and can be found on their website, www.iocdf.org.

Group Therapy

Clinician-led behavioral group therapy is a method that brings otherwise isolated patients with OCD together, many of whom may have never met another person with OCD. Rather than an insight-oriented model, group therapy for OCD is designed to be practical and applicable. Psychoeducation, setting ERP goals for the week, giving/getting feedback from the group leader and other group members about the goals, mutual assessment of progress or problems completing the ERP goals over the week, and reviewing relapse-prevention strategies are examples of what might be covered in group therapy (Kearns, Tone, Rush, & Lucey, 2010).

A meta-analysis consisting of twelve studies found group psychotherapy to be highly effective in reducing OCD symptoms (Schwartze, Barkowski, Burlingame, Strauss, & Rosendahl, 2016). A study by Wilson and colleagues (2014) found that group-based treatment led to significant reductions in symptoms from pre- to posttreatment, while another found similar results but that patients in individual therapy made treatment gains more quickly (Fals-Stewart, Marks, & Schafer, 1993).

Family Involvement

Family members are often drawn into the OCD web of altered household rules or demands to do or not do certain behaviors. The ways in which family members relate and interact with their loved one who has OCD are commonly affected by not knowing what is helpful or how to effectively respond to the OCD symptoms. The person with OCD may be a parent, child, significant other, or a caretaker. Integrating family members into helping execute the treatment plan by reducing accommodating behaviors results in better treatment outcome (Renshaw, Steketee, & Chambless, 2005).

OCD severity, family dynamics, and family accommodation strongly support the importance of having systematic and structured guidelines determined by the patient, family, and therapist for the family to practice their own response prevention (Burchi, Hollander, & Pallanti, 2018). Loved ones and family members may try to be patient, help with OCD rituals, or avoid triggering situations. Other reactions to the person with OCD, especially with compulsive reassurance seeking, may be frustration, anger, or avoidance of interacting with the person so as not to cause a trigger or be involved in the episode altogether. These traits and others comprise family accommodation, which has been identified as one of the most important factors that interferes with the course and outcome of a patient's treatment (Steketee, Van Noppen, Lam, & Shapiro, 1998).

Family accommodation describes changes that individuals make to their normal behavior in order to help their relative who has OCD and to avoid or alleviate distress related to the disorder (Lebowitz, Panza, & Bloch, 2016). The Family Accommodation Scale is a reliable and valid measure of the extent to which caregivers are a part of the system that maintains the patient's OCD functioning (Calvocoressi et al., 1999).

Calvocoressi and colleagues (1995) have identified several accommodating behaviors in OCD. Some of these are being involved in performing rituals (family members wash their hands when they come in the house or checking that doors are locked before leaving until the person with OCD feels "right"), assisting the person in avoiding triggers (driving routes that avoid cemeteries, not watching TV programs or movies with sexual or violent content), accommodating symptomatic behavior (buying only certain brands of food or clothing, waiting for person to complete their rituals even if means being late to events), excusing the person from participating in household chores (person is not responsible for helping clean the house, do laundry, put groceries away), and interfering in work/school functioning (finishing homework assignments or job tasks, checking to make sure the work is perfect).

Providing psychoeducation about why these accommodating behaviors do not work will alleviate some of the pressure and guilt that support people may feel when the OCD sufferer is in distress (Steketee et al., 1998). Accommodation interferes with treatment and recovery because it has the same effect as rituals performed by the person with OCD, can evoke hostility while the behaviors are carried out, and precludes the process of habituation to the person's triggers (Renshaw et al., 2005).

Behaviors supportive of helping the person with OCD cope with their symptoms include validating the person's distress while providing encouraging statements that highlight the person's strengths, keeping emotions in check, resisting temptations to do tasks that the person can do because it's easier, setting limits on providing reassurance, and recognizing when the person has done something challenging no matter how small it may seem (Lebowitz, 2018).

Once family members feel equipped to support and help a loved one, family interactions, communication styles, and the quality of relationships can be improved, and the severity and frequency of OCD episodes may diminish. Most important, family members can be taught to identify and minimize those behaviors that accommodate the OCD symptoms. When families function around the OCD symptoms, they are accommodating the OCD, which may unwittingly lead to the OCD becoming the head of the household. Once families learn how to provide support to their loved ones without being controlled by the OCD, they can feel confident that they are truly helping. Families can self-assess their accommodating behaviors using the Family Accommodation Scale (Pinto, Van Noppen, & Calvocoressi, 2013). An online version of the scale is available at http://www.dmertlich.com/assets/FAS.pdf.

Relapse Prevention

Recovering from OCD is a daily task. Relapse-prevention planning is conducted during the final phase of treatment. Highlighting areas of vulnerability for relapse and having plans for how to manage them can better ensure a stable recovery (Hiss, Foa, & Kozak, 1994). Empirically, having daily structure is the single most important factor for relapse prevention. Too much unstructured time leaves brain space for obsessions to fill. Boredom and lack of ongoing intellectual, emotional, and cognitive stimulation from isolating leads to overthinking and increased urges to ritualize.

People in recovery may feel they are doing so well that they go off their medication. They often do this on their own, not under the advice or supervision of their psychiatrist. While there is no need to stay on medication indefinitely, whatever symptoms they were helping will likely resurface. A well-planned-out schedule for titrating off medication according to medical advice will allow for resuming ERP therapy to address what symptoms emerge. This may take many months, but it will minimize the resurgence of sudden and overwhelming anxiety.

Staying busy is essential for maintaining recovery (Vaillant, 1988). For example, Jean had a good treatment outcome, and it was determined that he no longer needed weekly therapy appointments. Throughout the course of treatment, his therapist related her concern that there appeared to be a lot of downtime in his schedule. Jean said he was busy enough with going to the gym, meeting up with friends for lunch, spending time at the library, and visiting his sister and her kids. It was unclear if Jean was avoiding taking on more responsibilities such as work or taking classes to finish his bachelor's degree. Six months later, Jean called his therapist and said that he had relapsed. His therapist agreed to resume treatment under the condition that they start aftercare planning right away and that he should be actively looking into his options.

Ideally, patients have a more accepting attitude toward uncertainty, incomplete feelings, and imperfection. They are able to observe their obsessions rather than identify with them. Helping the patient to understand these concepts can create a mind-set of relapse prevention.

Aspects of life that cause vulnerability for relapse are illness, losses (death, unemployment), poor self-care and stress management (lack of sleep, unhealthy eating, lack of physical exercise), relationships, work, unexpected stressful events, and financial problems (Vaillant, 1988). Maintaining a healthy routine that emphasizes basic activities such as exercising, eating nutritiously, getting sufficient sleep, and balancing work and leisure will help set a lower stress baseline, which will help minimize the effects of challenges both planned and sudden.

For residual symptoms, daily ERP is recommended in a self-directed manner or under the supervision of a behavior therapist. Establishing and keeping engaged with a support system, whether it be personal, social, or community-based, helps with staying grounded and connected. Self-help support groups and social media platforms also provide opportunities for interacting with other OCD sufferers. By remaining mindful of their thoughts and actions, patients can regain a sense of power and control in their lives. They need not be defined or confined by their disease if they are able to seek support in managing their symptoms.

People who are in recovery should also be aware that a lapse is not a relapse (McKay, Todaro, Neziroglu, & Yaryura-Tobias, 1996). All-or-nothing thinking can lead to more distress when patients become more symptomatic and act out ritualistic urges. Creating a documented, structured relapse-prevention plan to which the person can refer will help to provide a concrete resource for implementing behavior strategies. Items on the list can include ways of conducting self-directed exposures, setting goals, enlisting the help of support people, and checking in with behavior therapists (Hiss et al., 1994).

References

Abramowitz, J. S. (2006). The psychological treatment of obsessive-compulsive disorder. *Canadian Journal of Psychiatry, 51*(7), 407–416.

Abramowitz, J. S., Deacon, B. J., Olatunji, B. O., Wheaton, M. G., Berman, N. C., Losardo, D., & Hale, L. R. (2010). Assessment of obsessive-compulsive symptom dimensions: Development and evaluation of the Dimensional Obsessive-Compulsive Scale. *Psychological Assessment, 22*(1), 180–198. doi:10.1037/a0018260

Adams, T. G., Riemann, B. C., Wetterneck, C. T., & Cisler, J. M. (2012). Obsessive beliefs predict cognitive behavior therapy outcome for obsessive compulsive disorder. *Cognitive Behaviour Therapy, 41*(3), 203–211.

Alonso, P., Cuadras, D., Gabriëls, L., Denys, D., Goodman, W., Greenberg, B. D., . . . Mallet, L. (2015). Deep brain stimulation for obsessive-compulsive disorder: A meta-analysis of treatment outcome and predictors of response. *PLoS ONE, 10*(7), e0133591.

Arrindell, W. A., de Vlaming, I. H., Eisenhardt, B. M., van Berkum, D. E., & Kwee, M. G. (2002). Cross-cultural validity of the Yale-Brown Obsessive Compulsive Scale. *Journal of Behavior Therapy and Experimental Psychiatry, 33*(3–4), 159–176.

Arumugham, S. S., Cherian, A. V., Baruah, U., Viswanath, B., Narayanaswamy, J. C., Math, S. B., & Reddy, Y. J. (2014). Comparison of clinical characteristics of familial and sporadic obsessive-compulsive disorder. *Comprehensive Psychiatry, 55*(7), 1520–1525.

Ayuso-Mateos, J. L. (2002). Global burden of obsessive-compulsive disorder in the year 2000. Retrieved from www.who.int/healthinfo/statistics/bod_obsessivecompulsive.pdf

Badour, C. L., Bown, S., Adams, T. G., Bunaciu, L., & Feldner, M. T. (2012). Specificity of fear and disgust experienced during traumatic interpersonal victimization in predicting posttraumatic stress and contamination-based obsessive-compulsive symptoms. *Journal of Anxiety Disorders, 26*(5), 590–598. doi:http://dx.doi.org/10.1016/j.janxdis.2012.03.001

Baer, L., & Greist, J. H. (1997). An interactive computer-administered self-assessment and self-help program for behavior therapy. *Journal of Clinical Psychiatry, 58*(Suppl 12), 23–28.

Bakhla, A. K., Verma, V., Soren, S., Sarkhel, S., & Chaudhury, S. (2013). An open-label trial of memantine in treatment-resistant obsessive-compulsive disorder. *Industrial Psychiatry Journal, 22*(2), 149–152. doi:10.4103/0972-6748.132930

Banks, G. P., Mikell, C. B., Youngerman, B. E., Henriques, B., Kelly, K. M., Chan, A. K., . . . Sheth, S. A. (2015). Neuroanatomical character-istics associated with response to dorsal anterior cingulotomy for obsessive-compulsive disorder. *JAMA Psychiatry, 72*(2), 127–135. doi:doi:10.1001/jamapsychiatry.2014.2216

Bhar, S. S., Kyrios, M., & Hordern, C. (2015). Self-ambivalence in the cognitive-behavioural treatment of obsessive-compulsive disorder. *Psychopathology, 48*(5), 349–356. Retrieved from http://www.karger.com/DOI/10.1159/000438676

Bloch, M. H., Landeros-Weisenberger, A., Rosario, M. C., Pittenger, C., & Leckman, J. F. (2008). Meta-analysis of the symptom structure of obsessive-compulsive disorder. *American Journal of Psychiatry, 165*(12), 1532–1542. doi:10.1176/appi.ajp.2008.08020320

Bloch, M. H., McGuire, J., Landeros-Weisenberger, A., Leckman, J. F., & Pittenger, C. (2009). Meta-analysis of the dose-response relationship of SSRI in obsessive-compulsive disorder. *Molecular Psychiatry, 15*(8), 850–855. doi:10.1038/mp.2009.50

Boulougouris, J. C., & Marks, I. M. (1969). Implosion (flooding)—A new treatment for phobias. *British Medical Journal, 2*(5659), 721–723. doi:10.1136/bmj.2.5659.721

Boyer, P., & Liénard, P. (2006). Why ritualized behavior?: Precaution sys-tems and action parsing in developmental, pathological and cultural ritu-als. *Behavioral and Brain Sciences, 29*(6), 595–613; discussion 613–550.

Buchholz, J. L., Abramowitz, J. S., Blakey, S. M., Reuman, L., & Twohig, M. P. (2019). Sudden gains: How important are they during exposure and response prevention for obsessive-compulsive disorder? *Behavior Therapy, 50*(3), 672–681. doi:10.1016/j.beth.2018.10.004

Bulli, F., Melli, G., Cavalletti, V., Stopani, E., & Carraresi, C. (2016). Comorbid personality disorders in obsessive-compulsive disorder and its symptom dimensions. *Psychiatric Quarterly, 87*(2), 365–376. doi:10.1007/s11126-015-9393-z

Burchi, E., Hollander, E., & Pallanti, S. (2018). From treatment response to recovery: A realistic goal in OCD. *International Journal of Neuropsychopharmacology, 21*(11), 1007–1013. doi:10.1093/ijnp/pyy079

Cain, C. K., Blouin, A. M., & Barad, M. (2003). Temporally massed CS presentations generate more fear extinction than spaced presentations. *Journal of Experimental Psychology: Animal Behavior Processes, 29*(4), 323–333.

Calvocoressi, L., Lewis, B., Harris, M., & Trufan, S. J. (1995). Family accommodation in obsessive-compulsive disorder. *American Journal of Psychiatry, 152*(3), 441–443.

Calvocoressi, L., Mazure, C. M., Kasl, S. V., Skolnick, J., Fisk, D., Vegso, S. J., . . . Price, L. H. (1999). Family accommodation of obsessive-compulsive symptoms: Instrument development and assessment of family behavior. *Journal of Nervous and Mental Disease, 187*(10), 636–642. doi:10.1097/00005053-199910000-00008

Chacon, P., Bernardes, E., Faggian, L., Batistuzzo, M., Moriyama, T., Miguel, E. C., & Polanczyk, G. V. (2018). Obsessive-compulsive symptoms in children with first degree relatives diagnosed with obsessive-compulsive disorder. *Brazilian Journal of Psychiatry, 40*(4), 388–393. doi:10.1590/1516-4446-2017-2321

Chapman, A. L. (2006). Dialectical behavior therapy: Current indications and unique elements. *Psychiatry (Edgmont), 3*(9), 62–68. Retrieved from https://www.ncbi.nlm.nih.gov/pubmed/20975829

Clark, D. A., & Inozu, M. (2014). Unwanted intrusive thoughts: Cultural, contextual, covariational, and characterological determinants of diversity. *Journal of Obsessive-Compulsive and Related Disorders, 3*(2), 195–204. doi:http://dx.doi.org/10.1016/j.jocrd.2014.02.002

Cromer, K. R., Schmidt, N. B., & Murphy, D. L. (2007). An investigation of traumatic life events and obsessive-compulsive disorder. *Behaviour Research and Therapy, 45*(7), 1683–1691. doi:10.1016/j.brat.2006.08.018

de Souza, F. P., Foa, E. B., MeyerI, E., NiederauerI, K. G., RaffinI, A. L., & Cordioli, A. V. (2007). Obsessive-compulsive inventory and obsessive-compulsive inventory-revised scales: Translation into Brazilian Portuguese and cross-cultural adaptation. *Revista Brasileira de Psiquiatria, 30*(1). doi:10.1590/S1516-44462006005000065

Denys, D., Mantione, M., Figee, M., van den Munckhof, P., Koerselman, F., Westenberg, H., . . . Schuurman, R. (2010). Deep brain stimulation of the nucleus accumbens for treatment-refractory obsessive-compulsive disorder. *Archives of General Psychiatry, 67*(10), 1061–1068. doi:10.1001/archgenpsychiatry.2010.122.

Derisley, J. (2008). *Breaking free from OCD: A CBT guide for young people and their families.* London and Philadelphia: Jessica Kingsley.

Dèttore, D., Pozza, A., & Andersson, G. (2015). Efficacy of technology-delivered cognitive behavioural therapy for OCD versus control conditions, and in comparison with therapist-administered CBT: Meta-analysis of randomized controlled trials. *Cognitive Behaviour Therapy, 44*(3), 190–211.

DeVeaugh-Geiss, J., Landau, P., & Katz, R. (1989). Preliminary results from a multicenter trial of clomipramine in obsessive-compulsive disorder. *Psychopharmacology Bulletin, 25*(1), 36–40.

Dougherty, D. D., Brennan, B. P., Stewart, S. E., Wilhelm, S., Widge, A. S., & Rauch, S. L. (2018). Neuroscientifically informed formulation and treatment planning for patients with obsessive-compulsive disorder: A review. *JAMA Psychiatry, 75*(10), 1081–1087. doi:10.1001/jamapsychiatry.2018.0930

Dubin, M. (2017). Imaging TMS: Antidepressant mechanisms and treatment optimization. *International Review of Psychiatry, 29*(2), 89–97. doi:10.1080/09540261.2017.1283297

Dunlop, K., Woodside, B., Olmsted, M., Colton, P., Giacobbe, P., & Downar, J. (2016). Reductions in cortico-striatal hyperconnectivity accompany successful treatment of obsessive-compulsive disorder with dorsomedial prefrontal rTM. *Neuropsychopharmacology, 41*(5), 1395–1403. doi:10.1038/npp.2015.292

Dykshoorn, K. L. (2014). Trauma-related obsessive–compulsive disorder: A review. *Health Psychology and Behavioral Medicine, 2*(1), 517–528. doi:10.1080/21642850.2014.905207

Ecker, W., Kupfer, J., & Gönner, S. (2014). Incompleteness as a link between obsessive-compulsive personality traits and specific symptom dimensions of obsessive-compulsive disorder. *Clinical Psychology & Psychotherapy, 21*(5), 394–402. doi:10.1002/cpp.1842

Eilertsen, T., Hansen, B., Kvale, G., Abramowitz, J. S., Holm, S. E. H., & Solem, S. (2017). The Dimensional Obsessive-Compulsive Scale: Development and validation of a short form (DOCS-SF). *Frontiers in Psychology, 8.* doi:10.3389/fpsyg.2017.01503

Esfahani, R. S., Motaghipour, Y., Kamkari, K., Zahiredin, A., & Janbozorgi, M. (2012). Reliability and validity of the Persian version of the Yale-Brown Obsessive-Compulsive Scale (Y-BOCS). *Iranian Journal of Psychiatry and Clinical Psychology, 17*(4), 297–303. Retrieved from http://ijpcp.iums.ac.ir/article-1-1453-en.html

Fals-Stewart, W., Marks, A. P., & Schafer, J. (1993). A comparison of behavioral group therapy and individual behavior therapy in treating obsessive-compulsive disorder. *Journal of Nervous and Mental Disease, 181*(3), 189–193. doi:10.1097/00005053-199303000-00007

Faria, M. A., Jr. (2013). Violence, mental illness, and the brain—A brief history of psychosurgery: Part 1—From trephination to lobotomy. *Surgical Neurology International, 4,* 49. doi:10.4103/2152-7806.110146

Fayad, S. M., Guzick, A. G., Reid, A. M., Mason, D. M., Bertone, A., Foote, K. D., . . . Ward, H. E. (2016). Six–nine year follow-up of deep brain stimulation for obsessive-compulsive disorder. *PLoS ONE, 11*(12), e0167875. doi:10.1371/journal.pone.0167875

Figee, M., de Koning, P., Klaassen, S., Vulink, N., Mantione, M., van den Munckhof, P., . . . Denys, D. (2014). Deep brain stimulation induces striatal dopamine release in obsessive-compulsive disorder. *Biological Psychiatry, 75*(8), 647–652. doi:10.1016/j.biopsych.2013.06.021

Foa, E. B. (2010). Cognitive behavioral therapy of obsessive-compulsive disorder. *Dialogues in Clinical Neuroscience, 12*(2), 199–207. Retrieved from https://www.ncbi.nlm.nih.gov/pubmed/20623924

Foa, E. B., Abramowitz, J. S., Franklin, M. E., & Kozak, M. J. (1999). Feared consequences, fixity of belief, and treatment outcome in patients with obsessive-compulsive disorder. *Behavior Therapy, 30*(4), 717–724.

Franklin, M. E., & Foa, E. B. (2011). Treatment of obsessive compulsive disorder. *Annual Review of Clinical Psychology, 7,* 229–243.

Gershuny, B. S., Baer, L., Radomsky, A. S., Wilson, K. A., & Jenike, M. A. (2003). Connections among symptoms of obsessive-compulsive disorder and posttraumatic stress disorder: A case series. *Behaviour Research and Therapy, 41*(9), 1029–1041. Retrieved from https://www.ncbi.nlm.nih.gov/pubmed/12914805

Goetter, E. M., Herbert, J. D., Forman, E. M., Yuen, E. K., Gershkovich, M., Glassman, L. H., . . . Goldstein, S. P. (2013). Delivering exposure and ritual prevention for obsessive-compulsive disorder via videoconference: Clinical considerations and recommendations. *Journal of Obsessive-Compulsive and Related Disorders, 2*(2), 137–145. doi:10.1016/j.jocrd.2013.01.003

Goodman, W. K., Price, L. H., Rasmussen, S. A., Mazure, C., Fleischmann, R. L., Hill, C. L., . . . Charney, D. S. (1989). The Yale-Brown Obsessive Compulsive Scale (YBOCS): Part I. Development, use, and reliability. *Archives of General Psychiaty, 46,* 1012–1016.

Harsanyi, A., Csigo, K., Demeter, G., Nemeth, A., & Racsmany, M. (2009). Hungarian translation of the Dimensional Yale-Brown Obsessive-Compulsive Scale and our first experiences with the test. *Psychiatria Hungarica, 24*(1), 18–59.

Hiranyatheb, T., Saipanish, R., Lotrakul, M., Prasertchai, R., Ketkaew, W., Jullagate, S., . . . Kusalaruk, P. (2015). Reliability and validity of the Thai self-report version of the Yale-Brown Obsessive-Compulsive Scale-Second Edition. *Neuropsychiatric Disease and Treatment, 11,* 2817–2824.

Hirschtritt, M. E., Bloch, M. H., & Mathews, C. A. (2017). Obsessive-compulsive disorder: Advances in diagnosis and treatment. *JAMA, 317*(13), 1358–1367.

Hiss, H., Foa, E. B., & Kozak, M. J. (1994). Relapse prevention program for treatment of obsessive-compulsive disorder. *Journal of Consulting and Clinical Psychology, 62*(4), 801.

Hitti, F. L., Vaughan, K. A., Ramayya, A. G., McShane, B. J., & Baltuch, G. H. (2018). Reduced long-term cost and increased patient satisfaction with rechargeable implantable pulse generators for deep brain stimulation. *Journal of Neurosurgery,* 1–8. doi:10.3171/2018.4 .Jns172995

Hussain, A., Dar, M. A., Wani, R. A., Shah, M. S., Jan, M. M., Malik, Y. A., . . . Margoob, M. A. (2015). Role of lamotrigine augmentation in treatment-resistant obsessive compulsive disorder: A retrospective case review from South Asia. *Indian Journal of Psychological Medicine, 37*(2), 154–158. doi:10.4103/0253-7176.155613

Jaisoorya, T. S., Janardhan Reddy, Y. C., Nair, B. S., Rani, A., Menon, P. G., Revamma, M., . . . Thennarasu, K. (2017). Prevalence and correlates of obsessive-compulsive disorder and subthreshold obsessive-compulsive disorder among college students in Kerala, India. *Indian Journal of Psychiatry, 59*(1), 56–62. doi:10.4103/0019-5545.204438

Kariuki-Nyuthe, C., Gomez-Mancilla, B., & Stein, D. J. (2014). Obsessive compulsive disorder and the glutamatergic system. *Current Opinion in Psychiatry, 27*(1), 32–37. doi:10.1097/yco.0000000000000017

Kearns, C., Tone, Y., Rush, G., & Lucey, J. V. (2010). Effectiveness of group-based cognitive-behavioural therapy in patients with obsessive-compulsive disorder. *Psychiatrist, 34*(1), 6–9. doi:10.1192/pb .bp.106.011510

Kim, C. H., Chang, J. W., Koo, M. S., Kim, J. W., Suh, H. S., Park, I. H., & Lee, H. S. (2003). Anterior cingulotomy for refractory obsessive-compulsive disorder. *Acta Psychiatrica Scandinavica, 107*(4), 283–290.

Kim, H. W., Kang, J. I., Kim, S. J., Jhung, K., Kim, E. J., & Kim, S. J. (2013). A validation study of the Korean version of the Dimensional Obsessive-Compulsive Scale. *Journal of Korean Neuropsychiatric Association, 52*(3), 130–142.

Kobak, K. A., Greist, R., Jacobi, D. M., Levy-Mack, H., & Greist, J. H. (2015). Computer-assisted cognitive behavior therapy for obsessive-compulsive disorder: A randomized trial on the impact of lay vs. professional coaching. *Annals of General Psychiatry, 14,* 10. doi:10.1186/s12991-015-0048-0

Lebowitz, E. R. (2018). Addressing family accommodation in childhood obsessive-compulsive disorder. In E. A. Storch, J. E. McGuire, & D. McKay (Eds.), *The Clinician's guide to cognitive-behavioral therapy for childhood* (pp. 243–261).

Lebowitz, E. R., Panza, K. E., & Bloch, M. H. (2016). Family accommodation in obsessive-compulsive and anxiety disorders: A five-year update. *Expert Review of Neurotherapeutics, 16*(1), 45–53. doi:10.15 86/14737175.2016.1126181

Li, B., & Mody, M. (2016). Cortico-striato-thalamo-cortical circuitry, working memory, and obsessive-compulsive disorder. *Frontiers in Psychiatry, 7,* 78. doi:10.3389/fpsyt.2016.00078

Li, F., Bai, X., & Wang, Y. (2013). The Scale of Positive and Negative Experience (SPANE): Psychometric properties and normative data in a large Chinese sample. *PLoS ONE, 8*(4), e61137. doi:10.1371/journal .pone.0061137

Lienard, P., & Boyer, P. (2008). Whence collective rituals: A cultural selection model of ritualized behavior. *American Anthropologist, 108*(4), 814–827. doi:doi.org/10.1525/aa.2006.108.4.814

Liu, H. B., Zhong, Q., & Wang, W. (2017). Bilateral anterior capsulotomy for patients with refractory obsessive-compulsive disorder: A multicenter, long-term, follow-up study. *Neurology India, 65*(4), 770–776.

Liu, J., Cui, Y., & Fang, M. (2008). Trans-cultural comparative research on symptoms of neuroses in China and Japan. *Chinese Mental Health Journal, 22*(1), 1–4.

López-Solà, C., Gutiérrez, F., Alonso, P., Rosado, S., Taberner, J., Segalàs, C., & Fullana, M. A. (2014). Spanish version of the Dimensional Obsessive-Compulsive Scale (DOCS): Psychometric properties and relation to obsessive beliefs. *Comprehensive Psychiatry, 55*(1), 206–214.

Markova, I. S., & Berrios, G. E. (1992). The meaning of insight in clinical psychiatry. *British Journal of Psychiatry, 160,* 850–860. doi:10.1192 /bjp.160.6.850

Mataix-Cols, D., Fernandez de la Cruz, L., Monzani, B., Rosenfield, D., Andersson, E., Perez-Vigil, A., . . . Thuras, P. (2017). D-cycloserine augmentation of exposure-based cognitive behavior therapy for anxiety, obsessive-compulsive, and posttraumatic stress disorders: A Systematic review and meta-analysis of individual participant data. *JAMA Psychiatry, 74*(5), 501–510.

Mataix-Cols, D., Rosario-Campos, M. C., & Leckman, J. F. (2005). A multidimensional model of obsessive-compulsive disorder. *American Journal of Psychiatry, 162*(2), 228–238. doi:10.1176/appi.ajp.162 .2.228

McKay, D., Todaro, J. F., Neziroglu, F., & Yaryura-Tobias, J. (1996). Evaluation of a naturalistic maintenance program in the treatment of obsessive-compulsive disorder: A preliminary investigation. *Journal of Anxiety Disorders, 10*(3), 211–217.

Melli, G., Avallone, E., Moulding, R., Pinto, A., Micheli, E., & Carraresi, C. (2015). Validation of the Italian version of the Yale-Brown Obsessive Compulsive Scale–Second Edition (Y-BOCS-II) in a clinical sample. *Comprehensive Psychiatry, 60*, 86–92.

Melli, G., Chiorri, C., Bulli, F., Carraresi, C., Stopani, E., & Abramowitz, J. S. (2015). Factor congruence and psychometric properties of the Italian version of the Dimensional Obsessive-Compulsive Scale (DOCS) across non-clinical and clinical samples. *Journal of Psychopathology and Behavioral Assessment, 37*(2), 329–339.

Mollard, E., Cottraux, J., & Bouvard, M. (1989). Version française de l'échelle d'obsession-compulsion de Yale-Brown. *L'encéphale: Revue de psychiatrie clinique biologique et thérapeutique, 15*(3), 335–341.

Nakajima, T., Nakamura, M., Taga, C., Yamagami, S., Kiriike, N., Nagata, T., . . . Hanada, M. (1995). Reliability and validity of the Japanese version of the Yale-Brown Obsessive-Compulsive Scale. *Psychiatry and Clinical Neurosciences, 49*(2), 121–126.

Nestadt, G., Samuels, J., Riddle, M., Bienvenu, O. J., Liang, K. Y., LaBuda, M., Walkup, J. Gardos, M., & Hoehn-Saric, R. A. (2000). A family study of obsessive-compulsive disorder. *Archives of General Psychiatry, 57*(4), 358–363. doi:10.1001/archpsyc.57.4.358

Nijensohn, D. E., & Goodrich, I. (2014). Psychosurgery: Past, present, and future, including prefrontal lobotomy and Connecticut's contribution. *Connecticut Medicine, 78*(8), 453–463.

Obsessive Compulsive Cognitions Working Group. (1997). Cognitive assessment of obsessive-compulsive disorder. *Behaviour Research and Therapy, 35*(7), 667–681.

Oestigaard, T. (2017). Holy water: The works of water in defining and understanding holiness. *WIREs Water, 4(3)*, e1205.

Ólafsson, R. P., Arngrímsson, J. B., Árnason, P., Kolbeinsson, Þ., Emmelkamp, P. M., Kristjánsson, Á., & Ólason, D. Þ. (2013). The

Icelandic version of the imensional Obsessive Compulsive Scale (DOCS) and its relationship with obsessive beliefs. *Journal of Obsessive-Compulsive and Related Disorders, 2*(2), 149–156.

Ólafsson, R. P., Snorrason, Í., & Smári, J. (2010). Yale-Brown Obsessive Compulsive Scale: Psychometric properties of the self-report version in a student sample. *Journal of Psychopathology and Behavioral Assessment, 32*(2), 226–235. doi:10.1007/s10862-009-9146-0

Oliver, G., Dean, O., Camfield, D., Blair-West, S., Ng, C., Berk, M., & Sarris, J. (2015). N-acetyl cysteine in the treatment of obsessive compulsive and related disorders: A systematic review. *Clinical Psychopharmacology and Neuroscience, 13*(1), 12–24.

Pallanti, S., Marras, A., Salerno, L., Makris, N., & Hollander, E. (2016). Better than treated as usual: Transcranial magnetic stimulation augmentation in selective serotonin reuptake inhibitor-refractory obsessive-compulsive disorder, mini-review and pilot open-label trial. *Journal of Psychopharmacology, 30*(6), 568–578. doi:10.1177/0269881116628427

Peng, Z.-w., Yang, W.-H., Miao, G.-D., Jing, J., & Chan, R. C. K. (2011). The Chinese version of the Obsessive-Compulsive Inventory–Revised Scale: Replication and extension to non-clinical and clinical individuals with OCD symptoms. *BMC Psychiatry, 11*, 129.

Pepper, J., Hariz, M., & Zrinzo, L. (2015). Deep brain stimulation versus anterior capsulotomy for obsessive-compulsive disorder: A review of the literature. *Journal of Neurosurgery, 122*(5), 1028–1037. doi:10.3171/2014.11.Jns132618

Pinto, A., Van Noppen, B., & Calvocoressi, L. (2013). Development and preliminary psychometric evaluation of a self-rated version of the Family Accommodation Scale for obsessive-compulsive disorder. *Journal of Obsessive-Compulsive and Related Disorders, 2*(4), 457–465. doi:10.1016/j.jocrd.2012.06.001

Pittenger, C., & Bloch, M. H. (2014). Pharmacological treatment of obsessive-compulsive disorder. *Psychiatric Clinics of North America, 37*(3), 375–391. doi:10.1016/j.psc.2014.05.006

Pittenger, C., Bloch, M. H., Wasylink, S., Billingslea, E., Simpson, R., Jakubovski, E., . . . Coric, V. (2015). Riluzole augmentation in treatment-refractory obsessive-compulsive disorder: A pilot placebo-controlled trial. *Journal of Clinical Psychiatry, 76*(8), 1075–1084. doi:10.4088/JCP.14m09123

Pittenger, C., Bloch, M. H., & Williams, K. (2011). Glutamate abnormalities in obsessive compulsive disorder: Neurobiology, pathophysiology, and treatment. *Pharmacology & Therapeutics, 132*(3), 314–332. doi:10.1016/j.pharmthera.2011.09.006

Polimeni, J., Reiss, J. P., & Sareen, J. (2005). Could obsessive-compulsive disorder have originated as a group-selected adaptive trait in traditional societies? *Medical Hypotheses, 65*(4), 655–664.

Port, R. F. (2000). Possible human instincts. First draft, fall, 1998. Retrieved from https://legacy.cs.indiana.edu/~port/teach/205/instincts.html

Reid, A. M., Garner, L. E., Van Kirk, N., Gironda, C., Krompinger, J. W., Brennan, B. P., . . . Elias, J. A. (2017). How willing are you?: Willingness as a predictor of change during treatment of adults with obsessive-compulsive disorder. *Depression and Anxiety, 34*(11), 1057–1064. doi:10.1002/da.22672

Renshaw, K. D., Steketee, G., & Chambless, D. L. (2005). Involving family members in the treatment of OCD. *Cognitive Behaviour Therapy, 34*(3), 164–175. doi:10.1080/16506070510043732

Rodriguez, C. I., Kegeles, L. S., Levinson, A., Feng, T., Marcus, S. M., Vermes, D., . . . Simpson, H. B. (2013). Randomized controlled crossover trial of ketamine in obsessive-compulsive disorder: Proof-of-concept. *Neuropsychopharmacology, 38*(12), 2475–2483. doi:10.1038/npp.2013.150

Rosengren, K. S., & French, J. A. (2013). Magical thinking. In M. Taylor (Ed.), *The Oxford handbook of the dvelopment of imagination* (pp. 42–60). New York: Oxford University Press.

Rosqvist, J., Egan, D., Manzo, P., Baer, L., Jenike, M. A., & Willis, B. S. (2001). Home-based behavior therapy for obsessive-compulsive disorder: A case series with data. *Journal of Anxiety Disorders, 15*(5), 395–400.

Rowa, K., Antony, M. M., Summerfeldt, L. J., Purdon, C., Young, L., & Swinson, R. P. (2007). Office-based vs. home-based behavioral treatment for obsessive-compulsive disorder: A preliminary study. *Behaviour Research and Therapy, 45*(8), 1883–1892.

Sansone, R. A., & Sansone, L. A. (2011). SNRIs pharmacological alternatives for the treatment of obsessive compulsive disorder? *Innovations in Clinical Neuroscience, 8*(6), 10–14. Retrieved from https://www.ncbi.nlm.nih.gov/pubmed/21779536; https://www.ncbi.nlm.nih.gov/pmc/articles/PMC3140892/

Schwartze, D., Barkowski, S., Burlingame, G. M., Strauss, B., & Rosendahl, J. (2016). Efficacy of group psychotherapy for obsessive-compulsive disorder: A meta-analysis of randomized controlled trials. *Journal of*

Obsessive-Compulsive and Related Disorders, 10, 49–61. doi:10.1016/j. jocrd.2016.05.001

Shah, D. B., Pesiridou, A., Baltuch, G. H., Malone, D. A., & O'Reardon, J. P. (2008). Functional neurosurgery in the treatment of severe obsessive compulsive disorder and major depression: Overview of disease circuits and therapeutic targeting for the clinician. *Psychiatry (Edgmont), 5*(9), 24–33.

Shapiro, L. J. (2014). *Understanding OCD: Skills to control the conscience and outsmart obsessive compulsive disorder.* Santa Barbara, CA: Praeger.

Sheth, S. A., Neal, J., Tangherlini, F., Mian, M. K., Gentil, A., Cosgrove, G. R., Eskandar, E. N., & Dougherty, D. D. (2013). Limbic system surgery for treatment-refractory obsessive-compulsive disorder: A prospective long-term follow-up of 64 patients. *Journal of Neurosurgery, 118*(3), 491–497.

Skriner, L. C., Freeman, J., Garcia, A., Benito, K., Sapyta, J., & Franklin, M. (2016). Characteristics of young children with obsessive-compulsive disorder: Baseline features from the POTS Jr. sample. *Child Psychiatry & Human Development, 47*(1), 83–93.

Spears, L. N. (2014). *An examination of magical beliefs as predictors of obsessive-compulsive symptom dimensions* (Doctoral dissertation). University of Kansas.

Steketee, G., Van Noppen, B., Lam, J., & Shapiro, L. J. (1998). Expressed emotion in families and the treatment of obsessive compulsive disorder. *In Session: Psychotherapy in Practice, 4*(3), 73–91.

Tarsy, D., Vitek, J. L., Starr, P., & Okun, M. (Eds.). (2008). *Deep brain stimulation in neurological and psychiatric disorders.* Totowa: Humana.

Telch, M. J., Cobb, A. R., & Lancaster, C. L. (2014). Exposure therapy. In P. Emmelkamp & T. Ehring (Eds.), *The Wiley handbook of anxiety disorders* (1st ed., pp. 717–756). Marblehead: John Wiley & Sons.

Tompkins, M. A. (2016). Nuts and bolts of imaginal exposure. Retrieved from http://www.sfbacct.com/exposure-therapy/59-nuts-and-bolts -of-imaginal-exposure

Vaillant, G. E. (1988). What can long-term follow-up teach us about relapse and prevention of relapse in addiction? *British Journal of Addiction, 83*(10), 1147–1157.

Van Ameringen, M., Turna, J., Khalesi, Z., Pullia, K., & Patterson, B. (2017). There is an app for that!: The current state of mobile applications (apps) for DSM-5 obsessive-compulsive disorder, posttraumatic stress disorder, anxiety and mood disorders. *Depression and Anxiety, 34*(6), 526–539. doi:10.1002/da.22657

Vega-Dienstmaier, J. M., Sal, Y. R. H. J., Mazzotti Suarez, G., Vidal, H., Guimas, B., Adrianzen, C., & Vivar, R. (2001). [Validation of a version in Spanish of the Yale-Brown Obsessive-Compulsive Scale]. *Actas Españolas de Psiquiatría, 30*(1), 30–35.

Washington, C., Norton, P., & Temple, S. (2008). Obsessive-compulsive symptoms and obsessive-compulsive disorder: A multiracial/ethnic analysis of a student population. *Journal of Nervous and Mental Disease, 196*(6), 456–461. doi:00005053-200806000-00003 [pii] 10.1097/NMD.0b013e3181775a62

Weck, F., Gropalis, M., Neng, J. M., & Witthoft, M. (2013). The German version of the H-YBOCS for the assessment of hypochondriacal cognitions and behaviors: Development, reliability and validity. *International Journal of Behavioral Medicine, 20*(4), 618–626. doi:10.1007 /s12529-012-9276-8

Wheaton, M. G., Galfalvy, H., Steinman, S. A., Wall, M. M., Foa, E. B., & Simpson, H. B. (2016). Patient adherence and treatment outcome with exposure and response prevention for OCD: Which components of adherence matter and who becomes well? *Behaviour Research and Therapy, 85*, 6–12. doi:10.1016/j.brat.2016.07.010.

Williams, M., Chapman, L. K., Simms, J. V., & Tellawi, G. (2017). Cross-cultural phenomenology of obsessive-compulsive disorder. In J. S. Abramowitz, D. McKay, & Storch (Eds.), *The Wiley handbook of obsessive compulsive disorders* (pp. 56–74). Hoboken: John Wiley & Sons.

Williams, M., Powers, M., Yun, Y. G., & Foa, E. (2010). Minority participation in randomized controlled trials for obsessive-compulsive disorder. *Journal of Anxiety Disorders, 24*(2), 171–177.

Wilson, R., Neziroglu, F., Feinstein, B., & Ginsberg, R. (2014). A new model for the initiation of treatment for obsessive-compulsive disorder: An exploratory study. *Journal of Obsessive-Compulsive and Related Disorders, 3*(4). doi:10.1016/j.jocrd.2014.08.003

Wootton, B. M., Dear, B. F., Johnston, L., Terides, M. D., & Titov, N. (2013). Remote treatment of obsessive-compulsive disorder: A randomized controlled trial. *Journal of Obsessive-Compulsive and Related Disorders, 2*(4), 375–384. doi:10.1016/j.jocrd.2013.07.002

Zhang, Q. J., Wang, W. H., & Wei, X. P. (2013). Long-term efficacy of stereotactic bilateral anterior cingulotomy and bilateral anterior capsulotomy as a treatment for refractory obsessive-compulsive disorder. *Stereotactic and functional neurosurgery, 91*(4), 258–261.

CHAPTER 8

Adjunctive Psychosocial Treatment and Coping Strategies

Self-Compassion

Self-compassion (SC) can go a long way for all of us! The following description of SC is based on Neff's book *Self-Compassion: The Proven Power of Being Kind to Yourself*. Neff (2011) has identified three components of SC: self-kindness, common humanity, and mindfulness. Rather than motivating us, our tendencies toward self-criticism and judgment only serve to hold us back. SC is useful for anyone with a mental disorder but especially for the toll intrusive thoughts take on the psyche of people with OCD.

Self-kindness allows us to be kind to ourselves in the very moments we are struggling the most. We tend to be down on ourselves and ruminate about our mistakes and imperfections. When we begin to become aware of our negative self-talk, we have the chance to change it. As Neff points out, if we talked to our friends the way we talk to ourselves, we wouldn't have many friends. She also states that we wouldn't treat even someone we don't like the way we treat ourselves. Paradoxically, if we talk to ourselves in the way we would to support a struggling friend, we can accept ourselves just as we are and be compassionate instead of critical. She differentiates SC from self-esteem, which is goal and achievement oriented. If we fail to meet our goals, we consider ourselves failures and become demoralized. Self-kindness is not self-indulgence or self-pity.

The human condition is one of suffering. The role of common humanity is to tap into our primitive need for connectedness at the very times
when we are tempted to isolate (Neff, 2011). Because we are mammals,
we are programmed to need intimate, family, and community relationships. We are also primed for danger. These survival instincts are driven
and maintained by neurochemical reinforcement. When we are faced
with danger or threat, our brains send off the fight-or-flight hormones
cortisol and adrenaline (Ranabir & Reetu, 2011), and we are physically
aroused to act for self-preservation. On the other hand, the emotion of
love and the need for connection activates the feel-good hormones of
oxytocin and endorphins (Dfarhud, Malmir, & Khanahmadi, 2014).
By nature, OCD sets off the fear hormones in a triggering situation
and the person feels a sense of threat in the absence of real danger. The
person can become very self-focused as the need and urgency for safety
becomes the primary goal. When the effort is made to plug in with
others instead of ritualizing, the social benefit provides an emotional
connection as well as a healthy distraction while the anxiety runs its
course.

Mindfulness connects us to the moment in which we are living. It is
a skill of observation, groundedness, openness, and objectivity (Keng,
Smoski, & Robins, 2011). We only have control over our immediate
moments. The past is over, and the future hasn't happened. We tend to
ruminate about past mistakes ("What could I have done better?") or
catastrophize about the future ("I need to prepare for any eventuality").
Unless we are faced with real urgency, we can accept that there will be
equilibrium from one moment to the next. We are clearer about our present reality and respond to it without negative reactivity. It's more of an
experiential practice than a thinking activity, subjective to and fraught
with emotions. When OCD patients practice mindfulness, they are not
trying to push their obsessions away; they notice them, accept them, and
stay focused on what they are doing.

Acceptance and Commitment Therapy (ACT) for OCD

Acceptance and commitment therapy is considered a "third wave" practice of behavior therapy. ACT seeks to train psychological flexibility,
which is the ability to distance oneself from problematic thoughts and
accept uncomfortable emotion in the service of engaging in personally
valued actions (Hayes, 2004). An important purpose of ACT is to accept
the obsessions and commit to changing the cognitive, behavioral, and

emotional relationship to them (Twohig et al., 2015). Ideally, accepting the obsession and *doing nothing* is the best practice. It should be noted that ACT is a successful coping approach for dealing with the OCD experience, but it should not be conducted instead of ERP. However, it may be useful for patients who have had difficulty engaging in ERP (Twohig, Hayes, & Masuda, 2006).

There are six core processes in ACT: acceptance, cognitive defusion, being present, self as context, values, and committed action. The following three of these appear to offer some augmenting benefit in treating OCD:

- Acceptance: The goal of acceptance is to help patients *welcome* unwanted obsessional thoughts, images, doubts, and anxiety.
- Cognitive defusion: Also referred to as *detachment*, it encourages patients to observe their distressing psychological experiences and to fully accept reality as it is in the moment.
- Values: Identifying, committing to, and taking action toward personal values help patients remember that the OCD is interfering with what is meaningful and that they are working hard in treatment to having a sense of these values in their lives.

ACT may also assist in preparing patients for in vivo exposure when they are too fearful to begin accepting their thoughts, psychological and physiological symptoms of distress, and decreasing cognitive avoidance. It should be made clear that ACT does not provide the neurobiological and psychological mechanisms of ERP that produce habituation.

Dialectical Behavior Therapy (DBT) for OCD

Strong emotions can interfere with recovery from OCD. The combination of being triggered by an obsessive fear, the urge to ritualize, and emotional dysregulation can lead to reinforcing the patient's distress and making the situation too difficult to manage.

Dialectical behavior therapy was initially developed to treat borderline personality disorder and combines standard cognitive behavioral techniques for emotion regulation, reality testing with concepts of distress tolerance, acceptance, and mindful awareness largely derived from Buddhist meditative practice (Linehan, 1993). DBT is not routinely incorporated into behavioral treatment but is effective for patients whose emotions interfere with the ability to focus on and habituate to the exposure task. Acquiring distress tolerance skills can help patients successfully engage in ERP (Allen & Barlow, 2009).

Emotion dysregulation can be an indication of trauma. People with OCD as the presenting problem who have a history of untreated trauma may appear treatment resistant or have poor treatment outcome (Gershuny et al., 2008). The OCD may have served as a protective mechanism that ERP begins to dismantle, and treatment response may result in an increase of trauma symptoms (Gershuny, Baer, Radomsky, Wilson, & Jenike, 2003). People may also experience a resurgence of trauma symptoms, especially if the symptoms are related to the event. Someone who was sexually assaulted may have symptoms of emotional or physiological contamination/disgust about bodily fluids or avoidance of environmental cues the person remembers from while the event was happening (decorative objects, TV show, songs, etc.).

DBT consists of four sets of skills:

- Mindfulness: How to be fully aware and present in this one moment
- Distress tolerance: How to tolerate pain in difficult situations, not change it
- Interpersonal effectiveness: How to ask for what you want and say no while maintaining self-respect and relationships with others
- Emotion regulation: How to change emotions that you want to change

If a traumatic event has not been identified during the assessment process but symptoms begin to emerge during exposure therapy, it is recommended that the person get treatment for trauma, often with the DBT model, and then reengage in ERP work (Ahovan, Balali, Shargh, & Doostian, 2016).

Assertiveness Training

Assertiveness is an effective communication, social, and stress management skill. People with OCD tend to feel guilty about the content of their intrusive thoughts as well as for the toll OCD takes on family and loved ones, and they often avoid causing conflict by not saying what they think or feel about things in general. Those with trait guilt (a higher baseline level than the norm) tend to want to please others and put their own needs aside, often resulting in anger or resentment (Shapiro, 2014).

People with trait guilt who are in an OCD episode have an especially hard time saying no to other's requests as they feel the need to compensate for any wrongs they may have committed. When people experience an OCD trigger, those with state guilt will also have an exaggerated need to fix the situation (Shapiro, 2014). They fear they may cause harm or offend someone, worry about negative social scrutiny, and try to be perfect. They may compulsively apologize, seek reassurance, go along with what they perceive others want, and have problems making decisions.

Being honest and not saying yes to favors or other things people ask is not only a matter of being genuine; in a practical sense, it helps manage stress. Assertive rights are not privileges, nor do they have to be earned. Rather, being assertive promotes autonomy and self-respect, and it garners respects from others. People can confuse assertiveness with aggression, since the feared outcome is confrontation. Assertive communication is expressed in an even tone so that the person can listen rather than react to strong emotions. Assertiveness helps reduce anger and blame, as individuals increase their ability to be more honest and be in control of their own behavior.

Basic assertive rights include the following:

- Being yourself
- Existing
- Acting in ways that promote your dignity and self-respect as long as others' rights are not violated in the process
- Being treated with respect
- Saying no, setting limits, and not feeling guilty
- Experiencing and expressing your feelings
- Taking time to slow down and think
- Changing your mind
- Asking for what you want
- Doing less than you are humanly capable of doing
- Asking for information
- Taking chances and making mistakes
- Feeling good about yourself
- Offering or accepting a workable compromise
- Offering no reasons or excuses for justifying your behavior
- Judging if you are or are not responsible for finding solutions to other people's problems
- Not feeling obligated or manipulated to fulfill others' needs
- Saying, "I don't know"
- Saying, "I don't understand"
- Respectfully disagreeing (Jakubowski & Lange, 1978; Smith, 1975)

Cognitive Distortions

We all have automatic negative thoughts (ANTs), assumptions, or biases of which we might not be aware. Some of them may be true, but if we catch ourselves in the moment, we can question their validity. Below are several types of ANTs compiled from two sources (Beck, 1976; Burns, 1980). They have overlapping themes:

- All-or-nothing or black-and-white thinking: Situations are thought of in a polarized manner, such as, "If I make a mistake, I have failed."
- Catastrophizing or fortune-telling: This occurs when someone is predicting the future negatively without considering other, more likely outcomes equally. This is characterized by starting a thought with, "What if?" Because people are imagining catastrophic outcomes, they are imposing stress and fear in the present about something that hasn't happened yet. Some people think they are mentally preparing themselves by doing so, but they are actually sacrificing the present quality of life over which they can have more control. This thinking includes statements such as, "What if I blank out during my presentation and people start leaving the room?"
- Disqualifying or discounting the positive or having a negative bias: This is the tendency to selectively notice things that are wrong and not to register things that are right. If the person is aware of some positive experiences, he or she may tell herself she was lucky or rationalize why it was the exception, such as, "I had a nice date last night, but it was because the other person was so nice."
- Mental filter or selective abstraction: This is similar to negative bias. Undue attention is paid to one negative detail instead of seeing the whole picture, such as, "I got a low rating on my job, so that means I'm doing a lousy job," even though the person scored higher on many items than last year.
- Magnification and minimization: Evaluations about oneself, another person, or a situation, are negatively magnified or positively minimized. Patients will exaggerate the importance of their problems and shortcomings and minimize the importance of their desirable qualities, such as, "People say I'm a nice person, but they don't know the real me."
- Negative predictions: Similar to catastrophizing, the person thinks pessimistically in new situations because of earlier experiences of failure. The person is closed minded about there being any kind of differing outcome, such as, "I remember when I tried to organize a family outing and it was a disaster."

- Overgeneralization: This includes sweeping conclusions with cognitive language like "always" or "never" that already rules out objective evidence in the gray area of reality, such as, "I always feel at my friend's house, and I'll never have a close relationship with her."
- Jumping to conclusions/mind reading/ fortune-telling: People interpret things negatively when there are no facts to support the conclusion. Without checking it out, they arbitrarily conclude that someone is reacting negatively to them, such as, "I noticed someone yawning when I was talking. That person must think I'm boring."
- Emotional reasoning: This is when people think something must be true because they feel as if it is and believe it so strongly, such as, "I feel so stupid and always wonder if I am offending someone. I can tell by the body language."
- Labeling: When people use labels, they make a judgment that tends to become fixed. When people go beyond labels, they recognize the complexity of things beyond the superficial, such as, "I'm such a loser because I got that answer wrong. I remember the last time that happened, I got so depressed about not being good enough." Labeling others might sound like, "Boy, that person gets on my nerves. What a jerk. I need to avoid him whenever I can." The label does not take into consideration the other qualities the person has that could be endearing.
- Fallacy of change: This involves expectations that other people will change to suit patients' needs if they just pressure or try to control them enough. Instead of being self-aware of what they can change to be happier, people externalize blame for their own unhappiness, such as, "If I work on that person, he will come around to my way of thinking."
- "Should," "must," "ought," and "have to" statements: These are also called *imperatives*. People may think they are motivating themselves by such imperatives. They feel they should do everything in their power in the proper way, as if there is a certain rule. "Should" statements that are directed against themselves lead to guilt and frustration; when they are made toward others, patients feel frustrated and a little angry, such as, "I shouldn't have made so many mistakes during that recital. I must practice more, or maybe I'm just not cut out for this."
- Rule following: People can have rigid rules about right and wrong, or they can take rules made to be guidelines literally. When such people break a rule, they feel as if they have failed and that they must be a bad person. When they sees others breaking rules, they judge them negatively or moralistically, such as, "I work hard to get to school on

time. That person's always late, and he gets away with it. I don't know if he is lazy or just doesn't care."

- Personalization and blame: This happens when people hold themselves personally responsible for something that isn't necessarily under their control. If someone rear-ends a car in front of a patient because that car stopped short, the patient will blame him or herself for not being more careful and not avoiding the accident and will think, "I'm such an idiot that I didn't see that coming." Some people do the opposite and blame others or their circumstances for their problems. They tend not to reflect on their responsibility in the situation or their control over their circumstances, such as, "The reason my marriage is so lousy is because my spouse is totally unreasonable."

Problem-Solving Skills Training

Another adjunctive cognitive treatment model helpful to people with OCD is problem-solving skills training. Problem-solving skills are effective in managing simple and complex problems. Because OCD provokes doubt, those with the disorder might be overwhelmed about how to make rational decisions about any number of typical lifestyle problems. For example, someone with OCD might want to change his job but become overwhelmed by the possibilities at hand, as well as how to organize a plan that will help him or her through the process. The following list of considerations may be used to navigate through problems:

- Goal setting: Patients should work with therapists to ensure that goals are realistic, achievable, measurable, and have an end point.
- Decision-making skills: Patients may attempt to find the "perfect" solution. Therapists should challenge the idea that there is a perfect solution or an obvious best choice, as this may lead to prolonged indecision. Therapists should encourage the patient's tolerance of benefits and drawbacks to each option and of there being no perfect way to decide.
- Fighting procrastination: Procrastination is often connected to indecision and perfectionism. Therapists can assist patients with breaking down tasks associated with the problem's resolution into substeps, emphasize the importance of getting started, and positively reinforce any response that approximates the desired response.
- Challenging perfectionism: Patients should be encouraged to actively value making small steps and being willing to risk making mistakes (Kaslow, Broth, Smith, & Collins, 2012).

Cognitive Restructuring

Cognitive restructuring can be helpful in addressing other types of cognitive distortions. A fundamental component of cognitive therapy is challenging the underlying thinking and beliefs that drive and maintain obsessions and compulsions in the individual's life. Hyman and Pedrick (2010) identify several dysfunctional beliefs that give rise to obsessions and compulsions that should be the target of cognitive restructuring interventions, including the following:

- Overestimating risk, harm, and danger
- Overcontrolling and perfectionism
- Catastrophizing minor events
- All-or-nothing thinking
- Magical thinking
- Taking responsibility for everyone and everything
- Pessimism
- Excessive worry about consequences of actions
- Intolerance of uncertainty
- Excessive worry about moral behavior

Coping Statements and Strategies

Supportive self-talk is different than self-reassurance. The focus and goal are to stay motivated through a trigger or an exposure session. It is not to reduce anxiety or for patients to tell themselves something that is not true such as, "No one will get sick if I don't wash my hands," since people get sick all the time. Here are some helpful self-talk coping statements and strategies (Foa & Wilson, 2001).

Supportive Coping Statements for Obsessions

- That thought isn't helpful right now.
- Now is not the time to think about it. I can think about it later.
- This is irrational. I'm going to let it go.
- I won't argue with an irrational thought.
- This is *not* an emergency. I can slow down and think clearly about what I need.
- This feels threatening and urgent, but it really isn't.
- I don't have to be perfect to be okay.
- I don't have to figure out this question. The best thing to do is just drop it.

- It's okay to make mistakes.
- I already know from my past experiences that these fears are irrational.
- I have to take risks in order to be free. I'm willing to take this risk.
- It's okay that I just had that thought/image, *and* it doesn't mean *anything*. I don't have to pay attention to it.
- I'm ready to move on now.
- I can handle being wrong.
- I don't deserve to suffer like this. I deserve to feel comfortable.
- That's not my responsibility.
- That's not my problem.
- I've done the best I can.
- It's good practice to let go of this worry. I want to practice. (Foa & Wilson, 2001, pp. 88–89)

Other Helpful Strategies

- Don't analyze obsessions.
- Obsessions are involuntary; the content is irrational.
- Accept the thoughts/obsessions. Fighting them will make them stronger.
- Change the way you obsess. Sing it; write it; change the picture; exaggerate it; make it a cartoon; turn down the volume; change the channel.
- Shift to a new/different activity.
- Make a collage of obsessive material. It can help externalize the thoughts and provide some emotional distance.
- Incorporate pleasurable pastimes/hobbies into daily routine (but don't let them get perfectionistic).
- Resist ritualizing by distracting yourself or removing yourself from the situation.
- Delay acting on the urge to ritualize. This will allow time for the urge to decrease or pass altogether.
- Change the ritual in some way. Change the order; eliminate a step; do it backward.
- Talk through it with someone.

Habit Reversal Therapy (HRT) for Problems with BFRBs, Tourette's, and Problems with Impulse Control

Habit reversal therapy is an effective behavior therapy for BFRBs, Tourette's, and other problems of impulse control (Azrin & Nunn, 1973). An initial strategy, Stimulus control, helps people to identify, change, and control the different triggers they notice in their routines, environments, and moods that lead to the impulsive behaviors.

HRT consists of doing the opposite behavior instead of repetitive impulsive urges. Habit reversal is a process that requires good motivation on the patient's part; it takes effort and practice, and progress generally tends to be slow. Lapses and relapses are not uncommon, but the best predictor of success is continued effort. Some people have trouble giving up their behavior compulsions because nothing healthy will replace the pleasure and gratification experienced during the episodes. There is sometimes a phase of high frustration and mourning the loss of what had been immediate and soothing relief from stress.

HRT has some applicability to OCD treatment because it teaches patients a set of alternative behaviors that can help them focus themselves, interrupt, and block compulsive behaviors. Some patients report that their rituals are almost automatic, such as walking into a room and putting things in perfect order.

The typical psychosocial treatment approaches include scheduled time for patients to express their tics. Medications have been very effective in treating Tourette's. Many people can control their tics for a certain amount of time, but the urges build and will need to be expressed.

Awareness training and developing a variety of competing physical responses are very effective in getting body-focused and non-body-focused behaviors under control. Awareness training starts with the person making a conscious effort to recognize urges that precedes the action. The person can log the frequency, sensations, and situations that provoke the urges. Sometimes awareness training actually has a natural effect in reducing the urges. When this happens, the person can gain more confidence, motivation, and belief that he or she can gain control over the behavior.

A component of habit reversal treatment is competing response training. This consists of performing behaviors that are, literally, opposite in manner and direction of the repetitive behavior. One example for someone who pulls her hair is to have her move her arms down beside her, on her lap, or under her legs or to hold on to an object with the hand she uses to pull. Some people keep fidgets (i.e., squishy balls) in places where they are vulnerable to pick or carry them with them throughout the day. This is effective and should be discreet and used in socially appropriate ways in order to avoid calling attention. At home, people also can use Bubble Wrap, do needlework, wear gloves, or use items with rough textures such as fabric or yarn. These are helpful in situations in which the person is vulnerable.

Habit inconvenience review is another component of habit reversal. An inventory is compiled of situations in which the behavior has caused inconveniences, embarrassment, and suffering. At some point, reviewing situations in which the behavior has significantly decreased or other positive aspects of eliminating the behaviors can be a fun and rewarding practice to see the changes the person has made.

To stop the impulsive behaviors from coming back, it is recommended to keep a list of all of the problems that were caused by their behavior. Parents and friends are also asked to provide support and feedback to patients for their accomplishments in getting their life back in better control.

When the person is feeling more confident, he or she is encouraged to resume enjoyable activities that were avoided because of being or embarrassed or ashamed. People can practice their new skills in a variety of situations, not just those that they have specifically addressed as part of their behavioral plan.

With regard to some BFRPs, accepting that periods of complete abstinence from the behavior is unrealistic will help reduce guilt and shame for when lapses, or even relapses, occur. People always have skin and hair on their bodies. Some non-BFRPs are somewhat easier to avoid, since they are more situationally based, such as casinos, stores, or porn sites, whereas the target BFRBs are impossible to avoid, since skin and hair are always present on the person's body.

The goal of treatment for Tourette's syndrome is to reduce tics to a level where people no longer cause a significant psychosocial or physical disturbance. It should not be expected that that they are able to constantly suppress their motor and phonic tics. Considering tics and individual comorbid symptoms as separate entities usually enables families and health care specialists to focus on individual needs more effectively. It should be recognized that the treatment of a child with Tourette's requires a steady commitment and, at times, a comprehensive multidisciplinary approach.

Classroom strategies of potential benefit include educating teachers and fellow students, providing optional study breaks, and eliminating unnecessary stressful situations. A variety of behavioral treatments (conditioning techniques, massed negative practice, relaxation training, biofeedback, awareness training, habit reversal, and hypnosis) have been proposed as alternative therapeutic approaches for tics. Relaxation therapy includes a variety of procedures, including the following:

- Progressive muscle relaxation
- Deep breathing

- Visual imagery
- Autogenic training (i.e., repetition of statements suggesting a relaxed state), which produce postures and activities characteristic of a relaxed state

Often enough, people with OCD may have a related disorder, or at least some traits of one, so it is worthwhile for clinicians and CBT therapists, specifically, to be aware of the differential treatment techniques that are effective for treating the wide range of symptoms. Many of these techniques are helpful in managing stress to protect against relapse. They are also helpful life skills that can improve communication and the quality of the relationship to oneself as well as others.

Coping Skills for OCD

For Obsessions

- Remember that obsessions are involuntary; people cannot control the thoughts they get.
- Resist analyzing them. Remind the person that the content is irrational and excessive.
- The emotions that accompany the disorder are like medication side effects. They are a product of the obsessive triggers. The person would not have the emotions were it not for OCD. Ask patients that if their OCD was cured, would they still react in the same way or would they react like others without OCD?
- Teach the person about paradoxical intention. When people have the thoughts on purpose, they are in control of their thoughts, and this strategy disempowers them.
- Suggest postponing obsessing until a specific and structured time. Allowing about ten minutes of focused time to intentionally obsess can help reduce the intensity.
- Help the person understand that accepting the thoughts will reduce anxiety and intensity and that fighting them will make them stronger.
- With a SUDS level below sixty, people can change the way they react to the thoughts by singing them, writing them down, dialing them down like a rheostat, exaggerating them, or making them a cartoon with a thought bubble.
- Have the person try distracting him or herself by engaging in a different activity if the SUDS level is on the manageable side.

- Have the person make a collage of the obsessive material by flipping through magazines or clipping images from the internet. It is a way of externalizing the thoughts and helping to desensitize to them.

For Rituals

- Explain that physically removing oneself from the trigger will help with response prevention. For mental rituals, the person can make alphabetical lists of categories (food, states, countries, etc.) while keeping the obsessive thought in awareness. Remind the patient that trying to use this strategy for obsessions will result in increasing them, due to the effort trying to avoid them.
- Delaying ritualizing by making a bargain to resist for X amount of time; this sets a concrete goal, and often the urge to perform the ritual will have passed. If urge has decreased but is still there, the person can renegotiate for delaying again. If urge passes, it can be let go.
- Changing the ritual in some way can break the rigidity and the specific order the person feels compelled to keep. For example, the person can skip a step, change the order, eliminate do it backward, or design other creative ways of disrupting it.
- If there is a support person available, the patient can talk it through with him or her.
- Use supportive self-statements. Have the patient write them on cue cards and keep with him or her.

References

Ahovan, M., Balali, S., Shargh, A. N., & Doostian, Y. (2016). Efficacy of dialectical behavior therapy on clinical signs and emotion regulation in patients with obsessive-compulsive disorder. *Mediterranean Journal of Social Sciences, 7*(4), 412–418.

Allen, L. B., & Barlow, D. H. (2009). Relationship of exposure to clinically irrelevant emotion cues and obsessive-compulsive symptoms. *Behavior Modification, 33*(6), 743–762. doi:10.1177/0145445509344180

Azrin, N. H., & Nunn, R. G. (1973). Habit-reversal: A method of eliminating nervous habits and tics. *Behaviour Research and Therapy, 11*(4), 619–628. doi:10.1016/0005-7967(73)90119-8

Beck, A. (1976). *Cognitive therapy and the emotional disorders.* New York: Penguin.

Burns, D. D. (1980). *Feeling good: The new mood therapy.* New York: Harper.

Dfarhud, D., Malmir, M., & Khanahmadi, M. (2014). Happiness & health: The biological factors. Systematic review article. *Iranian Journal of Public Health, 43*(11), 1468–1477. Retrieved from https://www.ncbi.nlm.nih.gov/pubmed/26060713; https://www.ncbi.nlm.nih.gov/pmc/articles/PMC4449495/

Foa, E. & Wilson, R. (2001). *Stop obsessing! How to overcome your obsessions and compulsions.* New York: Bantam.

Gershuny, B. S., Baer, L., Parker, H., Gentes, E. L., Infield, A. L., & Jenike, M. A. (2008). Trauma and posttraumatic stress disorder in treatment-resistant obsessive-compulsive disorder. *Depression and Anxiety, 25*(1), 69–71. doi:10.1002/da.20284

Gershuny, B. S., Baer, L., Radomsky, A. S., Wilson, K. A., & Jenike, M. A. (2003). Connections among symptoms of obsessive-compulsive disorder and posttraumatic stress disorder: A case series. *Behaviour Research and Therapy, 41*(9), 1029–1041. Retrieved from https://www.ncbi.nlm.nih.gov/pubmed/12914805

Hayes, S. C. (2004). Acceptance and commitment therapy, relational frame theory, and the third wave of behavioral and cognitive therapies. *Behavior Therapy, 35*(4), 639–665. doi:10.1016/S0005-7894(04)80013-3

Hyman, B. M. & Pedrick, C. (2010). *The OCD workbook: Your guide to breaking free from obsessive-compulsive disorder.* Oakland: New Harbinger Press.

Jakubowski, P. & Lange, A. A. (1978). *The assertive option.* Champagne: Research Press.

Kaslow, N. J., Broth, M. R., Smith, C. O., & Collins, M. H. (2012). Family-based interventions for child and adolescent disorders. *Journal of Marital and Family Therapy, 38*(1), 82–100.

Keng, S.-L., Smoski, M. J., & Robins, C. J. (2011). Effects of mindfulness on psychological health: A review of empirical studies. *Clinical Psychology Review, 31*(6), 1041–1056. doi:10.1016/j.cpr.2011.04.006

Linehan, M. M. (1993). *Cognitive behavioral treatment of borderline personality disorder.* New York: Guilford.

Neff, K. (2011). *Self-compassion: Stop beating yourself up and leave insecurity behind.* New York: William Morrow.

Ranabir, S., & Reetu, K. (2011). Stress and hormones. *Indian Journal of Endocrinology and Metabolism, 15*(1), 18–22. doi:10.4103/2230-8210.77573

Shapiro, L. J. (2014). *Understanding OCD: Skills to control the conscience and outsmart obsessive compulsive disorder.* Santa Barbara, CA: Praeger.

Smith, M. J. (1975). *When I say no, I feel guilty.* New York: The Dial Press.

Twohig, M. P., Abramowitz, J. S., Bluett, E. J., Fabricant, L. E., Jacoby, R. J., Morrison, K. L., & Smith, B. M. (2015). Exposure therapy for OCD from an acceptance and commitment therapy (ACT) framework. *Journal of Obsessive-Compulsive and Related Disorders, 6,* 167–173.

Twohig, M. P., Hayes, S. C., & Masuda, A. (2006). Increasing willingness to experience obsessions: Acceptance and commitment therapy as a treatment for obsessive-compulsive disorder. *Behavior Therapy, 37*(1). doi:10.1016/j.beth.2005.02.001

CHAPTER 9

In Society—Up Close

"Oh, That's Just My OCD!"

Quirks, Branding, Marketing, and the Media

OCD has had a lot of exposure in the media over the past few decades. The mixed message is, OCD is a mental illness that should be hidden and is weird, but it's also a cute way to reference having of certain personality "quirks." People don't want to have it, but they trivialize it as a way of making fun of themselves. Either way, social attitudes that are shaming or dismissive make it difficult to understand the humanity and the suffering caused by the disorder.

OCD has become so popular that it has found its way into mainstream culture. Modern society makes it easier to "do" OCD. Wherever you go in public, people can pump a handful of hand sanitizer. You can use "life hack" behaviors, shortcuts to make one's day-to-day behaviors or activities more efficient (Glowka, Barrett, & Barnhart, 2006), such as taking pictures of your door to remind yourself that it is locked or installing a portable video camera on the dashboard to make sure there was no hit-and-run accident while driving. A whole industry is devoted to getting rid of germs and bacteria by using bathroom and kitchen cleaners, and books like *The Secret* that reinforce the idea that your thoughts will made things happen.

An online study of those using the hashtag #OCD concluded that these social media users often overused humor, mocked symptoms, or used comical language to describe the condition (Pavelko & GallMyrick,

2015). One journal article described the perceived social attitude of OCD as a tragicomedy but noted that people were found to have an underlying sense of hostility toward the disorder based on the reactions viewers had while watching a video of a person with OCD performing extensive repeating rituals (Cefalu, 2009). Another example from a local community are comments made in Tracy Kidder's nonfiction book, *Hometown* (1999): "That's Alan Scheinman. Another local nut," says one person (109), and store clerks referred to him as "the germ-crazy lawyer" (117).

In 2015, the department store Target had a line of Christmas sweaters with "Obsessive Christmas Disorder" woven across the front. *Fortune* magazine ran the story with the headline "Target holds firm on selling 'OCD' sweaters" (Bukszpan, 2015). There were mixed reactions on social media to this campaign, but most people in the OCD community were outraged. One person asked if cancer would be commercialized in such a manner: "So disappointed in @asktarget. Would joke like this about cancer? It's not OK 2 trivialize mental illness" (Plicanic, 2015). Not only do we not joke about cancer, but also other mental illnesses, such as depression, are seldom, if ever, made light of.

One tweeter posted, "At what point did it become socially acceptable and even trendy to use obsessive-compulsive disorder (OCD) as an adjective for being particular, meticulous or organized?" (Greenstein, 2015). What started off as a small trend has turned into a part of everyday language. Companies even use it for branding; one beauty company has named itself Obsessive Compulsive Cosmetics. And social media and news sites use it to be entertaining, such as the Twitter profile OCD Things and Buzzfeed articles with titles like "33 Meticulous Cleaning Tricks For the OCD Person Inside You" and "5 Types of OCD Friends You Know and Love" (Greenstein, 2015).

There's even a market for OCD merchandise on popular e-tail websites. One blogger with OCD posted ten e-tail items for sale that she felt trivialized the disorder, including the Target sweater (Kranefuss, 2018). One popular website that markets handmade, vintage, and craft items had over twenty-three pages of OCD "gifts" (mugs, T-shirts, key chains, etc.). It appears that if you like things that start with the letter *c*, you can buy the item on the internet:

> obsessive chicken disorder, obsessive chess disorder, obsessive (Chicago) cubs disorder, obsessive cardinal (St. Louis) disorder, obsessive chiefs (Kansas City) disorder, obsessive corgi disorder, obsessive corvette disorder, obsessive cake disorder, obsessive

camping disorder, obsessive clown disorder, obsessive coffee disorder, obsessive coffee drinker, obsessive crochet disorder, obsessive carping disorder, obsessive crawfish disorder, obsessive crossfit disorder, obsessive coaching disorder, obsessive cannabis disorder, obsessive canine disorder, obsessive cheerleading disorder, obsessive cruise disorder, obsessive camera disorder, obsessive crafting disorder, obsessive canning disorder, obsessive chocolate disorder, obsessive cow disorder, obsessive chihuahua disorder, obsessive couponing disorder, obsessive Chevy disorder, obsessive cello disorder, obsessive champagne disorder, and obsessive cheese disorder (https://www.google.com/search?q=ocd+products+etsy&sxsrf =ACYBGNQj0f01SN7RLz_ZpCGyF42AeEHP9w:15801430 09930&source=lnms&tbm=isch&sa=X&ved=2ahUKEwi2hrS2m 6TnAhVxw1kKHQ6nDYQQ_AUoAnoECA0QBA&biw=1502& bih=821).

And there's the ever popular: I have CDO—it's like OCD but all the letters are in alphabetical order like they should be! (Retrieved from https://www.google.com/search?q=ocd+cdo&rlz=1C1GCEA _enUS856US856&oq=ocd+cdo&aqs=chrome..69i57j0l7 .7364j0j7&sourceid=chrome&ie=UTF-8)

Two sisters of media-famous family have jumped on the OCD fad. One sister airs a *K-C-D* series that provides tips on organizing (Pham, 2018), and the other sister commented that everything in her home "has to be immaculate" in order for her to accomplish everyday tasks. "I can't take a shower unless the bathroom is absolutely spotless; I think I'm totally OCD," she said. "I have a cleaner who comes three times a week, but I always do the cleaning on top of that" (Maslow, 2015).

Society is obsessed with OCD! It seems acceptable to make light of it when it's not a clinical problem and one doesn't have to experience all the serious downsides, including social stigma. Social stigma has been referred to as a "second disease," as it adds another level of challenge to having a mental disorder (Ociskova, Prasko, & Sedlackova, 2013). Sociocultural attitudes impacts sufferers' identities; they internalize the negative attitudes and label themselves as flawed, broken, or scary (Fennell & Liberato, 2007; Goffman, 1963). External stigmatization leads to self-stigmatization and self-prejudice, when people adopt society's stereotypes that cause lower self-esteem and lack of confidence in their abilities (Corrigan, Bink, Fokuo, & Schmidt, 2015).

In a blog article titled "What the Media Gets Wrong about OCD," Emily Ruth Verona (2018) wrote,

Mental health advocacy and education efforts such as *The OCD Stories* podcast are key in informing the media on what OCD is. *The OCD Stories* podcast is dedicated to inspiring people with OCD to seek proper treatment through thought-provoking and informative interviews with clinical specialists and OCD sufferers alike.

Then, a few years later, I caught an *NCIS* rerun that startled me. A character by the name of Nikki Jardine was introduced as having an aversion to germs. The way other characters looked at her made the word "quirky" immediately jump into my brain.

Lots of shows have normalized the way people laugh at OCD. *Friends*, which has always been one of my favorite comedies, used the condition for a throwaway laugh during season four, episode eleven ("The One With Phoebe's Uterus"), when one of Ross's cow-orkers introduces himself by saying, "I have to turn a light switch on and off 17 times before I leave the room or else my family will die." Additionally, Monica Geller, while never officially diagnosed on the series, exhibits a lot of this behavior for laughs. Cleaning. Organizing. Keeping everything just the way she "likes" it. *The Big Bang Theory*, another program I enjoy, walks this line a lot with Sheldon Cooper.*

OCD Stories

Truth into Fictional Narratives

The experience of having and overcoming OCD is so powerful that people take to writing their personal stories to depict what life is actually like living with it. As of this writing, there have been fifty-eight published memoirs of people's journey through recovery since the year 2000, not to mention the too-many-to-count YouTube personal videos.

Personal experience with OCD has made its way into Hollywood. Hannah, the protagonist in the TV series *Girls*, has OCD. Her character is considered a realistic portrayal since the award-winning show's writer and director, Leah Dunham, is an OCD sufferer herself. She wrote a piece in the *New Yorker* about growing up with OCD (Dunham, 2014) and has written her own memoir, *Not that Kind of Girl* (Dunham, 2015).

The movie writer and director of *Numb*, Jason Goode, has OCD and has two podcasts on *OCD Stories* (https://iocdf.org/blog/2017/11/02/how-the-media-gets-ocd-all-wrong-uk-based-podcast

---

-helps-ocd-sufferers-find-recovery/). One is titled *OCD in Hollywood*, and the other is *Relapse, Stress and Recovery*. He also published an article in the *Huffington Post* titled "Turning a Sudden Mental Disorder into a Film" that depicted his experiences with anxiety.

The feature film most emblematic of how one's station in life does not preclude the devastation OCD can cause is *The Aviator* (Scorsese et al., 2007). The movie was a representation of Howard Hughes's life as an aviation engineer, industrialist, film producer and director, one of the wealthiest people in the world, and an OCD sufferer. While never explicitly saying it, several scenes show how his OCD encroached upon his life. Because of his severe contamination symptoms, he began withdrawing from society, had people wear gloves to avoid having their germs spread on what they touched, hoarded his human waste in jars, neglected his self-care, and died weighing ninety pounds (Hack, 2007).

Documentaries, Videos, and TV Shows

Several documentaries about OCD have been produced in the recent past. *Living with Me and My OCD*, by Claire Watkinson (2017), is a personal documentary about her OCD journey. It highlights the struggles of living with OCD and dealing with stereotypical misconceptions of what OCD.

Unstuck is an inspirational and educational movie that features how six children overcame their OCD by facing their fears through ERP. The video also shows family involvement in the successful treatment process (Anderson, 2017).

The documentary *OCD: The War Inside* explores the daily reality of individuals living OCD. A young man had symptoms such as gnawing on walls, streets, and subway floors that were treated and got under control with behavioral therapy. One person hand washed until her hands were bloody, while another was unable to have people into her house (Hoffert & Pancer, 2001).

Television began to show interest in OCD, anxiety disorders, and hoarding disorder. *Obsessed* was a series that delved into lives affected by OCD, panic disorder, social anxiety disorder, and hoarding disorder and their treatment. The impact of these problems on families and friends were examined (Searer, Foy, LePlante, Sharenow, & Lonker, 2009).

The reality-based series *The OCD Project* was about six people living together in a southern California mansion while undergoing a twenty-one-day intensive ERP treatment with an OCD specialist. There were variable results, but the series revealed for the public true depictions of various types of OCD (Greener et al., 2010).

Lastly, *Hoarders* was a reality series showing the extent to which hoarding behavior takes over household and the impact it has on the families. Episodes depicted the emotional struggle and pain people with this problem experience when it comes to throwing away what most people would consider junk, useless, and meaningless. It also shows social ramifications of the disorder, such as eviction, kids being taken away, or jail (Severson et al., 2009).

Research on OCD in the Film Industry/Media

A research study identified thirty-six movies and one TV show with forty characters with OCD (Fennell & Boyd, 2014). There were several other characters that were not included in the study because they were not explicitly labeled as having it. The study was designed for fifty-four people with OCD to watch the movies and TV show and to communicate their perceptions about whether or not any stereotyping or stigma was portrayed. Many respondents reflected that movies like *As Good as It Gets* (Brooks, 1997) fosters stereotyping. The movie's character, Melvin Udall, has contamination OCD; he is characterized as cantankerous, controlling, and self-involved. The respondents also objected to the stereotypical portrayal of OCD as contamination, washing, and cleaning symptoms rather than depicting any of the many other types of OCD. They also stated when the term *OCD* was in the scripts, it was unclear if it was being used as a clinical term or being made light of. While some respondents felt invalidated, others appreciated being able to have people in their lives see more objectively how OCD functions (Fennell & Boyd, 2014).

An internet study was conducted using the hashtag #OCD to analyze increasing trivial language about OCD on Twitter. The findings indicated that social media users often used trivializing language when referring to the disorder. However, when the Twitter avatars identified themselves as having OCD, they were admired by the same people (Pavelko & Gall-Myrick, 2015). It appears that the social and cultural attitude toward OCD is that it is "quirky" but that when it becomes more personal, people have more respect and compassion.

Professional/Elite Performance

Superstition and Rituals

While numerous presentations of OCD symptoms are the subject of mockery and derision, others are inadvertently promoted by our society. For example, while society may negatively judge the average person, athletes seem to get a pass on their ritualistic behavior. Even fans have superstitious rituals, such as wearing a certain shirt, eating the same meals, and so on, that happened on a winning day for their team. In fact, major league baseball changed its rule about how long batters have to prepare their prepitch stances at home plate. Batters were taking up to a minute performing "just right" rituals by adjusting their gloves, helmet, feet, and grip while pitchers (perhaps by intention) waited (https://www.theglobeandmail.com/sports/baseball/mlbs-new-pace-of -play-rules-put-pressure-on-batters-to-adjust-rituals/article23256219/).

One batter's rituals consisted of stepping into the batter's box, adjusting gloves, brushing his lip, and tapping cleats with the bat to remove dirt. He also checked his helmet, tugged at his jersey, hitched up his pants, and checked his right thumb protector for every single pitch. Such behaviors now would likely cause him to be fined, due to new pace-of-play initiatives designed not only to speed up a game but also to keep fans from becoming bored and disinterested in the sport (Withers, 2018).

Socially Reinforced Perfectionism in a Performance-Driven Society

Practice makes perfect! It takes years of intense training to excel in one's chosen endeavor. Malcolm Gladwell, author of *Outliers,* claims that it takes about ten thousand hours of practice to achieve mastery in a field, which adds up to nine years of time (Gladwell, 2008)! In the meantime, how do people psychologically deal with the stress of competition? Do they stay focused or burn out? Are they driven or obsessive? How far is reaching too far? What does it take to have the "edge"? Do they resort to cheating behaviors such as athletes taking steroids or performing artists sabotaging their competitors? Because perfectionism involves overthinking, it can often lead to performance anxiety.

Excellence versus Perfectionism

Olympic and elite athletes, performing artists, and gifted students are vulnerable to being obsessive perfectionists. Researchers who have begun to examine the relationship between perfectionism and obsessiveness in sport and the performing arts found that study participants described extraordinary levels of dedication, meticulousness, and ruminative thoughts or overthinking as part of their performance process (Hill, Witcher, Gotwals, & Leyland, 2015). Other researchers who studied elite athletes identified the centrality of obsessive thoughts to the industriousness associated with perfectionism (Rice et al., 2016). Further, Hill and colleagues (2004) found evidence of a link between perfectionism and obsessive compulsive symptoms.

What differentiates these valued traits from being effective or dysfunctional? Striving for excellence is derived from an internal drive to realize one's potential rather than achieve a goal. The pursuer of excellence bases success on the effort or the willingness to try rather than the achievement of the goal (Drizinsky, Zülch, Gibbons, & Stahl, 2016; Greenspon, 2000). These authors go on to say that, on the other hand, perfectionists need to do things perfectly, not to feel the joy of accomplishment but to be acceptable, to maintain a sense of order in the world, and to have complete control over the outcome of their efforts.

Excellence is derived from an internal strength and confidence, while perfectionism may be socially reinforced. People with perfectionistic standards and performance in academics, athleticism, musicianship, and fine art performance receive accolades for the produced outcome. What may not be known is how much shame and criticism people might be avoid by engaging in compulsive, approval-seeking, mistake-avoidant behaviors.

The website Excel in Life has offered helpful ways to distinguish unhealthy perfectionism versus the characteristics of excellence, using ten points. She asks whether the person's mind-set is process oriented or outcome oriented. Someone who strives for excellence focuses on the process rather than the outcome. Goals are more performance than achievement based. A performance goal is more achievable because it can add new behaviors, rather than trying to approach a situation in the same old way, leading to failure.

A perfectionist's self-worth is measured by achievement. The odds of achieving perfection are poor to none. This results in a self-perception of worthlessness or failure because the person always falls short. On the other hand, a pursuer of excellence values him or herself based on the effort or willingness to try and not on the achievement of the goal. That person is unlikely to negatively label him or herself.

Perfectionists set unrealistic goals and standards that are too demanding and impossible to achieve. People setting out for excellence understands what realistic but challenging goals they can set that are clear, specific, and reachable. They understand their limits and can make decisions that challenge them to strive, sometimes in incremental steps. The perfectionistic counterparts set an imagined or ideal goal that they may not realize is a setup for failure.

The perfectionist thinks being self-critical is motivating. However, the pursuer of excellence is willing to self-examine performance and personal vulnerabilities and use them as lessons to improve in a more objective rather than emotional appraisal.

People who are perfectionists often seek external validation because they feel empty inside. Reaching a level of excellence is its own reward for people who are internally driven. They appreciate the praise and accolades they receive from others, but they are emotionally and psychologically fulfilled by an internal sense of satisfaction.

Willingness to risk and fail and avoidance of failure are very different learning processes. People who are willing to try and risk failure have nothing to lose and potentially everything to gain, because they are not held back by fear. People who have a perfectionistic attitude toward an endeavor limit ever reaching their potential level of performance, because trying to reach beyond their comfort zone feels too personally threatening.

Perfectionists sees others as competitors and adversaries to beat. They tend to be sore losers and blame others for what went wrong. Feedback is taken as criticism, and they have trouble taking responsibility for their part of the problem. The pursuer of excellence considers others as partners sharing in the achievement of their goals. They listen and accept feedback in a spirit of learning.

Another point of difference has to do with the need for instant gratification versus having patience. Perfectionists need the goal to be achieved immediately, or else they may have thoughts about giving up. They berate themselves for not succeeding and compare their performance those who did succeed. Those who seek excellence recognize the need for pacing, practice, and effort. They have a sense that there is always more to learn in order to hone their skills and sharpen their mind-set.

Finally, the pursuer of excellence finds enjoyment and fulfilment in the pursuit of goals, whereas perfectionists are usually unhappy or dissatisfied with how they experience their process. When their ego is on the line, perfectionists' sense of self may feel fragile. Those with a spirit of excellence accept that reaching their goals is challenging and achievable, and their identity is not caught up in failure or success. They are more likely to enjoy the challenge of getting to the goal than be too focused on the result. At times, the pursuit of excellence may just be about finishing a task, whereas perfectionism may be motivated by avoiding the challenging internal experience of having to struggle through what is experienced as tedious.

Athletes

Socially prescribed perfectionism has been characterized as the belief that striving for perfection and being perfect are important to others, that others expect them to be perfect, and that others will be highly critical of them if they fail to meet these expectations (Stoeber & Corr, 2015).

Elite athletes who are motivated by succeeding for others tend to suffer physical damage by playing through the pain (Hughes & Coakley, 1991) and winning at all costs (Demulier, Le Scanff, & Stephan, 2013). They may also resort to doping, since the need to succeed outweighs their health concerns (Lentillon-Kaestner, Hagger, & Hardcastle, 2012). One estimate of steroid use among elite athletes was 14–39 percent (De Hon, Kuipers, & van Bottenburg, 2015). Other issues of concern with perfectionism in athletes are depression (Demulier et al., 2013) and eating disorders, particularly in female athletes (Scoffier, Gernigon, & d'Arripe-Longueville, 2012).

Coaching style can also factor into the pressure to succeed no matter the cost. Those who are emotionally vulnerable may experience higher levels of stress and anxiety when they are criticized for making mistakes, and they may develop superstitious and compulsive behaviors (Swann, Moran, & Piggott, 2015). As is the case with many psychological issues, the willingness to be imperfect allows people to focus less on the outcome and more on their own motivation to challenge their limits (Terner, Pew, & Aird, 1978).

Perfectionism is also socially reinforced at fitness centers and gyms. Chapter 3 reviewed body appearance disorders related to OCD, such as BDD and muscle dysmorphia. Bodybuilders and avid fitness enthusiasts may engage in obsessive ideas about having perfect bodies and perform rigid ritualized workout routines. Results of bodybuilding competitions as well as physiques toned through routine workouts attract positive reinforcement when people admire how "cut" the person looks (Brian).

Musicians

High-performing musicians also suffer from socially reinforced perfectionism. Music is highly competitive, and there is little room for error, especially for concert performers and orchestra members. A life dedicated to training for the elite level of professionalism demands years of honing fine-motor dexterity and coordination, attention and memory, and personal aesthetic and interpretative skills (Kenny & Osborne, 2006). It also requires dedicated hours of solitary practice each day; often, playing passages or practicing a new skill is conducted in a repetitive manner. Musicians with OCD have trouble knowing when they have practiced enough to enhance their skills and stop rather than repeating the skill over and over until they have suffered physical pain or mental exhaustion.

Music performance anxiety can result from perceived external expectations of performing perfectly. A study of professional classical musicians found that those with higher personal standards of perfection and a high social standard of perfection experienced more debilitating anxiety (Mor, Day, Flett, & Hewitt, 1995). A study of university instrumental music students identified a significant relationship between dimensions of perfectionism (high concern over mistakes, high doubts about actions, and low personal standards) and performance anxiety (Sinden, 1999).

Hill and colleagues (2015) cited that participants in his study kept raising their standards of achievement and performance, had an "obsessive" approach to improvement, had a rigid and dichotomous thinking style, and experienced recurring dissatisfaction with their current performances. The participants stated that obsessiveness was a component of perfectionism and a means of motivation to do better. He found that the participants were consumed, if not "obsessed," with striving to constantly improve and had an "obsessive work ethic."

Parents

Like coaches, parents have a direct and personal impact on defining success and failure. Frost and colleagues (1990) define perfectionism as an excessive concern over making mistakes, high personal standards, perception of high parental expectations and high parental criticism, the doubting of the quality of one's actions, and a preference for order and organization. Parental criticism, expectations, and high expressed emotion predicted maladaptive perfectionism and overconcern over mistakes, and they were found to be associated with a performance-avoidance goal orientation (Madjar, Voltsis, & Weinstock, 2015). In reference to expressed emotion, perceived criticism and hostility create an atmosphere of distress and dysfunction. Some children may feel the need to be perfect in order to avoid negative attention.

Modern/Popular Cultural Figures

When you Google "people with OCD," several lists identify celebrities and other well-known people who have self-disclosed or are assumed to have OCD. It's unclear how reliable these lists are; they describe some behaviors that may be explained by personality traits without indicating a diagnosable disorder. People who self-disclose are committing acts of social justice and contributing to the destigmatization of OCD, as well as mental disorders more generally. One such person is Marc Summers, who was one of the first celebrities to out himself as having OCD. He hosted the children's game show *Double Dare* and had several other television roles. His book about his experience with OCD is titled *Everything in Its Place: My Trials and Triumphs with Obsessive Compulsive Disorder* (Summers, 1999).

Howie Mandel has also been public about having OCD. It is said that he invented the fist bump as a way of avoiding shaking hands with contestants on *Deal or No Deal* when he was the game show's host. He also wrote a memoir about having OCD, *Here's the Deal: Don't Touch Me* (Mandel & Young, 2009).

Other celebrities who are said to have come out as having OCD are, to name a few, Leonardo DiCaprio (who played Howard Hughes in *The Aviator*), Justin Timberlake, Megan Fox, Cameron Diaz, and Howard Stern.

It is safe to say that people who have OCD are in good company. OCD is more common than people think and is an equal-opportunity disorder. Because it is widely inherited, it can be considered a force of nature, not something that people can just "get over."

References

Anderson, K. (Writer). (2017). Unstuck: An OCD kids movie [Video]. In C. Baier (Producer). New York: Realistic Pictures, Inc.

Basamian, S. (Producer) & Hoffert, D., & Pancer, P. (Directors). (2001). OCD: The war inside [Documentary]. Canada: National Film Board of Canada.

Brian, D. The role of obsessive compulsive behaviour in sport and exercise. Retrieved from https://anxietyhouse.com.au/obsessive-compulsive -behaviour-in-sport-and-exercise/

Brooks, J. L., Johnson, B., Kavanaugh, M., Mark, L., Porter, A. L., Sakai, R., Schofield, J. D., Wilson, O., Zea, K., & Ziskin, L. (Producers) & Brooks, J. L. (Director). (1997). As good as it gets [Motion picture]. United States: TriStar Pictures.

Bukszpan, D. (2015). Target holds firm on selling "OCD" sweaters. *Fortune*. Retrieved from http://fortune.com/2015/11/12/target-ocd-sweaters/

Cefalu, P. (2009). What's so funny about obsessive-compulsive disorder? *PMLA, 124*(1), 44–58.

Corrigan, P. W., Bink, A. B., Fokuo, J. K., & Schmidt, A. (2015). The public stigma of mental illness means a difference between you and me. *Psychiatry Research, 226*(1), 186–191. doi:10.1016/j.psychres.2014.12.047

De Hon, O., Kuipers, H., & van Bottenburg, M. (2015). Prevalence of doping use in elite sports: A review of numbers and methods. *Sports Medicine, 45*(1), 57–69.

Demulier, V., Le Scanff, C., & Stephan, Y. (2013). Psychological predictors of career planning among active elite athletes: An application of the social cognitive career theory. *Journal of Applied Sport Psychology, 25*(3), 341–353. doi:10.1080/10413200.2012.736444

Drizinsky, J., Zülch, J., Gibbons, H., & Stahl, J. (2016). How personal standards perfectionism and evaluative concerns perfectionism affect the error positivity and post-error behavior with varying stimulus visibility. *Cognitive, Affective, & Behavioral Neuroscience, 16*(5), 876–887. doi:10.3758/s13415-016-0438-z

Dunham, L. (2014). Difficult girl: Growing up, with help. *New Yorker*, September 1.

Dunham, L. (2015). *Not that kind of girl: A young woman tells you what she's "learned."* New York: Random House.

Fennell, D., & Boyd, M. (2014). Obsessive-compulsive disorder in the media. *Deviant Behavior, 35*(9), 669–686. doi:10.1080/01639625.2013.872526

Fennell, D., & Liberato, A. S. Q. (2007). Learning to live with OCD: Labeling, the self, and stigma. *Deviant Behavior, 28*(4), 305–331. doi:10.1080/01639620701233274

Frost, R. O., Marten, P., Lahart, C., & Rosenblate, R. (1990). The dimensions of perfectionism. *Cognitive Therapy and Research, 14*(5), 449–468.

Gladwell, M. (2008). *Outliers: The story of success.* New York: Little, Brown and Co.

Glowka, W., Barrett, G., & Barnhart, D. K. (2006). Most useful word of the year. Retrieved from http://www.americandialect.org/Words_of _the_Year_2005.pdf

Goffman, E. (1963). *Stigma: Notes on the management of spoiled identity.* New York: Simon & Shuster.

Greener, A., Roth, J. D., Olde, J., Holmes, J., Assmus, M., Pollack, N., & Nelson, T. (Executive producers) & Jacobs, M. S. (Director). (2010). *The OCD Project* [television series episode]. New York: VH1.

Greenspon, T. (2000). "Healthy perfectionism" is an oxymoron!: Reflections on the psychology of perfectionism and the sociology of science. *Journal of Secondary Gifted Education, 11*(4), 197–208.

Greenstein, L. (2015). I'm so OCD. Retrieved from https://www.nami.org /Blogs/NAMI-Blog/October-2015/OMG,-I%E2%80%99m-So-OCD

Hack, R. (2007). *Hughes: The private diaries, memos, and letters; The definitive biography of the first american billionaire.* Beverly Hills, CA: Phoenix.

Hill, A., Witcher, C. S. G., Gotwals, J. K., & Leyland, A. F. (2015). A qualitative study of perfectionism among self-identified perfectionists in sport and the performing arts. *Sport, Exercise, and Performance Psychology, 4*(4), 237–253. doi:10.1037/spy0000041

Hill, R. W., Huelsman, T. J., Furr, R. M., Kibler, J., Vicente, B. B., & Kennedy, C. (2004). A new measure of perfectionism: The perfectionism inventory. *Journal of Personality Assessment, 82*(1), 80–91. doi:10.1207 /s15327752jpa8201_13

Hughes, R., & Coakley, J. (1991). Positive deviance among athletes: The implications of overconformity to the sport ethic. *Sociology of Sport Journal, 8,* 307–325.

Kenny, D. T., & Osborne, M. S. (2006). Music performance anxiety: New insights from young musicians. *Advances in Cognitive Psychology, 2*(2–3), 103–112. doi:10.2478/v10053-008-0049-5

Kidder, T. (1999). *Hometown.* New York: Washington Square Press.

Kranefuss, P. (2018). Ten times OCD was treated like a joke but we weren't laughing. Retrieved from http://www.treatmyocd.com/blog /ten-times-ocd-was-treated-like-a-joke-but-we-werent-laughing/

Lentillon-Kaestner, V., Hagger, M. S., & Hardcastle, S. (2012). Health and doping in elite-level cycling. *Scandinavian Journal of Medicine & Science in Sports, 22*(5), 596–606. doi:10.1111/j.1600 -0838.2010.01281.x

Madjar, N., Voltsis, M., & Weinstock, M. P. (2015). The roles of perceived parental expectation and criticism in adolescents' multidimensional perfectionism and achievement goals. *Educational Psychology, 35*(6), 765–778. doi:10.1080/01443410.2013.864756

Mandel, H., & Young, J. (2009). *Here's the deal, don't touch me.* New York: Bantam.

Maslow, N. (2015). 8 things you probably don't know about Kim Kardashian. Retrieved from https://www.popsugar.com/celebrity/photo -gallery/34746545/image/34752775/She-Has-Obsessive-Compul sive-Tendencies

Mor, S., Day, H. I., Flett, G. L., & Hewitt, P. L. (1995). Perfectionism, control, and components of performance anxiety in professional artists. *Cognitive Therapy and Research, 19*(2), 207–225. doi:10.1007 /BF02229695

Ociskova, M., Prasko, J., & Sedlackova, Z. (2013). Stigma and self-stigma in patients with anxiety disorders. *Activitas Nervosa Superior Rediviva, 55*(1–2), 12–18.

Pavelko, R. L., & GallMyrick, J. (2015). That's so OCD: The effects of disease trivialization via social media on user perceptions and impression formation. Author links open overlay panel. *Computers in Human Behavior, 49,* 251–258.

Pham, J. (2018). Khloé Kardashian slammed for exploiting OCD in a "cute" series for her website. Retrieved from https://stylecaster.com /khloe-kardashian-exploit-ocd-website/

Plicanic, K. [@kplicanic]. (2015). So disappointed in @asktarget. Would joke like this about cancer? It's not OK 2 trivialize mental illness. [*Fortune Magazine*]. Retrieved from fortune.com/2015/11/12 /target-ocd-sweaters/

Rice, S. M., Purcell, R., De Silva, S., Mawren, D., McGorry, P. D., & Parker, A. G. (2016). The mental health of elite athletes: A narrative systematic review. *Sports Medicine, 46*(9), 1333–1353.

Scoffier, S., Gernigon, C., & d'Arripe-Longueville, F. (2012). Effects of achievement goals on self-regulation of eating attitudes among elite female athletes: An experimental study. *Psychology of Sport and Exercise, 13*(2), 201–207.

Scorsese, M., Mann, M., Logan, J., DiCaprio, L., Blanchett, C., Beckinsale, K., . . . Channel, H. (2007). *The Aviator* [videorecording]. Burbank, CA: Distributed by Warner Home Video.

Searer, T., Foy, J., LePlante, R., Sharenow, R., & Lonker, S. (Producers). (2009). *Obsessed* [television series]. New York: A&E Network.

Severson, D., Berg, A., McKillop, D., Bryant, E. F., Butts, G., Morgan, J., . . . Kelly, M. (Executive producers). (2009). *Hoarders* [television series]. New York: A&E Network.

Sinden, L. M. (1999). *Music performance anxiety: Contributions of perfectionism, coping style, self-efficacy, and self-esteem* (Doctoral dissertation), Arizona State University. Retrieved from https:// www.worldcat.org/title/music-performance-anxiety-contributions -of-perfectionism-coping-style-self-efficacy-and-self-esteem/oclc /49334582

Stoeber, J., & Corr, P. J. (2015). Perfectionism, personality, and affective experiences: New insights from revised reinforcement sensitivity theory. *Personality and Individual Differences, 86,* 354–359.

Summers, M. (1999). *Everything in its place: My trials and triumphs with obsessive compulsive disorder.* New York: Jeremy P. Tarcher/ Putnam.

Swann, C., Moran, A., & Piggott, D. (2015). Defining elite athletes: Issues in the study of expert performance in sport psychology. *Psychology of Sport and Exercise, 16*, 3–14.

Terner, J. R., Pew, W. L., & Aird, R. A. (1978). *The courage to be imperfect: The life and work of Rudolf Dreikurs*. New York: Hawthorn.

Verona, E. R. (2018). What the media gets wrong about OCD. Retrieved from https://bust.com/living/195009-media-ocd.html

Watkinson, C. (Director). (2012, August 15). Living with me and my OCD [video file]. Retrieved from https://www.youtube.com/watch?v =m5SfUpEcpGI

Withers, T. (2018). MLB's pace-of-play rules force batters to adjust game rituals. *Globe and Mail*. Retrieved from https://www.theglo beandmail.com/sports/baseball/mlbs-new-pace-of-play-rules -put-pressure-on-batters-to-adjust-rituals/article23256219/

CHAPTER 10

At Work and School—Up Close

At Work

Prerna was a forty-five-year-old Indian female executive of a high technology firm. The stress of her company's recent financial problems had exacerbated her mild OCD symptoms, which had begun to impact her work performance. She was having trouble making decisions due to her fear that making a mistake would jeopardize the company's viability and cost people their jobs.

Lately, she had arrived late to work after having been up all night playing games on her phone and watching TV for hours. Sometimes, instead of going into her office, she sat in her car in the parking lot and took a nap. She then stayed late to make up for the lost time and to get some work done. She was mentally, physically, and emotionally exhausted when she got home, but she attended to her family. All the while she was reviewing her work challenges, and although she had some ideas about how to move forward, she was unable to commit to a decision because of potentially having to downsize, create layoffs, or restructure the business. She was especially upset about the impact it would have on her employees and their families.

Her symptoms began in childhood and consist of perfectionism, fear of making mistakes, symmetry, and ordering. Having done well in school, she was able to generalize her impeccable standards to work. In some ways, her perfectionism helped advance her career, as these traits were reinforced by getting promotions. However, like many perfectionists, she had reached a point of diminishing returns because of the inability to sustain her level of perfectionism indefinitely.

Prerna had a husband and two school-aged children. She already felt guilty about not being home for the children after school, but the problems at work made for longer hours there. She obsessed that the children were suffering from her not being around as much as they would like, that she might be considered neglecting her family, and that she had not been able to be intimate with her husband. Her husband hired a cleaning service to help maintain the housekeeping, but internally Prerna was never satisfied with what they did.

When she was at work, she checked her phone to make sure that she hadn't missed any calls from school needing her to pick up a child who was sick. When she was home, she checked her email to stay on top of any recent developments about the business.

Finally unable to cope, Prerna sought a referral from her primary care doctor for a psychiatrist, thinking that medication could help take the edge of the anxiety. Her psychiatrist prescribed an effective antidepressant commonly used for OCD, but she informed Prerna that it could take up to six to eight weeks before she noticed any effect. Prerna' psychiatrist referred her to a behavior therapist. She and Miles, her therapist, would work out a behavioral plan for managing her life as well as an ERP plan to target the perfectionism. Prerna was also educated about OCD being covered by the Americans With Disabilities Act of 1973. She was told that she could have some accommodations made for her schedule and that she should be allowed to go to mental health appointments.

It was a lot for her to absorb. How, under the current circumstance, was she going to explain to work that she needed to reduce her hours? How was she going to keep her email checking under control? What should she tell her family? Would they think less of her or think she was being dramatic?

Prerna's husband was glad that she was finally getting treatment and told her he would support her in whatever way he could so that she could to get control of her life back. She and her husband explained to the kids that there would be a change in routine and that their mother would be around the house more, about which they were happy. Her husband also told her not to feel pressured to tell the rest of the family until, or if, she wanted to. Miles explained to Prerna that sometimes keeping it a secret adds more stress to managing an episode and that there may be other family members who have OCD but also have not disclosed it.

Prerna was allowed to telecommute. She had some anxious thoughts about her work performance and if this change in her routine would produce inferior results. She was reassured by her colleagues that things were under control and that she should feel confident about her ideas and plans to execute them. She was able to resist asking them to tell her again that they weren't worried about her work ethic.

Meanwhile, she was able to see her therapist twice a week and brought her work in with her so that Miles could coach her through her thinking and work process in a more fluid manner. Prerna was encouraged to resist checking what she had already done and to be more spontaneous with her word choices. Prerna's anxiety level was at around a SUDS level of ninety, but she kept with her plan and was able to complete an assignment in about one-third of the time. Eventually she transitioned back to work and worked hard at maintaining her gains and practicing the kinds of self-care that prevents relapse.

At College

Grace was a nineteen-year-old premed student at a top-ranked college. When she was in eighth grade, she had difficulty getting to school on time. Before leaving the house, she lined up her stuffed animals and shoes in a perfect manner. She was afraid to raise her hand in class in case her answer was wrong, even though they were almost always right. She had limited interest in after-school activities because she was anxious to get home and get her homework completed perfectly. After that, she practiced her flute for hours, preparing for her lessons and band practice at school. These behaviors were reinforced by her parents and teachers as she excelled. As a result, she made few friends and was a bit socially behind. Throughout elementary, middle, and high school, Grace was very concerned with her academic performance and rarely socialized, choosing instead to spend her time on schoolwork. The social life she did have consisted of the community service in which she was involved.

After high school, Grace went on to a prestigious college, where academics were more challenging, as a premed student. She managed to get good grades but often went without sleep in order to memorize biology terms and other important information she would need to learn. During study groups, Grace would repeatedly ask clarifying questions, which caused frustration with the other students. At times, she would request a meeting with her professor to make sure that she understood the assignments in spite of the details being clearly outlined in the syllabus. She had trouble managing her time because she tried to attend every extra opportunity related to her program and became overwhelmed. When Grace received a B+ on one assignment, she burst into tears in class and asked for another meeting with the professor.

After sleepless nights, Grace was working in her chemistry lab and spilled some chemicals. People helped her clean them up, per the protocols, but she was so distressed from having made that mistake that she entertained the idea of not going back. Meanwhile, she was preoccupied about having chemical residue on her hands and avoided touching things as much as possible until she got home, where she scrubbed her hands with soap and hot water until they turned red. Then she worried that the lab had not been properly cleaned. She didn't know what she should do. She was afraid to go back to the lab because she might cause another accident, but she was also afraid of not going back to clean up the spill area again in case someone touched the chemicals without knowing.

Grace's situation was precarious. It was clear that something was interfering with her studies. She worried about not getting her work done, but she knew that she could not keep going on with the way things were. After the lab incident, her chemistry professor suggested that she talk to her advisor, who then recommended that she make an appointment at the student health center to address her anxiety. At the health center, she was diagnosed with OCD after relating her current and past history of how she did or didn't manage stress. She stated that she had always been anxious and thought it was just normal and that she had always found a way to get by.

The clinician explained to Grace that leaving home and going to college was a typical time for people with latent OCD to have their first episode. Grace felt doubly stigmatized about having a mental disorder and was especially worried about how it might affect her pursuit of dream to be a doctor. She already knew that the medical profession was not kind to "sick" doctors. She didn't know if the culture of the profession would provide support to students with a mental illness (after all, she couldn't be the first person to be in this situation) or if it would be used against her.

Grace qualified for academic accommodation per the Americans With Disabilities Act. Grace and her parents had to decide whether or not to take advantage of this support without knowing what the ramifications might be in the future. The choices presented were that Grace could power through like she always had, disclose to her school that she had OCD and was having trouble keeping up, or take a medical leave of absence to focus solely on treatment and symptom control. Grace and her parents decided that she would enter into twice-weekly behavior therapy, request a medical single room in a dorm at school, and wait for the medication to take effect.

Grace was referred to a psychiatrist and a behavior therapist to start treatment. The psychiatrist prescribed a medication and informed her of the side effects, as well as letting her know the limitations of medication treatment alone. He also told her that the medications might take up to six to eight weeks to start working and was glad to hear that she was entering into behavior therapy.

Sheila, Grace's behavior therapist, assessed her current and past symptoms using the Y-BOCS; she met criteria for perfectionism and not-just-right-experiences, as well as contamination. Sheila explained to Grace what perfectionism and NJREs were and gave several examples from the history she had collected going back to childhood. Grace now understood that being late for school because of lining up her stuffed animals and shoes in elementary school was an NJRE ritual. She had known it had never made sense, but she had been so anxious about it that her mother had allowed the behavior.

Grace's perfectionism and NJREs with her lifelong schoolwork was also presented as symptomatic of OCD. The praise for her excellent grades reinforced her need to excel in school so as not to disappoint people and let them down. Unfortunately, the people praising her had unwittingly reinforced her behavior and did not realize the extent of time and distress it took for Grace to succeed in achieving her accomplishments. Even her flute playing was perfectionistic and had stopped being enjoyable. Her music teacher had told her that she had special talent and that she could participate in competitions.

Finally, Grace expressed relief at now understanding the source of the pressure to perform at high standards and her high baseline anxiety. She was grateful that she would not have to live like this for the rest of her life!

Grace was motivated, but Sheila knew Grace might try to be the "perfect patient" and take on more challenging ERPs than she could manage. If Grace overchallenged herself and could not maintain the response prevention for the exposure task, she might feel like she failed and be discouraged. They decided the initial exposure would target her contamination symptoms at as SUDS level of sixty, out of one hundred.

Sheila worked in a group practice, and people in the office were used to unusual behaviors happening there. Grace agreed to shake hands with people and then cross-contaminate herself by touching all of her personal items, such as her cell phone, all the items in her backpack, and her hair and skin. After getting back to her dorm, Grace was to resist washing her hands and was to contaminate all the rest of the items in her room by touching them. After bathroom use or before eating, Grace could wash her hands in a normalized way (ten seconds), but then she had to recontaminate her hands by touching all of the items that were contaminated from before. In this way, she would get used to everything feeling dirty and then not have to organize her life around avoiding it.

Sheila wanted Grace to email her if she was having trouble following through; not hearing from her meant that Grace was on track. This was important, because Grace had trouble asking for help, and treatment effectiveness relied on the steady pace of facing the obsessive challenge.

Grace returned a few days later for their second session and reported that the contamination exposures were easier than she expected and that she would like to move up the hierarchy. She was still having trouble in the lab in spite of wearing protective gloves. Peroxide, a chemical used in the lab, was a trigger, and it could be easily purchased at the local CVS. Grace agreed to get rubbing alcohol and dab some on her hands and face and let it dry without washing her hands. Then she would do exposures to peroxide at a later time.

Unfortunately, she was still struggling to manage her time, getting her assignments done, and prepare for exams. Grace outlined the deadlines and exam schedule for the rest of the semester. They then organized a schedule to which Grace would adhere in order to pass. Would Grace be willing to do the work and hand it in to pass even if it meant less than perfect performance? Would she be willing to accept this change as a way of life going forward in service to reaching her goals? Would she accept failure as a possibility? Typically, this can be one of the most difficult challenges, since the risk of failure seems so high and how it may change her self-identity as no longer being seen as flawless by others.

Sheila helped Grace sort out the costs and benefits of continuing the same pattern and the high likelihood, given the competitive nature of acceptance to medical school, that she would not demonstrate the kind of reliability, flexibility, and effectiveness they would expect. When freed up from her obsessive fear, Grace might feel great relief and do well in school and in life. However, once the compulsive behaviors were under control, it might turn out that Grace had obsessive compulsive personality disorder.

Grace did well working up her contamination hierarchy, eventually touching the lab door handle, showering normally without avoiding the walls, and touching peroxide with her hands, all without washing her hands, as well as cross-contaminating all her belongings and possessions. She did her lab assignments, and her success with previous exposures generalized a bit so that her anticipatory and actual anxiety about doing the experiments lessened. Reaching the top of her hierarchy, Grace eliminated all subtle and observable contamination rituals, and she was able to focus on her work.

Regarding performance perfectionism, Grace began sending imperfect emails to family and friends, and she saw that no one cared or had any negative feedback about it. She attended study groups and did not ask reassurance-seeking clarifying questions and reduced her visits to her professors. Writing assignments still plagued her, and she still asked for extensions for a few of the papers. Sheila and Grace set absolute deadlines for the extended papers, perfect or not. Waiting for the grades on these papers was torture. She broke her perfect record with more than one A-, but she was relieved to have put them behind her and to move on to maintaining a workable study schedule.

Grace finished her first college semester well in spite of her anxiety and fears of failing or causing harm by chemical contamination. During her break, Sheila and Grace continued to process and set up perfectionism exposures so that she could be more spontaneous and freer to be herself. Grace would continue to be challenged by this symptom for some time, but it was under manageable control for now. Some cognitive therapy would be helpful in conjunction with behavioral work. She also felt that the medication was working and taking some of the edge off of her anxiety.

In Elementary School

Danny was a bright boy in the third grade, but he was having difficulty concentrating in class. He tapped his pencil in a rhythmic manner that drove the kids sitting near him crazy. When the teacher noticed, she would ask him to stop, and he would for a time. He also said words under his breath, which also called negative attention to himself. When he walked down the hall, some of the kids made fun of his behaviors.

The school contacted his parents, and a meeting was held with Danny, his parents, and his guidance counselor. Danny's parents, Amelia and Sam, were aware of his behaviors, and they disclosed that Danny had OCD. While Danny's behaviors were easily noticed, nobody was aware of his intrusive thoughts. Danny's obsessions had to do with the fear of offending God and being severely punished. The tapping rituals were performed in series of fours until he "felt right," and the talking under his breath were prayers promising God that he would try to be a good boy.

A psychiatrist had diagnosed Danny's OCD last year, and it had been getting gradually worse. Danny had been to an OCD child psychologist,

Pam, but he never told her about the fear-of-God obsessions because he felt it would be a betrayal of God's trust. She and Danny had successfully treated some mild contamination and hand washing symptoms, and he stopped seeing her. Then the tapping replaced the hand washing rituals.

Amelia and Sam were leery of medicating him. They were afraid of the side effects and were concerned about Danny being medicated at such an early age. The psychiatrist provided information about the pros and cons of using medication at Danny's age. On the one hand, he could resume behavior therapy with Pam and see if it would sufficiently help to get control over his symptoms, but on the other hand, Danny's academic and social development might suffer in the meantime. The psychiatrist ultimately left the decision up to his parents, who decided to have Danny resume behavior therapy.

Danny was still too afraid to disclose his fear-of-God obsessions to his therapist and wasn't really making progress with ERPs, since they weren't targeting the intrusive thoughts. His parents decided that it was time to consult the psychiatrist again, and Danny was prescribed an SSRI medication known to be effective for OCD. Danny was not happy with the decision and was afraid that God would consider taking them to be sinful.

Danny was not compliant with taking his medications every day. As a result, it never started working, and the behavior therapy was floundering. Danny's father had researched OCD resources and saw on the IOCDF website that there was a family support group in his local area that also had kid activities. Amelia and Sam were desperate to learn how other families coped with trying to help their child engage in behavior therapy, making decisions about medication, and knowing what to do if a child refuses to take them.

Danny and Pam developed a trusting relationship, and during one session, she asked him more about the purpose of his rituals. He broke into tears and was finally able to tell her about how he has been trying to please God and how afraid he was about failing. Danny told her that at church he was exposed to religious figures and had "bad" thoughts about how they could represent the devil. She said, "Oh, my dear! I had no idea how scared you must be!" Pam and Danny met with his parents, and Danny told them what his fears had been about.

Amelia felt guilty that she had insisted Danny go to church with her and Sam when he was adamant that he didn't want to go. She had seen how restless he was and how he sometimes muttered under his breath.

She reassured Danny that until he felt ready, he would not have to go back to church. Amelia trusted Pam to address this problem, and an appointment was set up for next week.

The issue now was about school and academics. Would Danny need an individual education plan (IEP) or just accommodations? The school psychologist would conduct an evaluation to assess whether he had special needs. Danny was upset that he needed to go through this and that things would be different for him than for his friends. When he was told he would have to take a test, he became anxious and was resistant. After the evaluation, a meeting was held with Danny, his parents, the school psychologist, and Danny's behavior therapist. The school psychologist shared the results of the evaluation; Danny was eligible for a 504 plan that can make adjustments in the classroom to facilitate his learning. The school began to arrange for accommodations that would meet Danny's needs such as sitting at the front of the class to reduce others noticing his "prayers" and tapping rituals.

For Danny and other children with mental health challenges, accommodations are meant to level the playing field so that there is equal parity to meet the demands of academic work. They are often temporary and adjusted once the symptoms are under better control. In the classroom, Danny would sit near the teacher, who could provide a nonverbal cue when Danny tapped or prayed under his breath. The teacher would not call on Danny when he looked visibly anxious. An understanding was made that his teachers would continue to carry on as normal even if Danny was engaging in rituals, to not try to stop them, and to avoid calling attention to him. The accommodations would be clearly stated so that there was consistency among teachers. A plan to review the efficacy of the accommodations would be scheduled in six months.

Other Interferences and Vocational Consequences

We have seen what OCD looks like on the job and at school. Other behavioral manifestations may be slowing down ordinary tasks due to not-right-feelings, having urges to check and recheck, wanting someone to use the bathroom frequently to wash their hands out of contamination fears, making someone late to work because of finishing rituals at home, and staying late to compensate for time missed. It also causes problems with time management. People may also get bogged down with the need to arrange things until they seem to be in their "proper place" or pause when asked a question in order to find the "right" and "perfect" words.

Social consequences at work or school may consist of misunderstandings between coworkers, employees, and supervisors (Arlington). Arlington suggests that a slow pace of work may give others the impression that the person is unmotivated, a procrastinator, or lazy. The stress of performance expectations can contribute to increasing symptoms and result in poor evaluations or disciplinary warnings.

One major problem is trying to keep the OCD a secret. But it can also be a risk to disclose having the disorder. In many situations, it is unclear what kind of attitude the employer has about mental illness, what kind of stigma may be attached to the person, or even what kind of discrimination may result. Even after deciding to disclose, many people are uncomfortable asking for help or special accommodations due to wanting to fit in. People may feel shame or be self-conscious about having something so personal out in the open and may fear ridicule or being socially isolated among their coworkers.

When the disorder is left undiagnosed, workers and their employers may misinterpret patterns such as calling in sick, arriving to work late, not meeting job requirements, and underperforming; they may assume those behaviors to indicate lack of motivation, laziness, poor work ethic, or not being qualified for the job. Support offered by some organizations may consist of extra job coaching or time management lessons, which are unlikely to change problematic work-related behaviors. The stress of not meeting work expectations and not understanding why typically increases the OCD behaviors, makes matters worse, and possibly results in being fired.

Thus, workers with undiagnosed OCD and their supervisors focus on the consequences of their compulsive behaviors, like absenteeism, chronic lateness, low productivity, or failure to complete work on time, rather than the compulsive behavior itself. As a result, most organizations will just refer the employee for coaching or time management classes, and the problems will persist. This can ultimately increase the worker's compulsions, which causes the employer to become frustrated and unsatisfied with the worker. In so many cases, the people end up being terminated.

The Americans With Disabilities Act

According to the U.S. Equal Employment Opportunity Commission (2008), the law defines a disability as "a physical or mental impairment that substantially limits one or more major life activities" under the ADA Amendments Acts. The Equal Employment Opportunity Commission has included OCD in its regulations as a condition that can substantially limit brain function and should qualify as a disability.

Reasonable accommodations are made when "any modification or adjustment to a job or the work environment that will enable a qualified applicant or employee with a disability to participate in the application process or to perform essential job functions. Reasonable accommodation also includes adjustments to ensure that a qualified individual with a disability has rights and privileges in employment equal to those of employees without disabilities" (Commission, 2008).

For people with OCD in the workplace, reasonable accommodations are the following:

- Making the environment conducive to concentrating for long stretches of time
- Modifying the environment to reduce or eliminate external stimuli
- Helping the person maintain stamina throughout the day
- Helping to manage time pressure and deadlines
- Initiating interpersonal contact
- Planning for how to focus on multiple tasks at the same time
- Creating an environment and communication style where the person can accept negative feedback (Matisik, 1996)

Whether or Not to Disclose

The question of whether or not to disclose having OCD can be complicated. There are risks and benefits to disclosing a mental health issue on the job. If symptoms are getting in the way of one's ability to do work, disclosing may become necessary in order to keep the job. One place to start is to contact the Job Accommodation Network (JAN), which is a resource under the U.S. Department of Labor. This service can provide advice about what and how to disclose, as well as what types of accommodations are usually offered based the needs of people with OCD. People can print download the information about accommodations and send it to their employer at the appropriate time.

Doing so is a proactive step that lets the employer know that employees are aware of their rights and provides them with a resource for determining what accommodations may be reasonable in this situation. JAN will also provide free consultation with employers and employees to work out reasonable accommodations upon request. The truth is that rituals and avoidances can be obvious, and people are apt to notice them anyway.

Other things to be kept in mind are the following:

- Securing documentation of the OCD diagnosis from the medical or mental health provider
- Being aware of the possible backlash of disclosure (stigma, judgment, coworker resentment)
- Checking the policies related to accommodations for disabilities through the human resources department
- Deciding on what specific reasonable accommodations will be helpful for job performance
- Learning how much information is necessary to disclose. Plan ahead for providing a few details about how and what accommodations will help the particular OCD challenges on the job, which will be discussed with a supervisor or human resources representative.

Employee Assistance Programs

Most companies have an employee assistance program (EAP), which is a dedicated confidential service for people to get help with any type of problem that interferes with work and quality of life. While EAP does not provide therapy, counselors may spend a few sessions assessing the problem and then provide appropriate referrals. Counselors typically follow up with the employees to see how they are doing as well as to ask about the quality of care they are receiving from the referral.

Human resources will help facilitate accommodations and the transition back to work from a leave. Some of the conditions that are found to be helpful are the following:

- Having a flexible start time
- Scheduling break times
- Providing retraining needs
- Providing reorientation and reintegration into the workplace, if necessary
- Implementing a gradual increase in hours and/or days worked if stamina is an issue
- Allowing for starting with the tasks the employee is most confident about completing successfully
- Mutually communicating about changes or modifications to tasks
- Providing clear directions and feedback (Melinert, 2014)

If people suspect that they are being discriminated against because of their OCD, there are recourses available. Discrimination may be subtle, such as being passed over for promotions, experiencing harassment or hostility because of "special" accommodations they receive, or an intolerance of mental health issues in general expressed by insensitive or inappropriate language. If legal action seems warranted, a complaint is filed with the Equal Employment Opportunity Commission, who contacts the employer. A "reasonable cause" may be determined, and the person can hire a lawyer and go forward with a claim in federal court.

With social and cultural attitudes changing from an increase in public awareness and companies preferring a more practical approach that does not affect their bottom line, human resource personnel can design supportive and mandatory mental health sensitivity trainings and develop proactive mental health policies. They can educate employees at large about how mental health issues are treated, presenting mental health as a public health issue (Arlington).

Mental health professionals know that OCD is an equal opportunity disorder affecting all walks of life. While there is no current literature on this topic, people who treat OCD have high-functioning physicians, psychologists, lawyers, business owners, and other professionals as patients. Support and destigmatization for such people are growing as well.

Why hire someone with OCD? The truth is that most people struggle with challenges. Many people with OCD have higher-than-average intelligence. OCD can be an asset to a business, because of intense dedication to work and attention to detail. It has been determined that the traits of obsessive-compulsive disorder, in moderation, have improved performance in police officers (DeCoster-Martin, Weiss, Davis, & Rostow, 2004). Given the level of imagination people with obsessions demonstrate, employees with OCD can use this skill to help anticipate real potential problems with a task or project. Empirically, when an actual problem arises in the lives of people with OCD, they respond in the same way that everybody else does because the situations are real and concrete.

References

Arlington, K. E. Mental illness on the job: The dilemma of obsessive compulsive disorder in the workplace & reducing the stigma. New York University. Retrieved from http://www.nyu.edu/classes/keefer/EvergreenEnergy/arlingtonk.pdf

Commission, USEEO. (2008). Summary of key provisions: EEOCs's notice of proposed rulemaking (NPRM) to implement the ADA Amendments Act of 2008 (ADAAA). Retrieved from https://www.eeoc.gov/laws/regulations/adaaa-summary.cfm

DeCoster-Martin, E., Weiss, W. U., Davis, R. D., & Rostow, C. D. (2004). Compulsive traits and police officer performance. *Journal of Police and Criminal Psychology, 19*(2), 64–71.

Matisik, E. N. (1996). The Americans With Disabilities Act and the Rehabillitation Act of 1973: Reasonable accommodation for employees with OCD [Pamphlet]. Milford: Obsessive-Compulsive Foundation.

Melinert, D. (2014, September). How to accommodate employees with mental illness. *Human Resources Magazine.* Retrieved from https://www.shrm.org/hr-today/news/hr-magazine/pages/1014-mental-health.aspx

CHAPTER 11

In Relationships—Up Close

Marriage/Committed Relationships

Drew began to have doubts about her marriage. Around six months ago, she started noticing how attractive other men were and became distraught that she might not be attracted to her husband, David, anymore. She started comparing his appearance to other men. She felt guilty about doing this, even though it wasn't exactly cheating on him, but since she found it somewhat pleasurable, part of her wondered if it meant her relationship could be in trouble. Having been raised Catholic, she was afraid that her lustful thoughts could be adulterous and sinful. She began asking herself, "I am looking at them too long?" and "Do I want their attention or to get signals that they find me attractive?"

She tried paying more attention to David as a way of feeling closer to him. When in public, she started averting her eyes. Neither of these attempts stopped the thoughts and images from coming into her head. She was afraid to talk to any of her friends about this because she was afraid they might disapprove of her and because she felt ashamed. She also started comparing her relationship to others' as a way of checking how they acted together in public.

Burdened by guilt, Drew began confessing her thoughts to David, even though she knew this might hurt him. After all, he did have the right to know. "David, I have something to tell you," she blurted out. "I can't help it, but I've been noticing how attractive other men are!" David had no idea what to think or what was happening, and he was caught off guard. She explained the instances that she remembered to him in as much detail as possible and felt relief after being honest with him.

When he thought about it for a second, David wasn't so concerned, since he never gave a second thought to noticing other women's beauty and told her it was natural to notice others. But as the days wore on and she kept confessing to him because of the relief it gave her, he became more upset and insecure about the relationship. The problem, though, wasn't the relationship! They both loved each other very much and were quite compatible. It was the effect of the increasing attention and focus of Drew's obsessive uncertainty that began taking over the quality of their relationship.

Drew started looking up relationship websites and took online tests to find some answers about what was going on, and not surprisingly, she got mixed messages. Yes, noticing how attractive other people are was normal. No, it didn't mean you were cheating on your husband. Yes, you could find people attractive without being attracted to them. Who can't help noticing how beautiful celebrities are? Is that okay or not? Some conservative websites said, "No, you shouldn't have those thoughts or feelings about those outside of your relationship. It is lustful to covet others."

She even came across terms such as *microcheating* and *mental cheating*. Drew read that microcheating, according to Lindsey Hoskins, is a set of behaviors that flirts with the line between faithfulness and unfaithfulness. Mental cheating is being attracted to someone else while you are in a relationship without acting on the attraction (cakescake, 2011). She had no idea how she could possibly know how to tell if this was what she was doing, but she did know that she was in trouble and felt that she was losing her mind, maybe even her husband.

Since Drew's real problem was OCD, people like her can get stuck on the literalness of the religious or moral law because OCD polarizes them into all good/bad, right/wrong, or black/white thinking. Being in the ambiguous gray area doesn't feel "right" and is intolerable. Drew had the obsessive need to know and be sure about the status of heir fidelity, but she would never get any definitive proof that would put her at ease.

Drew's example is one form of Relationship OCD (RO). The real problem involves the domains of cognitive dysfunctional beliefs specific to OCD (Obsessive Compulsive Cognitions Working Group, 1997). The specific cognitive domains involved in RO are intolerance of uncertainty and nagging doubts ("Am I with the right person?"), perfectionism and not-just-right-experiences over trivial traits ("I don't like the way she laughs"), overimportance of thoughts ("My doubting thoughts must mean she and I have lost our spark and passion"), and overimportance of controlling thoughts ("I shouldn't be having these thoughts if I love her").

People may also doubt that their partner loves them. Associated behaviors may be reading more into body language, asking endless reassurance questions, checking their partners' schedules or electronic activities, checking credit card statements, or snooping around for any evidence of out-of-relationship activity. This is not a form of jealousy but the obsessive need to know and be sure. For the OCD sufferer, RO may increase clinging and dependent behaviors and increase fear of abandonment, guilt, and shame. For the other partner, RO may reinforce feelings of anger and frustration as well as withdrawal and rejecting behaviors; these behaviors might challenge mutual trust, increase abandonment fears, and turn off the partner due to the repetitiveness of the OR partner's behaviors (Cunningham, Shamblen, Barbee, & Ault, 2005; Doron, Derby, & Szepsenwol, 2014).

In this example, we can see that OCD has become a "third person" in the relationship that creates a dysfunctional triangle pitting people against each other instead of toward the disorder. Once a clear diagnosis is made, plans for how to take control together can keep it at bay.

Other obsessions that are characteristic of RO are the following:

- "How do I know if he is the one?"
- "Maybe my doubts mean I'm not ready to be in a committed relationship even though I love her."
- "Is my anxiety getting in the way of my sexual performance, or am I not really attracted to him?"
- "This just doesn't seem to feel right."
- "How will I know if she really loves me? I know she's sick of me asking."

The Relationship Obsessive Compulsive Inventory assesses the severity of OCD symptoms in intimate relationships and measures how people with OCD feel about their partners, their perceptions about how their partner feels about them, and the "rightness" of how the relationships feels (Doron, Derby, Szepsenwol, & Talmor, 2012a). These authors also developed the Partner-Related Obsessive-Compulsive Symptom Inventory, which examines six clinically important factors that affect the quality of relationships when OCD is the third party (Doron et al., 2012b): physical appearance, sociability, morality, emotional stability, intelligence, and competence. The authors also looked at constructs such as relationship-centered OC symptoms, typical OC symptoms and beliefs, negative affect, low self-esteem, relationship dissatisfaction, and attachment insecurity.

Social allergies, such as hypersensitivity, annoyance, and disgust about partner's behaviors (Cunningham et al., 2005), may also play a role in partner-focused OC symptoms. The repetition of being exposed to the "flawed behaviors" of the partner may create a heightened awareness and anticipation of their occurrence. Being preoccupied with one's own deficits may further strengthen and maintain partner-focused obsessions and compulsive behaviors (Doron, Derby, Szepsenwol, & Talmor, 2012a).

Single/Dating

Charlie suffered a serious breakup last year and had his heart broken. "No one will ever be as good as my ex," he thought. He had been in therapy and had made enough progress to get back in the dating scene. He went on a couple of dates but was having trouble not comparing any potential boyfriend to his ex-partner, Jake. He didn't find them as interesting, smart, or attractive. He knew it wasn't fair to make comparisons, but he didn't want to waste his time with someone who didn't have the qualities he liked. Charlie wondered if his pickiness was a sign of perfectionistic, rigid, or unreasonable standards, or if he just wanted to find the right person. He was very social at the gym, at bars, and at parties, and had been fixed up with other men, but nothing had panned out.

Because of feeling lonely, Charlie decided to take his friends' advice and started to develop an online dating profile. Charlie knew he was average in terms of his looks but felt good about his personality and his career, and he supported himself well. He wanted to be truthful about himself but also "marketable." Being a little scrupulous, he wanted to be completely honest in describing himself, but he also thought about portraying an image according to what men *he* would like to attract. "Should I be honest about being a little overweight?" he thought. Then, there were so many apps to choose from! He asked himself, "Which ones do I use? Do I sign up for the free ones? Is it worth the time and expense of some of the others?" He was having trouble deciding because of choice overload. He ended up deciding to take his friends' feedback about what to include in his profile and signed up for the four apps they recommended.

Charlie took a deep breath and uploaded his profile. After a few minutes, he began checking to see if anyone had responded. Nothing. Being anxious, he checked again and still nothing. On one hand, he was impatient and disappointed that no one had yet responded, and on the other, there was a kind of excitement at the anticipation that something could happen. If continuing to check his phone made him more anxious about his prospects, why did he keep doing it? He was compulsively checking because of the OCD, but there is something else called *intermittent variable reward*, a reinforcement with the anticipation of something exciting happening, which is a common behavior with dating apps (van Velthoven, Powell, & Powell, 2018).

According to MacPherson (2018), "Human nature enjoys anticipation. Anticipation adds energy and electricity to any experience. . . ."

Because our brains' pleasure centers are activated in anticipation of a sensation, we tend to keep repeating actions that are not considered pleasurable in and of themselves, but that occur immediately before a pleasurable sensation takes place. Our brains find the anticipation enjoyable.

So, while Charlie was obsessive and picky about finding the perfect "right one" and was experiencing the mental compulsive acts that go along with it, he was also experiencing the feeling of excited anticipation that set off by dopamine.

Turner (2018) explains, "We maximally text, email, and upload content on social media because it increases our likelihood of receiving a digital interaction and the resulting dopamine reward. We maximally check texts, emails, and social media notifications in anticipation of the reward, because that allows us to most quickly get the reward and respond to the digital interaction." Sadly, the excited anticipation Charlie initially felt from this activity turned into anxiety-ridden compulsive phone checking. His felt like there was a battle between the release of feel good neurotransmitters about the idea of potential dates and the onslaught of obsessive doubt and anxiety from neurochemicals set off by the OCD.

Charlie wanted to continue using the dating apps, but he knew he had to figure out a way to manage his anticipatory anxiety and checking behaviors so that his OCD did not ruin the quality of his life or get in the way of being able to focus on his dates. He resumed working with his outpatient behavior therapist, and together they worked out a behavioral plan to normalize the frequency of phone checking as well as used cognitive therapy and mindfulness to rein in his anticipatory anxiety.

Family, Child, and Parental Issues

Nobody does or should suffer from OCD alone, including family members. Loved ones' suffering is an often unnoticed or undertreated problem. OCD suffering is all-inclusive because recognizing and treating family problems in communication, style, and interactions can contribute to better treatment outcome and recovery.

What happens when a parent or a child has OCD? Families and loved ones of the OCD sufferer burn out. They may start out trying to make light of the obsessions in a friendly way meant to help allay their loved one's fears. Then they may start saying things with a little less patience like, "That's ridiculous," or "Come on, you don't really believe that, do you?" Then things might take a turn for the worse, as frustration builds from how the OCD is encroaching on relationships and the household. People can start showing more negative affect and say things like, "Get over it" or "Why can't you just stop it!"

How people communicate their feelings toward a person with a psychiatric disorder can be understood by the clinical construct of *expressed emotion* (EE). Research has shown that the level of EE within the household can predict the outcome of treatment (Steketee, Van Noppen, Lam, & Shapiro, 1998). High EE consists of criticism, hostility, and emotional overinvolvement, while low EE communicates supportive, nurturing, and accepting emotions (Wuerker, 1996).

With high EE, family members may tell the OCD sufferer that they can't stand them anymore, that he or she is sick or crazy. Other characteristics of high EE are loved ones feeling a sense of sacrifice about how the OCD is taking away from quality of life, having emotional overreactions toward the OCD sufferer during flare-ups, and feeling intrusiveness when a family member is communicating in a hostile manner (Renshaw, Chambless, & Thorgusen, 2017). Parents, in particular, can be highly critical, antagonistic, negative, and harsh; can express a sense of disgust; and can be less emotionally responsive to their loved one's emotional needs (Renshaw et al., 2017).

By contrast, low EE has been related to the absence of psychopathology and to a more functional family environment (Hibbs et al., 1993). Families with low EE are more supportive, communicative, accepting, and nurturing (Villard & Whipple, 1976). In a spirit of caring, empathy, and compassion, people may offer support by saying, "I know you're struggling. Is there anything I can do to help?" or "This has happened before, and you've gotten through it."

Codependency is another family and relationship dynamic that affects OCD treatment and recovery. It is defined as family members being drawn into bizarre enabling behaviors to pacify their ill relatives and developing a high tolerance for inappropriate behavior (Cooper, 1995). The model considers these families as normal feeling people who are trying to cope with unremitting stress but lacks effective skills to cope with the illness and their own self-care. Clinical vignettes illustrate how these families are similar to families of alcoholics in their management of emotions and in their dysfunctional behaviors. Recommendations are offered for practitioners who work with families of mentally ill people.

Sometimes a loved one of a person with OCD needs the person to stay sick in order to maintain the homeostasis of the relationship. The loved one can feel threatened that as the person with OCD improves, there may be a fear that the person in recovery will come to realize how dysfunctional the relationship is. Sometimes a loved one needs to be needed, which can often be a way that the person deflects from his or her own problems.

When a Child Has OCD

Most children have a phase of ritualized repetitive behaviors that are performed to create order or control over their lives, but when does the phase end and OCD begin? Some children like to arrange their stuffed animals on their bed in a certain way. Some children like having certain predictable and ordered routines. Under normal circumstances, a child will be able to cope with changes in these routines, but a child with OCD can become dysregulated and need to have the order restored before moving on to another task (Leonard, Goldberger, Rapoport, Cheslow, & Swedo, 1990).

Thus, early onset OCD can have an impact on a child's emotional and psychological development (Leckman, Bloch, & King, 2009). Domains of social, academic, vocational, or family dysfunction can be affected even after treatment of an episode (Hollander et al., 1997).

Depending on the family dynamics, a child with OCD may be called names and be shamed. Rituals might disrupt family routines such as dinner and getting ready for school or may make the family wait when going to family, social, or leisure events. They may also cause school tardiness, absences, scapegoating by classmates, or incomplete homework assignments.

Family interventions for helping a child cope with OCD symptoms can be taking the "third person" approach. Rather than calling the child a name, the child and his family can give the OCD a silly name or disarming word. The emotional focus is better turned toward the OCD behaviors rather than being critical of the child.

The Parent with OCD

Parents are the single most important role models in a child's life (https://www.aacap.org/aacap/families_and_youth/facts_for_families /fff-guide/children-and-role-models-099.aspx). How parents behave influences their children's ideas, beliefs, and behavioral choices about how to treat people and make decisions.

A parent with OCD may model dysfunctional behavior that the child will assume is normal and to be emulated. For example, Austin was invited to a play date at his friend's house after school. When he and his friend, Jake, arrived at Jake's house and went inside, Austin began taking off his clothes. When Jake's mother went to greet them, she was a bit surprised and asked him what he was doing. "What do you mean? This is the first thing we are supposed to do when we get home from school," Austin said. "Well, you don't have to do that here," said Jake's mother.

Austin's behavior may be interpreted as normal, given his family circumstances, and he may be showing his mother that he loves her by conforming. But what happens when he begins to have more autonomy and learns how abnormal the rules of his life have been? If a parent is anxious in certain situations, a child will learn to be afraid of that situation. If a child sees a parent overwashing, checking, or having perfectionistic standards, the child will learn that those are appropriate behaviors. A parent may ask the child to perform checking rituals or provide reassurance in triggering situations.

Parenting style is another factor that influences children's behavior. Baumrind (1971) has identified three parental authority styles: permissive, authoritative, and authoritarian. They are characterized as being either high or low on the two parenting dimensions of warmth and control. Baumrind operationalized the permissive parenting style as high on warmth and nurturing, but low on behavioral control; generally, children are allowed to do what they want without behavioral limits. Authoritarian parenting is considered the opposite, in that it is low on warmth and nurturance and very high on behavioral control. Parents tend to be rigid and expect strict adherence to rules without teaching why in ways that are emotionally distant. Authoritative parenting is high on both warmth and control and provides reasonable guidelines while still providing a loving and nurturing environment.

With respect to parents with OCD, they tend to have an authoritarian parenting style (Timpano et al., 2010). An association has been made between the authoritarian parental style of control and greater rates of child anxiety (Ballash, Leyfer, Buckley, & Woodruff-Borden, 2006).

Siblings

Siblings may feel ignored, left out, angry, and compassion overloaded and may bear witness to scenes that they may not be ready to handle emotionally. This is especially true when there is high EE in the family. Siblings may also be put in the precarious position of accommodating their sibling's OCD by engaging in rituals even though they may do so unwillingly.

A study was conducted on the consequences of OCD on siblings with and without the disorder. The sibling without the disorder reported experiencing codependency, feeling or being abandoned, checking on how their sibling is coping, and having less autonomy than the sibling with OCD (Baz, 2019). The author recommended further research be conducted that compares the outcome of treatment with and without including a sibling component. The aim is to delineate whether decreased sibling accommodation may be a consequence of symptom reduction in the child with OCD following treatment, or whether the inclusion of a sibling component in treatment may facilitate such changes in family members themselves (Barrett, Healy-Farrell, & March, 2004).

Family Accommodation and Family Roles

Most families are trying to cope as best as they can under difficult circumstances. Wanting to alleviate a loved one's suffering is the most natural instinct people have when it comes to feeling compassion. However, family members may actually be enabling the OCD in a spirit of wanting to be helpful. Family interactions around OCD depend on where the person with OCD is in the course of his or her illness, what his or her family role is (child, parent, spouse, sibling), and what the stress tolerance level of family members and the personalities of all involved are. When families learn what their role is and how they interact with the OCD, they can feel better equipped in knowing how to support and help a loved one and can improve negative family interactions and communication styles; the OCD episode can improve, and the quality of relationships can improve as a result.

Family accommodation of OCD has been found to be a predictor in treatment outcome (Albert, Baffa, & Maina, 2017). Examining the role that family members play in the OCD system can help deconstruct dysfunctional family dynamics and behaviors. Who is the sufferer? Is the sufferer a young child, an adult child, a parent, a spouse? Did the person disclose that he or she had OCD before the marriage, or did the onset occur already into the marriage? Did the onset occur pre- or postnatally? Is the family a single parent who suffers from OCD or has a child with it? Is the sufferer a teenager who has to hide it from friends to avoid being teased but can't control the symptoms at home? How is a sibling suffering, and what are his or her feelings about the OCD taking over the attention and functioning of the household? Do the sibling's needs get met, or are they neglected? How long has the OCD been active in the family? Has it been newly diagnosed, and is the family sorting out how to manage it in healthy ways? Has it been in the family for years, maybe even decades, and is the family set in their ways of responding to it? How flexible are people in the family to change? How much do people want to meet halfway to make communication go better in the face of OCD? How willing are people to end the cycle of blaming that only prevents change from happening?

According to Gravitz (1998), other role assignments family members may have are the following:

- The responsible one, who takes over or covers up the duties and responsibilities of the person with OCD. If the responsible one is a child, he or she may learn to become overly responsible and learn to put others' needs ahead of his or her own.
- The adjuster, who has a way of ignoring or denying the OCD and may self-isolate from the rest of the family. Even with that type of coping, the adjuster does notice and is affected by the OCD. Playing this role may hinder his or her ability to learn how to manage his or her own stresses if denial is used as a defense.
- The lost one, who makes no demands on anyone and tries to stay below the radar so as not to be a burden in the family. These people may have trouble connecting with others and may tend to ignore their own needs as they may perceive them to be less important due to the OCD demands on the family.
- The placater, a people pleaser who is motivated to help avoid conflict. Someone in this role may not develop self-awareness or learn effective interpersonal skills for asserting his or her needs.
- The mascot, who is like the class clown and uses joking and levity to distract away from the stress in the house. These people may deny their own emotions since they are taking care of everyone else's needs with incongruent humor.

Families and therapists can assess their accommodation using the patient or parent version of the Family Accommodation Scale (Lebowitz, Panza, Su, & Bloch, 2012; Pinto, Van Noppen, & Calvocoressi, 2013). These authors have provided the following list of family accommodating behaviors:

- Participating in rituals (using hand sanitizer unnecessarily)
- Assisting in avoidance behavior (not driving by cemeteries or playgrounds)
- Keeping track of the body parts the person with OCD has washed
- Facilitating symptomatic behavior (buying excessive amounts of cleaning products for the person with OCD)
- Modifying the family's routine (waiting until the person completes rituals)
- Taking on extra responsibilities (doing the person's laundry)
- Modifying leisure activities (declining invitations due to emotional contamination symptoms)
- Interfering in work/school functioning (completing assignments that are due, reassuring that performance is perfect)

Accommodating behaviors do not work because they do the following:

- Interfere with the ability of the individual with OCD to experience normalized behaviors
- Cause resentment, hostility, and criticism
- Create a new dysfunctional "normal" in the household, as family members feel guilty when they cause a trigger
- Can be agreed by the person with OCD as not helpful

Instead of accommodating behaviors, family members can do the following:

- Make supportive and encouraging statements to help the person challenge his or her obsessive triggers
- Resist their own urges to participate in rituals just to placate the OCD
- Direct anger and frustration at the illness rather than the person
- Practice tolerance and patience in response to the distress experienced by the person with OCD
- Remember that giving more attention to the person with OCD isn't always better
- Find ways of kindly communication limits around participating in rituals
- Agree on and create a plan for reasonable behavioral expectations (being on time for meals, limiting the amount of water for showers)
- Find ways to encourage the person with OCD to complete chores and tasks around the house

- Create mutually agreed upon words or phrases that will indicate that reassurance will not be provided
- Decline to answer repetitive questions that have already been answered
- Give praise for small gains by recognizing and acknowledging improvements

Issues in Recovery

Eng and Emily were legally separated due to OCD burnout. Emily was resentful because their relationship revolved around the OCD. She claimed that when her husband's symptoms subsided, he didn't seem to need her or want to be around her as much. They entered into couple's therapy to try to work on the relationship and improve their communication. Eng was pleased with the progress he made with exposure therapy. However, Emily had old anger and resentment about what she been through during Eng's prolonged OCD episode.

This is a common pattern in treatment: the OCD sufferer feels relief from decrease in symptoms, but family is still in a resentful and angry phase due to how much their lives may have been affected by accommodating the OCD. Emily entered into individual therapy with someone skilled in OCD and family issues. She found this helpful and was able work through her anger and improve her current relationship with her husband. Because they wanted the relationship to work out, she began to soften and be more open as she now had a place to work on her own issues.

Guidelines of General Support

Is it ever okay to provide reassurance? Sometimes it's a judgment call. No one will ever say outright that it's okay, but situations may arise where it is the lesser of evils. Sometimes in public, it may be the merciful thing to do, but make it known that it is the exception and not the rule.

Families are unsure if they should wait for the person to finish ritualizing when they are on their way out the door to an event. Since no one can ever be sure how long it will take for the person to finish, it becomes another judgment call. We know in treatment that if patients know they can get away with ritualizing, they will. On the other hand, if they see that there are direct consequences such as the family leaving without them, they may decide the next time that missing out on the event is more important than ritualizing. It may take a few times of following through on this to show that this plan is serious, but it is surprising how effective it can be. There may be a lot of guilt about leaving the person behind, but it is often the most effective response to putting limits on how OCD controls family functioning. Some families often make idle threats about leaving and never do. If families agree that this is the best option, they must be strong and keep their word. Otherwise, the person with OCD won't take this or any other kind of plan seriously.

Family behavior therapy can be very effective in getting control of the OCD. This involves setting behavioral contracts with a designated family member who coaches the sufferer through exposures and help keeps limits on specific behaviors in order to keep things functioning as normally as possible in the household. Working with a therapist to set up and follow through on a weekly plan is helpful to problem solve unexpected situations that may arise. If the family has high EE, this type of situation is contraindicated. It will only make matters worse.

Family support groups may be available in communities, often established with the assistance of the IOCDF. If there are no support groups in a local area, rather than reinventing the wheel, the IOCDF has starter information at https://iocdf.org/ocd-finding-help/supportgroups /how-to-start-a-support-group/. Families often feel uncertain about how to manage around the OCD and can offer and receive support to others in similar situation.

Traditional family or marital therapy may be helpful for issues outside of the OCD that may be complicating family relationships. Life and relationship issues are challenging at best, and working with a professional trained to sort out where the OCD ends and other family problems begin can be very important. One couple channeled their energy into their symptomatic child as a distraction from their own marital problems. This not only served to irresponsibly deflect from their issues and use the child as a scapegoat; the child's life with OCD was collaterally made worse. When child therapists become aware of this dynamic, a recommendation should be made for the parents to enter into marital therapy not only to explore whether or not the relationship can get on a better track but also more importantly to understand how they are keeping their child from getting better.

In another type of situation, the father had OCD, and his parenting credibility was undermined due to the lack of support from his wife in the presence of the children. Even when he attempted to set appropriate and healthy with limits them, neither his wife nor his children took him seriously. Again, in this case, couple's therapy was useful to sort out the ramifications of this pattern of parenting and functioning.

Remind the OCD sufferer and family members that recovery can have an up-and-down course. A bad day does not mean a relapse, and a good day does not mean a cure. Families can often overlook how much the person continues to struggle on a daily basis with symptoms when the person seems to be doing better. There are times when people with OCD can get in their own way by hanging on to symptoms to show that they still need family support. Family members are advised to check in and ask how patients are doing, validate how hard they continue to work to maintain their recovery, and offer praise when a behavior that had been ritualistic becomes normalized.

Some helpful guidelines are provided for helping families develop a healthy household environment even though OCD challenges may exist. Guidelines can help family members find ways of not being reactionary when there is an OCD flare-up, since emotions can cause impulsive and regrettable responses in the moment. Instead, families can create proactive and emotionally even responses during these occurrences, such as validating the person's anxiety and reminding him or her that it will pass. Keeping an organized and ordered household will be conducive to reducing a sense of chaos. Families can also lead with a spirit of love and mutual respect by listening and seeing what constructive ways there may be to address the problem of the moment.

OCD can be a very demanding problem for everyone. Helping people get outside of the OCD system and staying interested in how *all* family members are doing, as well as affirming that what they are doing is important, will help equalize family participation and connectedness. Sometimes OCD creates an emotional one-way street, and the very people the person with OCD wants to protect by performing rituals actually become hurt by the disorder. Keeping a line of open communication in all directions is critical.

References

Albert, U., Baffa, A., & Maina, G. (2017). Family accommodation in adult obsessive-compulsive disorder: Clinical perspectives. *Psychology Research and Behavior Management, 10*, 293–304. doi:10.2147/PRBM.S124359

Ballash, N., Leyfer, O., Buckley, A. F., & Woodruff-Borden, J. (2006). Parental control in the etiology of anxiety. *Clinical Child and Family Psychology Review, 9*(2), 113–133.

Barrett, P., Healy-Farrell, L., & March, J. S. (2004). Cognitive-behavioral family treatment of childhood obsessive-compulsive disorder: A controlled trial. *Journal of the American Academy of Child and Adolescent Psychiatry, 43*(1), 46–62. doi:10.1097/00004583-200401000-00014

Baumrind, D. (1971). Current patterns of parental authority. *Developmental Psychology, 4*(1pt2), 1.

Baz, A. (2019). A comparative examinataion of the relationship between early maladaptive schemas and symptom dimensions in patient with obsessive compulsive disorder, uneffected siblings of patients and healthy controls. *Klinik Psikofarmakoloji Bulteni, 29*, 38–38.

cakescake. (2011). Mental cheating. Retrieved from https://www.urbandictionary.com/define.php?term=mental%20cheating

Cooper, M. (1995). Applying the codependency model to a group for families of obsessive-compulsive people. *Health & Social Work, 20*(4), 272–278. doi:10.1093/hsw/20.4.272

Cunningham, M. R., Shamblen, S. R., Barbee, A. P., & Ault, L. K. (2005). Social allergies in romantic relationships: Behavioral repetition, emotional sensitization, and dissatisfaction in dating couples. *Personal Relationships, 12*(2), 273–295. doi:10.1111/j.1350-4126.2005.00115.x

Doron, G., Derby, D. S., & Szepsenwol, O. (2014). Relationship obsessive compulsive disorder (ROCD): A conceptual framework. *Journal of Obsessive-Compulsive and Related Disorders, 3*(2), 169–180. doi:10.1016/j.jocrd.2013.12.005

Doron, G., Derby, D. S., Szepsenwol, O., & Talmor, D. (2012a). Flaws and all: Exploring partner-focused obsessive-compulsive symptoms. *Journal of Obsessive-Compulsive and Related Disorders, 1*(4), 234–243.

Doron, G., Derby, D. S., Szepsenwol, O., & Talmor, D. (2012b). Tainted love: Exploring relationship-centered obsessive compulsive symptoms in two non-clinical cohorts. *Journal of Obsessive-Compulsive and Related Disorders, 1*(1), 16–24. doi:10.1016/j.jocrd.2011.11.002

Ducharme, J. (2018). Micro-cheating could be ruining your relationship. Here's what to do about it. Retrieved from https://time.com/5332013/micro-cheating/

Gravitz, H. L. (1998). *Obsessive compulsive disorder: New help for the family.* Santa Barbara, CA: Healing Visions.

Hibbs, E. D., Hamburger, S. D., Kruesi, M. J., & Lenane, M. (1993). Factors affecting expressed emotion in parents of ill and normal children. *American Journal of Orthopsychiatry, 63*(1), 103–112.

Hollander, E., Stein, D. J., Kwon, J. H., Rowland, C., Wong, C. M., Broatch, J., & Himelein, C. (1997). Psychosocial function and economic costs of obsessive-compulsive disorder. *CNS Spectrums, 2*(10), 16–25.

Lebowitz, E. R., Panza, K. E., Su, J., & Bloch, M. H. (2012). Family accommodation in obsessive-compulsive disorder. *Expert Review of Neurotherapeutics, 12*, 229–238.

Leckman, J. F., Bloch, M. H., & King, R. A. (2009). Symptom dimensions and subtypes of obsessive-compulsive disorder: A developmental perspective. *Dialogues in Clinical Neuroscience, 11*(1), 21–33. Retrieved from https://www.ncbi.nlm.nih.gov/pubmed/19432385; https://www.ncbi.nlm.nih.gov/pmc/PMC3181902/

Leonard, H. L., Goldberger, E. L., Rapoport, J. L., Cheslow, D. L., & Swedo, S. E. (1990). Childhood rituals: Normal development or obsessive-compulsive symptoms? *Journal of the American Academy of Child & Adolescent Psychiatry, 29*(1), 17–23. doi:10.1097/00004583-199001000-00004

MacPherson, L. (2018, November 8). A deep dive on variable rewards and how to use them. *Designli*. Retrieved from https://designli.co/blog/a-deep-dive-on-variable-rewards-and-how-to-use-them/

Obsessive Compulsive Cognitions Working Group. (1997). Cognitive assessment of obsessive-compulsive disorder. *Behaviour Research and Therapy, 35*(7), 667–681.

Pinto, A., Van Noppen, B., & Calvocoressi, L. (2013). Development and preliminary psychometric evaluation of a self-rated version of the family accommodation scale for obsessive-compulsive disorder. *Journal of Obsessive-Compulsive and Related Disorders, 2*(4), 457–465.

Renshaw, K. D., Chambless, D. L., & Thorgusen, S. (2017). Expressed emotion and attributions in relatives of patients with obsessive-compulsive disorder and panic disorder. *Journal of Nervous and Mental Disease, 205*(4), 294–299. doi:10.1097/NMD.0000000000000636

Steketee, G., Van Noppen, B., Lam, J., & Shapiro, L. (1998). Expressed emotion in families and the treatment of obsessive compulsive disorder. *In Session: Psychotherapy in Practice, 4*(3), 73–91. doi:10.1002/(sici)1520-6572(199823)4:3<73::Aid-sess6>3.0.Co;2-9

Timpano, K., Keough, M. E., Mahaffey, B., Schmidt, N. B., & Abramowitz, J. (2010). Parenting and obsessive compulsive symptoms: Implications of authoritarian parenting. *Journal of Cognitive Psychotherapy, 24.* doi:10.1891/0889-8391.24.3.151

Turner, A. N. (2018, February 19). Dating apps are obsessive [Hackernoon]. Retrieved from https://hackernoon.com/understanding-dating-apps-and-obsession-ae4f7303afb7

van Velthoven, M. H., Powell, J., & Powell, G. (2018). Problematic smartphone use: Digital approaches to an emerging public health problem. *Digital Health, 4*, 1–9. doi: 10.1177/2055207618759167

Villard, K., & Whipple, L. J. (1976). *Beginnings in relational communication*. New York: John Wiley & Sons.

Wuerker, A. M. (1996). Communication patterns and expressed emotion in families of persons with mental disorders. *Schizophrenia Bulletin, 22*(4), 671–690. doi:10.1093/schbul/22.4.671

Glossary

accommodation

When others enable or participate in rituals or change their behavior to avoid causing undue stress on the person or to avoid emotional conflicts related to how the OCD controls household or social activities.

avoidance behavior

Any behavior that is done with the intention of avoiding a trigger in order to avoid anxiety. Avoidance behaviors are treated as a ritual.

compulsions/rituals

Compulsions, also known as rituals, are repetitive behaviors or thoughts that conform to rigid rules as far as number, order, and so on, that function as an attempt to reduce anxiety brought on by intrusive thoughts.

distraction

A strategy used primarily outside ERP to enhance one's ability to resist rituals. One does another activity (playing a board game, watching TV, taking a walk, etc.) while triggered in order to cope with anxiety without ritualizing.

exposure and response prevention (ERP)

The behavioral treatment of choice for OCD, during which a person with OCD purposefully triggers an obsession and blocks his or her rituals in order to create habituation. ERP is initially done with a behavioral coach, who assists the person with OCD to resist rituals. Eventually the coaching is faded, as the person with OCD becomes more able to resist rituals without help.

generalization

The transfer of learning from one environment to another, or from one stimulus to a broader range of stimuli in the same category.

habit reversal

Therapy for doing the opposite action than urges provoked by body-focused repetitive behaviors.

habituation

The process of getting used a situation that at first was uncomfortable and caused distress.

insight

The belief that obsessions are excessive worry and that rituals are not reasonable behaviors. People with good insight have the same level of belief about the obsessive trigger as the general population.

mental ritual

A mental act done in response to an unwanted obsession that is completed in order to reduce anxiety. Often a mental ritual must be repeated multiple times. It can be a prayer, a repeated phrase, a review of steps taken, a self-reassurance, and so on. Often a mental ritual is repeated so often that the individual barely has any awareness of the thought.

mindfulness

A focus on the present moment that prevents worries about the past and the future.

neutralization

When an individual with OCD "undoes" a behavior or thought that is believed to be dangerous by neutralizing it with another behavior or thought. This behavior is also considered a ritual.

not-just-right-experiences (NJREs)

A feeling that something is wrong or doesn't feel right with no obsessive fear attached to it. People have trouble focusing on tasks until a ritual is performed until the "just right" feeling is achieved.

obsessions

Obsessions are repetitive intrusive thoughts or images that dramatically increase anxiety. The obsessions are so unpleasant that the person with OCD tries to control or suppress the fear. The more the person attempts to suppress the fear, the more entrenched and ever-present it becomes.

overvalued ideation

A higher level of belief about the validity of an obsession, which is not delusional.

perfectionism

Unrealistically high expectations about one's performance on any task. Failure is catastrophic and unbearable. Anything less than 100 percent perfection is considered a failure. Consequently, perfectionists are paralyzed and sometimes unable to begin a task until the last minute or are sometimes unable to complete a task.

reassurance seeking

When a person with OCD asks others' questions repetitively to reduce his or her anxiety, such as "Do you think this food is spoiled?" or "Do you think I will get sick?" Sometimes a person with OCD can get reassurance merely from watching another's facial expression and/or body posture. All reassurance seeking is considered a ritual.

relapse prevention

A set of skills, both cognitive and behavioral, aimed at preventing an individual with OCD from slipping back into old compulsive behaviors.

response prevention

Resisting the urge to perform rituals.

Subjective Units of Distress Scale (SUDS)

This is a scale from either one to ten or one to one hundred, in which the person with OCD rates his or her anxiety, one being the least anxious and ten or one hundred being the most anxious. The scale is each individual person's sense of his or her own anxiety.

Source: Developed by Carol Hevia, PsyD. Used by permission.

For Further Reading

For Professionals

Abramowitz, Jonathan, & Jacoby, Ryan. (2015). *Obsessive-Compulsive disorders in adults and children*. Boston: Hogrefe.

Foa, Edna & Kozak, Michael J. (2004). *Mastery of obsessive-compulsive disorder: A cognitive-behavioral approach* (Therapist Guide). Oxford: Oxford University Press.

Foa, Edna, Yadin, Elna, & Lichner, Tracey K. (2012). *Treatments that work*. Oxford: Oxford University Press.

Hudak, Robert, & Dougherty, Darin (Eds.). (2011). *Clinical obsessive-compulsive disorders in adults and children*. Cambridge: Cambridge University Press.

McKay, Matthew, & Steketee, Gail (1998). *Overcoming obsessive-compulsive disorder: A behavioral and cognitive protocol for the treatment of OCD*. Oakland, CA: New Harbinger.

Rego, Simon A. (2016). *Treatment plans and interventions for obsessive-compulsive disorder (Treatment plans and interventions for evidence-based psychotherapy)*. New York: Guilford.

Shapiro, Leslie J. (2015). *Understanding OCD: Skills to control the conscience and outsmart obsessive compulsive disorder*. Santa Barbara, CA: Praeger.

Steketee, Gail S. (1996). *Treatment of obsessive compulsive disorder (Treatment Manuals for Practitioners)*. New York: Guilford.

Wagner, Aureen Pinto (2003). *Treatment of OCD in children and adolescents: A cognitive-behavioral therapy manual*. Lighthouse Press.

Weg, Alan (2011). *Storytelling: A strategy for successful therapy*. Oxford: Oxford University Press.

Wilhelm, Sabine, & Steketee, Gail S. (2006). *Cognitive therapy for obsessive-compulsive disorder: A guide for professionals*. Oakland, CA: New Harbinger.

Williams, Monnica T., & Wetterneck, Chad T. (2019). *Sexual obsessions in obsessive-compulsive disorder: A step-by-step, definitive guide to understanding, diagnosis, and treatment*. New York: Oxford University Press.

For People with OCD and Loved Ones

Gravitz, Herbert L. (1998). *Obsessive compulsive disorder: New help for the family*. Santa Barbara, CA: Healing Visions.

Hershfield, Jon (2015). *When a family member has OCD*. Oakland, CA: New Harbinger.

Hershfield, Jon (2018). *Overcoming harm OCD: Mindfulness and CBT tools for coping with unwanted violent thoughts*. Oakland, CA: New Harbinger.

Hershfield, Jon, & Corboy, Tom (2013). *The mindfulness workbook for OCD: A guide to overcoming obsessions and compulsions using mindfulness and cognitive behavioral*. Oakland, CA: New Harbinger.

Landsman, Karen J. (2005). *Loving someone with OCD*. Oakland, CA: New Harbinger.

Winston, Sally M., & Seif, Martin N. (2017). *Overcoming unwanted intrusive thoughts: A CBT-based guide to getting over frightening, obsessive, or disturbing thoughts*. Oakland, CA: New Harbinger.

Resources

Anxiety in the Classroom, https://anxietyintheclassroom.org/
For teachers and educators, this website offers information for people who work in the school system, parents, and students.

Body Dysmorphic Disorder, https://bdd.iocdf.org/
A symptom-specific web page found on the IOCDF website, it outlines the subtypes of BDD, provides epidemiological information, describes treatment, and provides input from experts in the field.

Body-Focused Repetitive Behaviors, http://www.trich.org/
The goal of this website for trichotillomania, skin picking, is to connect individuals and their families with each other to help end isolation and provide a community of support. They refer people to treatment providers, services, and educational resources, and conduct outreach to health care providers and educators, teaching them how to recognize these disorders.

Homosexual Obsessions, http://www.ocdtypes.com/test.php and https://ocdla.com/gay-ocd-hocd-test https://www.intrusivethoughts.org
A very helpful website, it addresses what can seem like a sensitive topic for some OCD sufferers.

The International Obsessive Compulsive Disorders Foundation (IOCDF), www.iocdf.org
The mission of the International OCD Foundation is to help those affected by obsessive compulsive disorder and related disorders to live full and productive lives. Their aim is to increase access to effective treatment through research and training, foster a hopeful and supportive

community for those affected by OCD and the professionals who treat them, and fight stigma surrounding mental health issues. The foundation is an international membership-based organization serving a broad community of individuals with OCD and related disorders, their family members and loved ones, and mental health professionals and researchers around the world. There are affiliates in twenty-five states and territories in the United States, in addition to global partnerships with other OCD organizations and mental health nonprofits around the world.

Misophonia Association, www.misophonia-association.org/home.html
The expressed mission of the Misophonia Association is to educate, advocate, conduct research, and provide support for sufferers and families of this difficult problem.

The National Alliance on Mental Illness, https://www.nami.org/Learn -More/Mental-Health-Conditions/Obsessive-compulsive-Disorder /Support
The National Alliance on Mental Illness is the nation's largest grassroots mental health organization dedicated to building better lives for the millions of Americans affected by mental illness. Their mission is to educate and provide support for individuals, families, and educators. Their website has an OCD-specific section informing the public about diagnosis, symptoms, causes, treatment, and related disorders.

Self-Compassion, https://self-compassion.org/
An educational, clinical, and research resource for people who want to learn the practice with are videos, exercises, and meditations that guide people through skills' application.

Index

About the Author

LESLIE J. SHAPIRO, LICSW, has been treating OCD and related disorders since 1989. She has been a staff behavior therapist at the OCD Institute, the flagship residential level of care for severe OCD, since its inception in 1997. She is the author of *Understanding OCD: Skills to Control the Conscience and Outsmart Obsessive Compulsive Disorder.* Shapiro was awarded the first interdisciplinary career-development research grant at McLean Hospital to support her pilot project on conscience-elated factors in OCD. She continues this research at the Office of Clinical Assessment and Research at the OCD Institute.

Shapiro has authored several online OCD continuing-education courses and has lectured on OCD in professional, academic, and community settings. Her other roles have included committee membership for Partners for Research Advancement in Nursing and Social Work at McLean Hospital, adjunct professor at the Boston University School of Social Work, and teaching, supervising, and training students and staff at the OCD Institute.

Printed in the USA
CPSIA information can be obtained
at www.ICGtesting.com
LVHW011421010424
776073LV00002B/2